Updates in Surgery

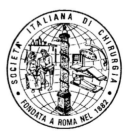

Andrea Renda

Multiple Primary Malignancies

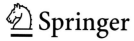
Springer

Andrea Renda
Surgical, Anesthesiology-rianimative
and Emergency Sciences Department
Federico II University
Naples, Italy

The publication and the distribution of this volume have been supported by the Italian Society of Surgery

The Editor acknowledges the educational contribution offered by Johnson & Johnson Medical S.p.A.

Library of Congress Control Number: 2008936505

ISBN 978-88-470-1094-9 Springer Milan Berlin Heidelberg New York
e-ISBN 978-88-470-1095-6

Springer is a part of Springer Science+Business Media
springer.com
© Springer-Verlag Italia 2009

This work is subject to copyright. All rights are reserved, whether the whole or part of the material is concerned, specifically the rights of translation, reprinting, re-use of illustrations, recitation, broadcasting, reproduction on microfilms or in other ways, and storage in data banks. Duplication of this publication or parts thereof is only permitted under the provisions of the Italian Copyright Law in its current version, and permission for use must always be obtained from Springer. Violations are liable for prosecution under the Italian Copyright Law.

The use of general descriptive names, registered names, trademarks, etc., in this publication does not imply, even in the absence of a specific statement, that such names are exempt from the relevant protective laws and regulations and therefore free for general use.
Product liability: The publisher cannot guarantee the accuracy of any information about dosage and application contained in this book. In every individual case the user must check such information by consulting the relevant literature.

Cover design: Simona Colombo, Milan, Italy
Typesetting: Graphostudio, Milan, Italy
Printing and binding: Arti Grafiche Nidasio, Assago, Italy

Printed in Italy
Springer-Verlag Italia S.r.l. – Via Decembrio 28 – I-20137 Milan

*In loving memory of Gaetano Renda,
Giuseppe Zannini and Simone Renda*

Foreword

In 2006, when my colleague Andrea Renda proposed multiple primary malignancies (MPM) as the subject of the Biennial Report to the 2008 Congress of the Italian Society of Surgery, I, together with the Steering Committee, quickly agreed. Recent progress in our understanding of the etiopathology of these neoplasms has led to innovative and significant progress on the clinical level. Importantly, the incidence of the onset of two or more tumors in the same patient suggests a more than casual relationship. Furthermore, the occurrence of MPM derives from several different mechanisms—viral, iatrogenic, immunologic, environmental, and hereditary—such that any form of treatment must take into account the etiology of these tumors.

After an epidemiological introduction, this monograph analyzes various aspects of multitumoral syndromes based on the experience of the Department of Surgical Sciences, along with that of other clinical departments of the University Federico II of Naples. In the discussion of inherited tumors, reference is made to the series of patients treated at the Department of Surgery at the University of Siena. The many topics that comprise this volume range from carcinogenesis to diagnostic strategies, and from epidemiology to innovations in imaging and endoscopic techniques. Among the clinical aspects, particular emphasis is given to sporadic and hereditary syndromes, as these patients are frequently treated by general surgery departments. The correlation between molecular tests and clinical behaviors of MPM is highly relevant, since the diagnostic, therapeutic, and surveillance strategies for more than a few of these syndromes are strongly influenced by the underlying genetics.

Despite its wealth of information, this work does not claim to be conclusive. The interesting clinical trials proposed by the authors will no doubt bring further insights and new perspectives regarding the pathogenesis and clinical approach to MPM.

I am proud that Italian surgery has been able to provide a relevant contribution to this extremely interesting field, one that will benefit not only surgeons, but also many different research and clinical specialists.

Rome, October 2008

Roberto Tersigni
President, Italian Society of Surgery

Preface

Many surgeons are confronted with cancer patients who have already been treated for another malignant neoplasm or who have a lesion formerly considered to be a metastasis but subsequently recognized as a new primary tumor. In other cases, individuals who have been cured of one cancer (i.e., of the digestive tract or breast) may later present with leukemia or lymphoma. In every surgeon's series there are also patients with inherited disease in which there are multiple tumors. In our experience, in studies of familial adenomatous polyposis and colorectal cancer, we have seen many patients with multiple primary tumors.

These observations lead to several questions: What is the real incidence of multiple primary malignancies? What are their most frequent causes? Is there a relationship or a dependence among them? How do we best approach their diagnosis and prevention? Is the optimal prophylactic therapy surgical or medical?

In this volume, we have tried to answer these questions through in-depth discussions and literature reviews. To this end, I have been greatly assisted by the Board of Società Italiana di Chirurgia (SIC), which I sincerely thank, in its choice of this subject as the focus of a 2-year study. The aim here is not to produce an exhaustive monograph, but to point out topics under investigation. Experts in the field, mostly from the University Hospital Federico II in Naples but also from other institutes in Campania, as well as other guest authors have been invited to relate their own experience and thus to approach the problem from different points of view. I would therefore like to thank all those who took part in this study for their much-appreciated and crucial cooperation.

The monograph is divided into three parts: the first mainly concerning the history and the nosography of multiple primary malignancies; the second based on the etiology and the more frequent tumoral associations seen in general surgery; and the third on the clinical concepts.

I hope I have succeeded in my intention and apologize for any, inadvertent, omissions.

Naples, October 2008 *Andrea Renda*

Contents

Contributors XV

Chapter 1 - Nosography 1
Andrea Renda, Nicola Carlomagno

Chapter 2 - Epidemiology: Data from Cancer Registries 7
Maurizio Montella, Carlotta Buzzoni, Anna Crispo

Chapter 3 - Bioinformatics in MPM: Using Decision Trees To Predict a Second Tumor Site 27
Alberto Cavallo, Concetta Dodaro

Chapter 4 - Carcinogenesis 51
Nicola Carlomagno, Francesca Duraturo, Gennaro Rizzo, Cristiano Cremone, Paola Izzo, Andrea Renda

Chapter 5 - Iatrogenic Second Tumors 63
Pietro Lombari, Loredana Vecchione, Antonio Farella, Sebastiano Grassia, Fernando De Vita, Giuseppe Catalano, Marco Salvatore, Andrea Renda

Chapter 6 - Immunodeficiency and Multiple Primary Malignancies 83
Michele Santangelo, Sergio Spiezia, Marco Clemente, Andrea Renda, Arturo Genovese, Giuseppe Spadaro, Concetta D'Orio, Gianni Marone, Stefano Federico, Massimo Sabbatini, Eliana Rotaia, Pierluca Piselli, Claudia Cimaglia, Diego Serraino

Chapter 7 - Multiple Primary Malignancies and Human Papilloma Virus Infections 97
Stefania Staibano, Massimo Mascolo, Lorenzo Lo Muzio, Gennaro Ilardi, Loredana Nugnes, Concetta Dodaro, Andrea Renda, Gaetano De Rosa

Chapter 8 - The Hereditary Syndromes 107
Nicola Carlomagno, Luigi Pelosio, Akbar Jamshidi, Marius Yabi, Francesca Duraturo, Paola Izzo, Andrea Renda

Chapter 9 - Multifocal and Multicentric Tumors 129
Carlo de Werra, Ivana Donzelli, Mario Perone, Rosa Di Micco,
Gianclaudio Orabona

**Chapter 10 - The Cancer Spectrum Related to Hereditary and
Familial Breast and Ovarian Cancers** 143
Matilde Pensabene, Rosaria Gesuita, Ida Capuano, Caterina Condello,
Ilaria Spagnoletti, Eleonora De Maio, Flavia Carle, Stefano Pepe,
Alma Contegiacomo

**Chapter 11 - The Role of Genetic Predisposition and Environmental
Factors in the Occurrence of Multiple Different Solid Tumors.
The Experience of the University Hospital of Sienna** 157
Francesco Cetta, Armand Dhamo, Annamaria Azzarà, Laura Moltoni

**Chapter 12 - "Sporadic" Colorectal Tumors in Multiple
Primary Malignancies** 179
Concetta Dodaro, Enrico Russo, Giuseppe Spinosa, Luigi Ricciardelli,
Andrea Renda

**Chapter 13 - Multiple Primary Malignancies:
"Non-codified" Associations** 195
Alessandro Scotti, Alessandro Borrelli, Gioacchino Tedesco,
Francesca Di Capua, Cristiano Cremone, Michele Giuseppe Iovino, Andrea
Renda

**Chapter 14 - Laboratory for Patients at Risk of
Multiple Primary Malignancies** 211
Marcello Caggiano, Angela Mariano, Massimiliano Zuccaro, Sergio Spiezia,
Marco Clemente, Vincenzo Macchia

**Chapter 15 - Multiple Primary Malignancies: Role of Advanced
Endoscopy To Identify Synchronous and Metachronous
Tumors of the Digestive Tract** 221
Giuseppe Galloro, Luca Magno, Giorgio Diamantis, Antonio Pastore,
Simona Ruggiero, Salvatore Gargiulo, Marcello Caggiano

**Chapter 16 - Diagnostic Imaging Techniques for Synchronous
Multiple Tumors** 231
Vincenzo Tammaro, Sergio Spiezia, Salvatore D'Angelo, Simone Maurea,
Giovanna Ciolli, Marco Salvatore

Chapter 17 - "DNA-Guided" Therapy 245
Nicola Carlomagno, Luigi Pelosio, Akbar Jamshidi, Francesca Duraturo, Paola
Izzo, Andrea Renda

Chapter 18 - Chemoprevention 267
Pietro Lombari, Gaetano Aurilio, Fernando De Vita, Giuseppe Catalano

Conclusions 281
Andrea Renda

Subject Index 285

Contributors

Gaetano Aurilio
Medical Oncology, Department of Clinical and Experimental Medicine "F. Magrassi – A. Lanzara"; Second University of Naples, Naples, Italy

Annamaria Azzarà
Department of Surgery, University of Sienna, Sienna, Italy

Alessandro Borrelli
Surgical, Anesthesiology-rianimative and Emergency Sciences Department, Federico II University, Naples, Italy – Surgical Sciences and Diagnostic and Therapeutic Advanced Technologies Ph.D. Course, Federico II University, Naples

Carlotta Buzzoni
AIRTUM and Epidemiology Clinical and Descriptive Unit CSPO, Florence, Italy

Marcello Caggiano
Surgical, Anesthesiology-rianimative and Emergency Sciences Department, Federico II University, Naples, Italy

Ida Capuano
Unit of Screening and Follow-up for Hereditary and Familial Cancer, Department of Molecular and Clinical Endocrinology and Oncology, Federico II University, Naples, Italy

Flavia Carle
Centro di Epidemiologia, Biostatistica e Informatica Medica, Università Politecnica delle Marche, Ancona, Italy

Nicola Carlomagno
Surgical, Anesthesiology-rianimative and Emergency Sciences Department, Federico II University, Naples, Italy

Giuseppe Catalano
Medical Oncology, Department of Clinical and Experimental Medicine "F. Magrassi – A. Lanzara", Second University of Naples, Naples, Italy

Alberto Cavallo
Department of Engineering of Informations, Second University of Naples, Naples, Italy

Francesco Cetta
Department of Surgery, University of Sienna, Sienna, Italy

Claudia Cimaglia
Department of Epidemiology, INMI L. Spallanzani IRCCS, Rome, Italy

Giovanna Ciolli
Surgical, Anesthesiology-rianimative and Emergency Sciences Department, Federico II University, Naples, Italy – Surgical Sciences and Diagnostic and Therapeutic Advanced Technologies Ph.D. Course, Federico II University, Naples

Marco Clemente
Surgical, Anesthesiology-rianimative and Emergency Sciences Department, Federico II University, Naples, Italy

Caterina Condello
Unit of Screening and Follow-up for Hereditary and Familial Cancer, Department of Molecular and Clinical Endocrinology and Oncology, Federico II University, Naples, Italy

Alma Contegiacomo
Unit of Screening and Follow-up for Hereditary and Familial Cancer, Department of Molecular and Clinical Endocrinology and Oncology, Federico II University, Naples, Italy

Cristiano Cremone
Surgical, Anesthesiology-rianimative and Emergency Sciences Department, Federico II University, Naples, Italy

Anna Crispo
Epidemiology Unit, INT, Naples, Italy

Salvatore D'Angelo
Surgical, Anesthesiology-rianimative and Emergency Sciences Department, Federico II University, Naples, Italy

Contributors

Concetta D'Orio
Department of Clinical Medicine, Cardiovascular ed Immunologic Sciences, Federico II University, Naples, Italy

Gaetano De Rosa
Department of Biomorfological and Functional Sciences, Unit of Pathology, Federico II University, Naples, Italy

Fernando De Vita
Medical Oncology, Department of Clinical and Experimental Medicine "F. Magrassi – A. Lanzara", Second University of Naples, Naples, Italy

Carlo de Werra
General, Oncological, Geriatrical and Advanced Technology Department, Federico II University, Naples, Italy

Armand Dhamo
Department of Surgery, University of Sienna, Sienna, Italy

Francesca Di Capua
Surgical, Anesthesiology-rianimative and Emergency Sciences Department, Federico II University, Naples, Italy

Eleonora De Maio
Unit of Screening and Follow-up for Hereditary and Familial Cancer, Department of Molecular and Clinical Endocrinology and Oncology, Federico II University, Naples, Italy

Rosa Di Micco
General, Oncological, Geriatrical and Advanced Technology Department, Federico II University, Naples, Italy

Giorgio Diamantis
General, Oncological, Geriatrical and Advanced Technology Department, Federico II University, Naples, Italy

Concetta Dodaro
Surgical, Anesthesiology-rianimative and Emergency Sciences Department, Federico II University, Naples, Italy

Ivana Donzelli
General, Oncological, Geriatrical and Advanced Technology Department, Federico II University, Naples, Italy

Francesca Duraturo
Department of Biochemistry and Biomedical Technologies, Federico II University, Naples, Italy

Antonio Farella
Department of Biomorfological and Functional Sciences, Unit of Diagnostic Imaging and Radiotherapy, Federico II University, Naples, Italy

Stefano Federico
Department of Systematic Pathology, Faculty of Medicine, Federico II University, Naples, Italy

Giuseppe Galloro
General, Oncological, Geriatrical and Advanced Technology Department, Federico II University, Naples, Italy

Salvatore Gargiulo
Surgical, Anesthesiology-rianimative and Emergency Sciences Department, Federico II University, Naples, Italy

Arturo Genovese
Department of Clinical Medicine, Cardiovascular ed Immunologic Sciences, Federico II University, Naples, Italy

Rosaria Gesuita
Unit of Screening and Follow-up for Hereditary and Familial Cancer, Department of Molecular and Clinical Endocrinology and Oncology, Federico II University, Naples, Italy

Sebastiano Grassia
Surgical, Anesthesiology-rianimative and Emergency Sciences Department, Federico II University, Naples, Italy

Gennaro Ilardi
Department of Biomorfological and Functional Sciences, Unit of Pathology, Federico II University, Naples, Italy

Michele Giuseppe Iovino
Surgical, Anesthesiology-rianimative and Emergency Sciences Department, Federico II University, Naples, Italy

Paola Izzo
Department of Biochemistry and Biomedical Technologies, Federico II University, Naples, Italy

Contributors

Akbar Jamshidi
Surgical, Anesthesiology-rianimative and Emergency Sciences Department, Federico II University, Naples, Italy

Lorenzo Lo Muzio
Department of Biomorfological and Functional Sciences, Unit of Pathology, Federico II University, Naples, Italy

Pietro Lombari
Surgical, Anesthesiology-rianimative and Emergency Sciences Department, Federico II University, Naples, Italy

Vincenzo Macchia
Department of Clinical Pathology, Faculty of Medicine, Federico II University, Naples, Italy

Luca Magno
General, Oncological, Geriatrical and Advanced Technology Department, Federico II University, Naples, Italy – Surgical Sciences and Diagnostic and Therapeutic Advanced Technologies Ph.D. Course, Federico II University, Naples

Angela Mariano
Department of Clinical Pathology, Faculty of Medicine, Federico II University, Naples, Italy

Gianni Marone
Department of Clinical Medicine, Cardiovascular ed Immunologic Sciences, Federico II University, Naples, Italy

Massimo Mascolo
Department of Biomorfological and Functional Sciences, Unit of Pathology, Federico II University, Naples, Italy

Simone Maurea
Department of Biomorfological and Functional Sciences, Unit of Diagnostic Imaging and Radiotherapy, Federico II University, Naples, Italy

Laura Moltoni
Department of Surgery, University of Sienna, Sienna, Italy

Maurizio Montella
Epidemiology Unit, INT, Naples, Italy

Loredana Nugnes
Department of Biomorfological and Functional Sciences, Unit of Pathology,
Federico II University, Naples, Italy

Gianclaudio Orabona
General, Oncological, Geriatrical and Advanced Technology Department,
Federico II University, Naples, Italy

Antonio Pastore
General, Oncological, Geriatrical and Advanced Technology Department,
Federico II University, Naples, Italy

Luigi Pelosio
Surgical, Anesthesiology-rianimative and Emergency Sciences Department,
Federico II University, Naples, Italy

Matilde Pensabene
Unit of Screening and Follow-up for Hereditary and Familial Cancer, Department
of Molecular and Clinical Endocrinology and Oncology, Federico II University,
Naples, Italy

Stefano Pepe
Unit of Screening and Follow-up for Hereditary and Familial Cancer, Department
of Molecular and Clinical Endocrinology and Oncology, Federico II University,
Naples, Italy

Mario Perone
General, Oncological, Geriatrical and Advanced Technology Department,
Federico II University, Naples, Italy

Pierluca Piselli
Department of Epidemiology, INMI L. Spallanzani IRCCS, Rome, Italy

Andrea Renda
Surgical, Anesthesiology-rianimative and Emergency Sciences Department,
Federico II University, Naples, Italy – Centre of Excellence for Innovative
Technologies in Surgery

Luigi Ricciardelli
Surgical, Anesthesiology-rianimative and Emergency Sciences Department,
Federico II University, Naples, Italy

Gennaro Rizzo
Surgical, Anesthesiology-rianimative and Emergency Sciences Department,
Federico II University, Naples, Italy

Eliana Rotaia
Department of Systematic Pathology, Faculty of Medicine, Federico II University, Naples, Italy

Simona Ruggiero
General, Oncological, Geriatrical and Advanced Technology Department, Federico II University, Naples, Italy

Enrico Russo
Surgical, Anesthesiology-rianimative and Emergency Sciences Department, Federico II University, Naples, Italy – Molecular Imaging Ph.D. Course, Federico II University, Naples

Massimo Sabbatini
Department of Systematic Pathology, Faculty of Medicine, Federico II University, Naples, Italy

Marco Salvatore
Department of Biomorfological and Functional Sciences, Unit of Diagnostic Imaging and Radiotherapy, Federico II University, Naples, Italy

Michele Santangelo
Surgical, Anesthesiology-rianimative and Emergency Sciences Department, Federico II University, Naples, Italy

Alessandro Scotti
Surgical, Anesthesiology-rianimative and Emergency Sciences Department, Federico II University, Naples, Italy

Diego Serraino
SOC Epidemiology & Biostatistics, CRO - IRCCS, Aviano (PN), Italy

Giuseppe Spadaro
Department of Clinical Medicine, Cardiovascular ed Immunologic Sciences, Federico II University, Naples, Italy

Ilaria Spagnoletti
Unit of Screening and Follow-up for Hereditary and Familial Cancer, Department of Molecular and Clinical Endocrinology and Oncology, Federico II University, Naples, Italy

Sergio Spiezia
Unit of Screening and Follow-up for Hereditary and Familial Cancer, Department of Molecular and Clinical Endocrinology and Oncology, Federico II University, Naples, Italy

Giuseppe Spinosa
Surgical, Anesthesiology-rianimative and Emergency Sciences Department,
Federico II University, Naples, Italy

Stefania Staibano
Department of Biomorfological and Functional Sciences, Unit of Pathology,
Federico II University, Naples, Italy

Vincenzo Tammaro
Surgical, Anesthesiology-rianimative and Emergency Sciences Department,
Federico II University, Naples, Italy

Gioacchino Tedesco
Surgical, Anesthesiology-rianimative and Emergency Sciences Department,
Federico II University, Naples, Italy

Loredana Vecchione
Medical Oncology, Department of Clinical and Experimental Medicine "F. Magrassi – A. Lanzara", Second University of Naples, Naples, Italy

Marius Yabi
Surgical, Anesthesiology-rianimative and Emergency Sciences Department,
Federico II University, Naples, Italy

Massimiliano Zuccaro
Surgical, Anesthesiology-rianimative and Emergency Sciences Department,
Federico II University, Naples, Italy

Chapter 1
Nosography

Andrea Renda, Nicola Carlomagno

Ever since Billroth's report, in 1889, of a patient with multiple tumors, a gastric carcinoma that developed after the removal of a spinocellular epithelioma of the right ear; multiple primary malignancies (MPM) have been an object of medical curiosity. Until 1932, when Warren and Gates classified 1259 such patients from literature reports and post mortem examinations [1], only a few such cases had been recognized. MPM were defined as presenting the following clinical and histological characteristics: (1) malignant tumors based on histopathologic criteria, (2) topographic distinct without connection via submucosal or intra-epithelial alterations (skip metastasis), and (3) ruling out that the second tumor was not a metastasis of the first.

In 1961, Moertel [2] classified MPM as being simultaneous, synchronous, or metachronous, depending on whether diagnosis of the second tumor was contemporary or was made within or after 6 months of the first ("index tumor") .

The incidence of MPM is increasing and is expected to continue to do so. The increase has been ascribed to several factors, such as increases in the incidence of many forms of cancer; the longer mean lifetime, mostly in western populations; treatments at initial tumor staging; the quality of oncologic follow-up; and the better prognosis of many neoplasms [3].

Improvements in oncologic (medical and surgical) therapies have resulted in unprecedented recoveries and survivals (5-year survival: children 79% and adults 66%). In Italy, there have been relevant improvements in survival for all cancers, with a certain degree of geographic variability, especially for men. Five-year survival for male patients in in northern-central Italy increased from 25% in the period 1978–1982 to 42% in 1992–1994. This corresponds to an annual rate of about 3%. In the southern part of the country, the annual increase was about 2%, with survival reaching 36% in 1992–1994. For women, survival increased at the same rate (2%) in northern-central and southern Italy, from 42 to 56% and 38 to 52%, respectively [4].

Notwithstanding the improvement in oncologic therapy, the incidence of cancer is increasing (1,444,920 new cancer cases and 559,650 deaths estimated in the USA in 2007) [5]. In Italy, cancer remains a leading cause of death and the

A. Renda (ed.), *Multiple Primary Malignancies.*
©Springer-Verlag Italia 2009

number of affected individuals is increasing in our country and, specifically, in Campania, the region where our institute is located. An analysis of data from ISTAT, available on the World Wide Web, indicated that cancer mortality in Italy and in Campania is increasing at a rate that is higher than that for death due to other pathologies and/or to traumatic accidents (Fig. 1.1).

We have often observed that some patients recovering from malignant tumors and/or others who are healthy and have survived for 5 or more years after treatment develop other tumors, either inexplicably (at least on the strength of today's biomedical knowledge) or because of well-known predisposing factors (genetic, environment, hormones, immunology, iatrogenetic, viral).

In some cases, an inherited syndrome can be identified through detailed genetic studies, but there are also associations of malignant tumors that are not nosographically recognized.

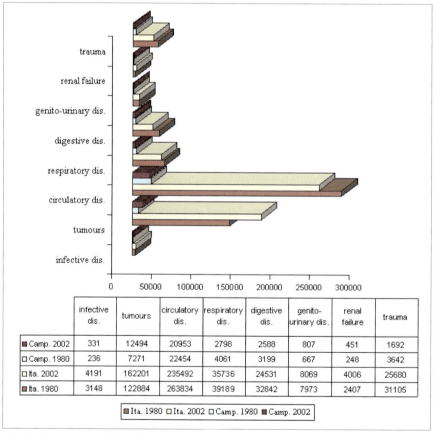

Fig. 1.1 Main causes of death in Italy and in the Campania region in 1980 and 2002. Data are from the ISS (Office of Statistics) website, in cooperation with Informatics department of the SIDBAE-ISS. Description of national and regional (Campania) mortality. Data from ISTAT reports on death certificates

A review of the main scientific studies that have examined MPM revealed numerous retrospective cases or post-mortem reports, but definitive conclusions about the incidence of MPM and its clinical and prognostic implications could not be reached. Retrospective studies are particularly difficult for those cases in which either the index tumor far preceded the second tumor or there is incomplete clinical information.

In order to better understand MPM, cases described in the literature and those comprising our own series were evaluated. We mainly studied those cases that are more frequently observed in general surgery departments. Accordingly, cases of basaloma were excluded, due to the biological peculiarities of this malignancy.

The aim of this monograph was to address the following topics concerning MPM:
1. Nosography: definition, classification, incidence and epidemiology
2. Pathogenesis: etiological mechanisms
3. Clinical features: identification of specific syndromes and, especially, diagnosis and therapy, including preventive/prophylactic surgery, chemoprevention, and follow-up

MPM

Two or more malignant primary tumors arising in the same patient is the well-accepted definition of MPM (except cutaneous basaloma). Multifocal tumors (for example hepatocellular carcinoma) are considered a single neoplastic event, while familial adenomatous polyposis (FAP), with or without colorectal cancer at diagnosis, should in any case be considered a malignant tumor.

Some pathologies are often associated in our memories with the celebrities who were affected or died from them [7–12]. There is a long-standing belief that the actions of public figures influence popular behavior. In spite of their exclusive position in society, many famous patients did not have a better prognosis than their contemporaries. For example, in 2004, Susan Sontag, an American author, died at the age of 71. She was initially diagnosed with advanced breast cancer but later developed a form of leukemia traceable to the massive doses of radiotherapy and chemotherapy she received to treat the breast disease. Shortly before dying, she was diagnosed with a rare form of uterine cancer, which, however, did not appear to play any role in her demise.

Barbara Bel Geddes, an American actress, survived breast cancer in 1972, but died of lung cancer in 2005, at age 83. Ruth Mosko Handler, (American creator of Barbie) survived breast cancer in the 1970s but died following surgery for colon cancer. Henny van Andel-Schipper (born in the Netherlands; world's oldest person until her death in 2005) was successfully treated for breast cancer at age 100 but died at age 115 of an unrelated gastric cancer. Former US president Ronald Reagan had been operated on for colon and epithelial cancer but died in 2004 with Alzheimer's disease at age 93. John Wayne, the famous American actor, died of a gastric cancer in 1964, 15 years after recovering from lung cancer. He represents an interesting case of a man totally engaged with all his family in fighting cancer. In this connection, it might be useful to quote some lines from a text by John Wayne's Foundation (http://www.jwcf.org) even to pay homage to this extraordinary actor, to his brave fight against cancer and to his relatives' following activity: "During his long fight with cancer he became very passionate about wanting to help others fight this terrible disease. In fact, in his final days, he charged his family to help support others fighting cancer and to help find a cure. John Wayne was a model of true grit, individualism and courage who pursued his life with enthusiasm and generosity. Like its namesake, the John Wayne Cancer Foundation is not afraid to challenge conventional approaches and fund new, innovative solutions. Along with the impressive movie career that made John Wayne a popular figure in our American culture, a commitment to support the fight against cancer is an ongoing part of the Wayne legacy."

There is a growing interest on the part of the scientific community in MPM. A search of the National Library's website showed that, between 2005 and 2007, scientific output regarding MPM was nearly the same as for some of the most frequently observed neoplasms (breast, colon, lung, gastric, pancreas) (Figs. 1.2, 1.3). Nonetheless, most MPM studies differ in that they are retrospective or are based on case reports, with all the associated limits (Fig. 1.4). In particular, conclusions drawn from retrospective studies are compromised by, e.g., the long latency period between two neoplastic events or treatment of the same patient at

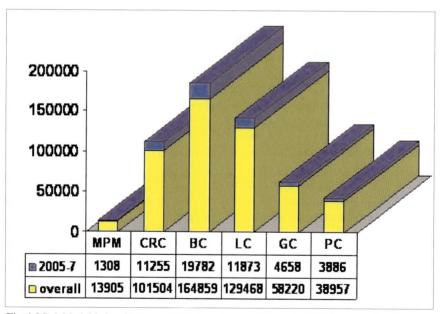

Fig. 1.2 Pub Med (National Library of Medicine) query (November 2007) concerning the number of overall and recent (last 2 years) publications on MPM compared with those addressing more common tumors, i.e., breast (BC), colorectal (CRC), lung (LC), stomach (SC), and pancreas (PC)

1 Nosography

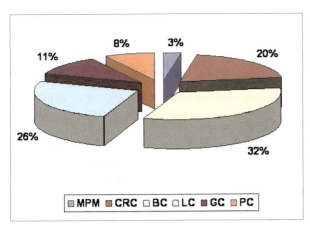

Fig. 1.3 Pub Med (National Library of Medicine) query (November 2007) concerning the percentage of publications in the last 2 years on MPM compared with those addressing more frequent tumors, i.e., breast (BC), colorectal (CRC), lung (LC), stomach (SC), and pancreas (PC)

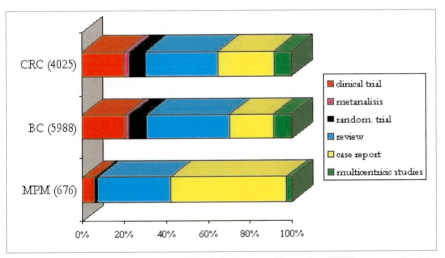

Fig. 1.4 Pub Med (National Library of Medicine) query (November 2007): source of publications on MPM, breast cancer (BC), and colorectal cancer (CRC)

two different centers; thus, it is often very hard or even impossible, to obtain complete and valid clinic data (staging, histology, immunohistochemistry, treatments, etc.).

Classification

The correct classification of MPM must consider the relationship between different parameters, such as time, histology, anatomo-topography, and anatomo-function. As noted above, temporal classification describes MPM as simultaneous, synchronous, or metachronous, depending on whether the second neoplasia was contemporary with the first one, or occurred within or after 6 months following the diagnosis of the index tumor. Staging of the primary and successive neoplasms is as important a consideration as time. The histological classification must take into account the histotype of the first tumor and of subsequent or collateral tumors (hematopoietic, epithelial, connective-tissue, etc.). Anatomo-topography refers to whether a single organ or different organs or tissues are affected. Anatomo-functional classification studies MPM affecting the body's different systems (respiratory system, digestive tract, endocrine glands, etc.). While there may be clear relationships with respect to the above parameters, the synchronous or metachronous diagnosis of the second neoplasm sometimes poses many problems because of the time elapsed. Guidelines arrived at through, for example, a consensus conference must clarify those aspects of diagnostic priority (time, histology, solid tumor, number of tumors, etc.) and their prognostic value. They could then be applied to compare different patient experiences and to analyze large series or national and regional tumor registers in order to identify the prognostic implications of specific parameters.

References

1. Warren S, Gates O (1932) Multiple primary malignant tumors. Am J Cancer 10:1358–1414
2. Moertel CG, Dockerty MB, Beggenstoss AH (1961) Multiple primary malignant neoplasms. Tumors of multicentric origin. Cancer 14:238–248
3. De Angelis R, Grande E, Inghelmann R et al (2007) Cancer prevalence estimates in Italy from 1970 to 2010. Tumori 93:392–397
4. Grande E et al (2007) Regional estimates of all cancer malignancies in Italy. Tumori 93:345–351
5. Jemal A, Siegel R, Ward E et al (2007) Cancer statistics, 2007. CA Cancer J Clin 57:43–66
6. Mydlík M, Derzsiová K (2005) The disease of Franz Kafka. Prague Med Rep 106(3):307–313
7. Sirven JI, Drazkowski JF, Noe KH (2007) Seizures among public figures: lessons learned from the epilepsy of Pope Pius IX. Mayo Clin Proc 82(12):1535–1540
8. Gerstenbrand F, Karamat E (1999) Adolf Hitler's Parkinson's disease and an attempt to analyse his personality structure. Eur J Neurol 6(2):121–127
9. Diamant H (1998) Franz Kafka, Sigmund Freud and Markus Hajek. A connection in life and death. Wien Klin Wochenschr 110(15):542–545
10. Folz BJ, Ferlito A, Weir N et al (2007) A historical review of head and neck cancer in celebrities. J Laryngol Otol 121(6):511–520
11. Lugli A, Zlobec I, Singer G et al (2007) Napoleon Bonaparte's gastric cancer: a clinicopathologic approach to staging, pathogenesis, and etiology. Nat Clin Pract Gastroenterol Hepatol 4(1):52–57
12. Nattinger AB, Hoffmann RG, Howell-Pelz A, Goodwin JS (1998) Effect of Nancy Reagan's mastectomy on choice of surgery for breast cancer by US women. JAMA 279:762–766

Chapter 2
Epidemiology: Data from Cancer Registries

Maurizio Montella, Carlotta Buzzoni, Anna Crispo

Introduction

Recent advances in the cancer treatment and the resulting increase in patient survival have led to greater scientific interest in multiple primary malignancies (MPM). It is now recognized that longer survival combined with the administration of active but toxic therapeutic regimens has made patients more prone to develop a "second primary cancer," as a consequence of therapy (e.g., thyroid cancer in lymphoma patients treated with radiotherapy) or of longer exposure to risk factors [1].

The frequency of MPM depends on the length of the observation period, applied diagnostic and prognostic criteria, exposure to environmental factors, genetically defined individual susceptibility, diagnostic accuracy, follow-up, and administered treatment. The diagnosis is strictly related to the length of patient follow-up: the longer the follow up period, the higher the chance of occurrence, and therefore the diagnosis of MPM. Conversely, a poor prognosis, as defined by morphological and clinical parameters, correlates with a shorter patient survival time, decreasing the chance of a patient developing MPM [1].

The IARC/IACR coding system is widely used, in particular by cancer registries. It is based on a topographic criterion that assigns to any incident cancer a three character-code according to the ICDO-3 classification based on the primary site, without taking into account the time interval between subsequent primary cancer diagnoses. If two tumors arise from the same primary site (muticentric), the considered code will be the first at assignment for both, unless they belong to different morphological categories [2–4]. Incidence and survival data are collected worldwide by cancer registries according to highly standardized protocols. Herein we report and discuss data extrapolated from the Italian Cancer Registry Network (AIRTUM), the European Cancer Registry (EUROCARE), and the USA (Surveillance Epidemiology and End Results, SEER) [4–7].

A. Renda (ed.), *Multiple Primary Malignancies.*
©Springer-Verlag Italia 2009

AIRTUM

The AIRTUM database, compiled by the ISS (Istituto Superiore di Sanità) in Rome, consists of all cancer data collected from each accredited registry. It is the largest Italian archive and currently contains information on more than 1 million cancer patients (1,389,425 malignant tumors diagnosed between 1978 and 2003) and over a half million cancer-related deaths (520,440 deaths occurred in the same period). Around 15,000,000 people (26% of the overall population) live in areas covered by the Italian Cancer Registry Network (AIRTUM). The population covered by a registry varies considerable: some regions are completely (e.g. Umbria) or partially (e.g. Veneto) represented by registry activity whereas in others the registry is responsible for a smaller area, such as an entire city or part of one, e.g., Turin and ASL-Napoli 4, respectively. Unfortunately coverage is not homogeneously distributed throughout Italy, as northern regions are better represented than southern ones (37% vs. 12%), while in central Italy coverage is 26%. Currently (early 2008), 1,291,585 primary tumors and 90,391 secondary tumors have been recorded; 6,909 patients were reported to have three tumors. Tables 2.1 and 2.2 list the overall distribution according to site, age, and gender. Tables 2.3–2.8 describe the distribution with respect to the second tumor: colon, rectum, breast, lung, Hodgkin and non-Hodgkin lymphomas, and are stratified by gender.

Table 2.1 AIRTUM 1998–2002. Distribution of second tumor according to first cancer (index tumor) and sex: observed/expected ratio (*O/E*)

Index tumor site	Male Observed	O/E	Female Observed	O/E
All sites excluding skin melanoma	5,033	1.00	2,428	0.97
Stomach	207	0.86*	112	1.07
Colon	532	0.90*	256	0.89
Rectum	218	0.80*	117	1.03
Liver and bile ducts (intrahepatic)	89	0.75*	22	0.75
Lung	440	0.92	77	1.06
Melanoma	100	1.06	74	1.11
Breast			764	0.80*
Ovary			82	1.23
Prostate	1,220	0.78*		
Testis	4	0.49		
Bladder	790	1.41*	91	1.26*
Brain and CNS	20	0.88	10	0.72
Thyroid	34	1.22	72	1.22
Lymphoma (Hodgkin)	15	1.21	11	1.53
Lymphoma (non-Hodgkin)	182	1.12	109	1.15
Myeloma	82	1.02	45	1.01
Leukemia	107	0.99	49	0.96

*$p < 0.05$

2 Epidemiology: Data from Cancer Registries

Table 2.2 AIRTUM 1998–2002. Distribution of second malignancies according to sex and age: observed/expected ratio (O/E)

Sex	Male								Female							
Age	00–49		50–74		75+		Total		00–49		50–74		75+		Total	
Site/tumor	Obser.	O/E	Obser.	O/E	Obser.	O/E	Obser.	O/E	Obser.	O/E	Obser.	O/E	Obser.	O/E	Obser.	O/E
All subsequent cancers	111	2.57*	3.194	1.05*	1.728	0.87*	5.033	1	194	1.26*	1.446	1.04	788	0.83*	2.428	0.97
Oral/pharynx	6	2.22	130	1.60*	35	1.07	171	1.47*	4	2.04	23	1.29	17	1.42	44	1.38*
Esophagus	8	15.10*	48	1.40*	18	1.08	74	1.43*	2	7.96	11	1.87	5	0.89	18	1.53
Stomach	5	2.56	177	1.03	150	0.99	332	1.02	6	2	62	1.03	70	0.87	138	0.96
Colorectal	9	1.76	439	1.04	269	0.91	717	0.99	17	1.62	200	1.02	131	0.76*	348	0.92
Liver	3	2.05	126	0.94	47	0.67*	176	0.86*	3	4.86*	29	0.87	18	0.58*	50	0.77
Gallbladder	0	0	6	0.56	8	0.9	14	0.71	0	0	8	0.55	11	0.84	19	0.68
Pancreas	6	6.59*	95	1.21	48	0.82	149	1.08	5	3.60*	46	1.05	48	0.96	99	1.04
Lung	22	4.32*	645	1.15*	278	0.86*	945	1.07	13	2.60*	144	1.65*	53	0.89	210	1.38*
Bone	0	0	0	0	2	1.31	2	0.44	0	0	4	2.31	0	0	4	1.3
Connective-tissue	2	4	12	1.28	6	0.92	20	1.22	1	1.06	9	1.55	5	1.44	15	1.47
Skin (melanoma)	1	0.36	44	0.99	25	1.27	70	1.05	3	0.44	28	0.99	12	0.91	43	0.89
Breast									52	0.72*	281	0.66*	112	0.62*	445	0.66*
Cervix									3	0.51	12	0.61	9	1	24	0.69
Endometrium									19	3.05*	128	1.62*	33	1.12	180	1.57*
Ovary									8	1.27	76	1.57*	19	0.72	103	1.27*

continue →

continue **Table 2.2**

Sex Age	Male 00-49 Obser.	O/E	50-74 Obser.	O/E	75+ Obser.	O/E	Total Obser.	O/E	Female 00-49 Obser.	O/E	50-74 Obser.	O/E	75+ Obser.	O/E	Total Obser.	O/E
Prostate	1	0.67	483	0.76*	313	0.72*	797	0.74*								
Testis	1								3	0.51	1.1		1.14	5		0.9
Bladder	7	2.97*	284	1.21*	188	1.12	479	1.18*	0	0	41	1.36	39	1.26	80	1.29*
Kidney and urinary tract	10	4.40*	151	1.47*	59	1.18	220	1.42*	11	4.41*	76	2.14*	36	1.60*	123	2.04*
Brain	3	2.01	36	0.93	9	0.52*	48	0.83	1	0.48	25	1.06	11	0.82	37	0.95
Thyroid	1	0.73	28	1.84*	11	2.69*	40	1.94*	15	1.4	39	1.18	12	1.72	66	1.30*
Lymphoma	7	1.7	104	1.11	47	0.86	158	1.03	5	0.82	43	0.74	34	0.92	82	0.81
Lymphoma (Hodgkin)	1	1.04	4	0.7	3	1.28	8	0.89	0	0	2	0.61	3	2.07	5	0.82
Lymphoma (non-Hodgkin)	6	1.9	100	1.13	44	0.84	150	1.04	5	1.05	41	0.75	31	0.88	77	0.81
Multiple myeloma	2	3.72	38	0.97	24	0.85	64	0.94	0	0	22	0.98	14	0.75	36	0.85
Leukemia	6	4.11*	62	1	46	0.86	114	0.97	7	2.92*	35	1.22	29	0.99	71	1.17
Mesothelioma	0	0	21	1.15	11	1.06	32	1.1	1	4.24	6	1.59	1	0.46	8	1.3
Kaposi's sarcoma	0	0	13	2.47*	10	2.12*	23	2.24*	0	0	1	0.69	2	1.1	3	0.9
Skin (non-melanoma)	15	1.82*	668	1.31*	488	1.17*	1,171	1.25*	38	2.03*	300	1.33*	232	1.13	570	1.27*

*$p <0.05$

Table 2.3 AIRTUM 1998–2002. Colon cancer, distribution of second tumor: observed/expected ratio (*O/E*)

Second tumor site	Male Observed	Male O/E	Female Observed	Female O/E
All sites	645	0.92*	322	0.94
All sites excluding non-melanoma skin cancer	532	0.90*	256	0.89
Buccal cavity and pharynx	14	1.06	2	0.55
Esophagus	11	1.86	1	0.69
Stomach	24	0.62*	10	0.54*
Rectum	41	1.58*	13	1.02
Liver and bile ducts (intrahepatic)	21	0.89	3	0.37
Gallbladder	0	0	2	0.58
Pancreas	17	1.05	15	1.23
Lung	84	0.82	22	1.22
Bone	0	0	0	0
Soft tissue	2	1.05	1	0.89
Skin melanoma	7	0.93	5	1.02
Breast			76	1.09
Cervix uteri			1	0.29
Corpus uteri			17	1.4
Ovary			17	1.91*
Prostate	125	0.99		
Testis	1	1.97		
Bladder	56	1.2	8	1.02
Kidney and urinary tract	30	1.67*	15	2.12*
Brain and CNS	3	0.46	3	0.68
Thyroid	4	1.74	5	1.15
Lymphoma	21	1.19	7	0.61
Lymphoma (Hodgkin)	2	2.08	0	0
Lymphoma (non-Hodgkin)	19	1.14	7	0.64
Myeloma	9	1.13	4	0.78
Leukemia	13	0.95	6	0.81
Mesothelioma	2	0.59	0	0
Kaposi's sarcoma	2	1.67	1	2.38
Skin (non-melanoma)	113	1.01	66	1.21

*$p < 0.05$

Table 2.4 AIRTUM 1998–2002 Rectal cancer, distribution of second tumor: observed/expected ratio (*O/E*)

Second tumor site	Male Observed	O/E	Female Observed	O/E
All sites	269	0.83*	134	1
All sites excluding skin	218	0.80*	117	1.03
Buccal cavity and pharynx	7	1.11	4	2.82
Esophagus	2	0.73	2	3.59
Stomach	15	0.84	9	1.21
Colon	37	1.37	10	0.75
Liver and bile ducts (intrahepatic)	6	0.55	1	0.32
Gallbladder	0	0	0	0
Pancreas	4	0.54	4	0.86
Lung	35	0.73	13	1.85
Bone	0	0	0	0
Soft tissue	1	1.11	0	0
Melanoma	2	0.55	4	2.02
Breast			29	1.03
Cervix uteri			0	0
Corpus uteri			4	0.82
Ovary			6	1.68
Prostate	37	0.64*		
Testis	1	3.92		
Bladder	27	1.24	4	1.31
Kidney and urinary tract	11	1.29	7	2.52*
Brain and CNS	0	0	0	0
Thyroid	1	0.89	4	2.22
Lymphoma	8	0.99	3	0.66
Lymphoma (Hodgkin)	1	2.09	1	4.34
Lymphoma (non-Hodgkin)	7	0.92	2	0.46
Myeloma	1	0.27	1	0.5
Leukemia	5	0.79	3	1.02
Mesothelioma	2	1.33	1	3.72
Kaposi's sarcoma	1	1.88	0	0
Skin (non-melanoma)	51	1.01	17	0.81

*$p < 0.05$

Table 2.5 AIRTUM 1998–2002. Breast cancer, distribution of second tumor: observed/expected ratio (*O/E*)

Second tumor site	Male Observed	O/E	Female Observed	O/E
All sites	27	1.39	965	0.86*
All sites excluding skin	26	1.59*	764	0.80*
Buccal cavity and pharynx	1	2.77	12	0.97
Esophagus	0	0	2	0.46
Stomach	6	5.67*	59	1.17
Colon	0	0	92	0.91
Liver and bile ducts (intrahepatic)	1	1.4	41	1.05
Gallbladder	0	0	24	1.03
Pancreas	0	0	8	0.79
Lung	1	2.24	33	0.96
Bone	3	1.06	72	1.25
Soft tissue	0	0	2	1.73
Melanoma	0	0	7	1.77
Breast	0	0	14	0.73
Cervix uteri			16	1.13
Corpus uteri			104	2.26*
Ovary			31	0.97
Prostate	8	2.35*		
Testis	0	0		
Bladder	1	0.78	23	1.02
Kidney and urinary tract	1	2.02	42	1.84*
Brain and CNS	0	0	17	1.14
Thyroid	0	0	30	1.38
Lymphoma	0	0	31	0.81
Lymphoma (Hodgkin)	0	0	2	0.85
Lymphoma (non-Hodgkin)	0	0	29	0.81
Myeloma	1	4.55	13	0.84
Leukemia	0	0	26	1.18
Mesothelioma	2	18.92*	2	0.83
Kaposi's sarcoma	0	0	0	0
Skin (non-melanoma)	1	0.33	201	1.20*

*$p < 0.05$

Table 2.6 AIRTUM 1998–2002. Lung cancer, distribution of second tumor: observed/expected ratio (*O/E*)

Second tumor site	Male Observed	Male O/E	Female Observed	Female O/E
All sites	514	0.91*	95	1.11
All sites excluding skin	440	0.92	77	1.06
Buccal cavity and pharynx	28	2.48*	2	2.17
Esophagus	7	1.43	0	0
Stomach	34	1.15	3	0.71
Colon	47	1.01	15	1.86*
Rectum	26	1.24	4	1.3
Liver and bile ducts (intrahepatic)	14	0.69	2	1.02
Gallbladder	1	0.53	0	0
Pancreas	15	1.17	5	1.79
Lung	0	0	0	0
Bone	2	1.31	0	0
Soft tissue	8	1.28	1	0.75
Melanoma			20	1.03
Breast			1	1.05
Cervix uteri			4	1.18
Ovary			1	0.43
Prostate	67	0.67*		
Testis	0	0		
Bladder	68	1.75*	3	1.64
Kidney and urinary tract	21	1.4	4	2.2
Brain and CNS	5	0.89	0	0
Thyroid	8	3.86*	0	0
Lymphoma	16	1.1	1	0.34
Lymphoma (Hodgkin)	0	0	0	0
Lymphoma (non-Hodgkin)	16	1.17	1	0.35
Myeloma	3	0.47	1	0.79
Leukemia	11	1.02	2	1.14
Mesothelioma	0	0	0	0
Kaposi's sarcoma	1	1.03	0	0
Skin (non-melanoma)	74	0.85	18	1.37

*$p < 0.05$

Table 2.7 AIRTUM 1998–2002. Hodgkin lymphoma, distribution of second tumor: observed/expected ratio (O/E)

Second tumor site	Male Observed	O/E	Female Observed	O/E
All sites	19	1.31	16	1.92*
All sites excluding skin	15	1.21	11	1.53
Buccal cavity and pharynx	0	0	1	11.28
Esophagus	1	7.25	0	0
Stomach	0	0	1	3.31
Colon-rectum	3	1.76	1	1.14
Liver and bile ducts (intrahepatic)	0	0	1	6.94
Gallbladder	0	0	0	0
Pancreas	2	6.29	0	0
Lung	1	0.49	0	0
Bone	0	0	0	0
Soft tissue	0	0	0	0
Melanoma	0	0	0	0
Breast			1	0.45
Cervix uteri			0	0
Corpus uteri			1	3.2
Ovary			0	0
Prostate	1	0.44		
Testis	0	0		
Bladder	0	0	0	0
Kidney and urinary tract	1	2.36	1	6.47
Brain and CNS	0	0	0	0
Thyroid	0	0	0	0
Lymphoma	2	3.68	3	8.19*
Lymphoma (non-Hodgkin)	2	4.58	3	10.84*
Myeloma	0	0	0	0
Leukemia	2	6.27	1	6.26
Mesothelioma	0	0	0	0
Kaposi's sarcoma	1	28.83	0	0
Skin (non-melanoma)	4	1.86	5	4.30*

*$p < 0.05$

Table 2.8 AIRTUM 1998–2002. Non Hodgkin lymphoma, distribution of second tumor: observed/expected ratio (*O/E*)

Second tumor site	Male Observed	Male O/E	Female Observed	Female O/E
All sites	237	1.23*	141	1.26*
All sites excluding skin	182	1.12	109	1.15
Buccal cavity and pharynx	4	0.99	1	0.83
Esophagus	1	0.59	0	0
Stomach	23	2.25*	7	1.31
Colon	25	1.09	16	1.11
Liver and bile ducts (intrahepatic)	14	2.13*	5	1.97
Gallbladder	1	1.65	0	0
Pancreas	2	0.46	3	0.83
Lung	32	1.12	12	2.04*
Bone	0	0	0	0
Soft tissue	2	3.57	0	0
Melanoma	4	1.66	6	3.31*
Breast			21	0.83
Cervix uteri			0	0
Corpus uteri			4	0.92
Ovary			2	0.65
Prostate	27	0.8		
Testis	0	0		
Bladder	10	0.79	6	2.55
Kidney and urinary tract	3	0.58	7	2.99*
Brain and CNS	2	1.01	3	2.01
Thyroid	0	0	3	1.61
Lymphoma	1	0.19	2	0.5
Lymphoma (Hodgkin)	0	0	0	0
Myeloma	1	0.46	1	0.61
Leukemia	10	2.67*	1	0.44
Mesothelioma	2	2.17	2	8.06
Kaposi's sarcoma	2	5.75	0	0
Skin (non-nmelanoma)	55	1.85*	32	1.88*

*$p < 0.05$

EUROCARE

In the EUROCARE-4 study, 82 cancer registries in 23 European countries collected data according to a standardized protocol [7]. The study included information on 3,032,852 tumors incident in the resident population of most western European countries and two eastern European countries during the period 1995–1999. Of these, 170,006 (5.6%) were MPM; their proportion ranged from 2% in the Flemish registry (Belgium) to 11.8% in the Norway registry. These registries were started in 1997 and 1959, respectively (Table 2.9). For cancer registries operating <10 years, there was a strong relationship between running time of the registry and the proportion of MPM. For "older" registries, no such association was seen (Table 2.9).

The quality of case ascertainment was measured by the percentage of microscopically verified tumors, and its completeness by the percentage of cases identified with a death certificate only (DCO). A high percentage of DCO can affect both the possibility of correctly detecting subsequent tumors and survival estimates. Completeness of case ascertainment varied greatly across registries, but was limited (DCO >10%) to only a few registries (Austria, Thames, and Wales) for first cancers. By contrast, both quality and completeness were better for subsequent tumors for the majority of registries. The number of patients lost to follow-up also affects the likelihood of detecting subsequent tumors. Among the registries considered in the present study, the overall percentage of cases lost to follow-up was rather low (0.3%). For a few registries (Haut-Rhin, Herault, Somme, Salerno and Geneva) between 5 and 8% of the cases were lost to follow-up after diagnosis of the first cancer. Although for multiple primaries the percentages of such cases was mostly rather low, for the registry of Kielce (Poland) it was 26.7%, which can strongly influence survival estimates.

The practice of autopsy can influence the proportion of multiple primaries that were incidentally found. In general, the percentages of cases detected at autopsy was low, with the exception of the registries of West Bohemia (Czech Republic), Friuli Venezia Giulia (Italy), and Basel (Switzerland) (11.7, 12.0, and 16.8%, respectively).

Table 2.10 shows the distribution (%) of subsequent tumors by site and registry. The incidence is usually higher not only for frequently occurring tumors (e.g., lung), but also for those associated with a long survival time (breast, prostate, and colorectal).

In the most recently established registries, the percentage of diagnosed multiple cancers was lower, ranging from about 12% in the oldest registries to <1% in the most recent ones.

SEER

The SEER (Surveillance Epidemiology and End Results) Program represents a unique population-based resource for evaluating the risk of subsequent cancers

Table 2.9. Distribution of cases by sequence number, country, and registry (patients age 15–99, Eurocare period 1995–1999)

Country	Reg[a]	Y	OPO %	1st [B] %	2nd %	3rd %	4th %	1st + N	OPO %	Sub. N	prim %	All N	%
Austria	Austria	1983	91.5	3.5	4.8	0.2	0.0	164,348	95.0	8,702	5.0	173,050	100.0
	Tyrol	1988	91.3	2.7	5.7	0.2	0.0	12,889	94.0	818	6.0	13,707	100.0
Belgium	Flemish	1997	94.5	3.5	2.0	0.0	0.0	79,765	98.0	1,641	2.0	81,406	100.0
Czech Republic	West Bohemia	1988	90.4	4.5	4.8	0.3	0.0	18,757	94.9	1,011	5.1	19,768	100.0
Denmark	Denmark	1953	92.0	1.9	5.9	0.2	0.0	103,540	93.9	6,754	6.1	110,294	100.0
Finland	Finland	1959	89.2	3.8	6.6	0.4	0.0	95,276	93.0	7,140	7.0	102,416	100.0
France	Herault	1995	95.9	2.0	2.0	0.0	0.0	10,210	97.9	215	2.1	10,425	100.0
	Isere	1989	92.1	2.2	5.5	0.2	0.0	11,680	94.2	713	5.8	12,393	100.0
	Manche	1994	94.4	2.5	3.1	0.0	0.0	6,033	96.9	192	3.1	6225	100.0
	Somme	1989	92.9	2.2	4.7	0.2	0.0	6,124	95.1	316	4.9	6440	100.0
	Tarn	1989	91.2	2.4	5.9	0.4	0.0	4,601	93.7	311	6.3	4912	100.0
Germany	Saarland	1968	89.0	4.3	6.3	0.3	0.0	26,236	93.3	1,887	6.7	28,123	100.0
Iceland	Iceland	1955	82.9	6.4	9.8	0.9	0.1	4,601	89.3	554	10.7	5155	100.0
Ireland	Ireland	1994	93.2	3.9	2.8	0.1	0.0	61,388	97.1	1,836	2.9	63,224	100.0
Malta	Malta[a]	1993	97.2	1.4	1.4	0.0	0.0	5,871	98.6	82	1.4	5953	100.0
Netherland	North Neth.	1995	90.9	5.2	3.8	0.2	0.0	40,010	96.1	1,640	3.9	41,650	100.0

continue →

continue **Table 2.9**

Country	Reg[a]	Y	OPO %	1st [B] %	2nd %	3rd %	4th %	1st + N	OPO %	Sub. N	prim %	All N	%
Northern Ireland	Northern Ireland[a]	1993	94.1	2.4	3.4	0.0	0.0	30,308	96.6	1,081	3.4	31,389	100.0
Norway	Norway[a]	1959	81.9	6.3	11.8	0.0	0.0	85,547	88.2	11,460	11.8	97,007	100.0
Poland	Warsaw[a]	1989	92.3	3.4	4.3	0.0	0.0	28,767	95.7	1,295	4.3	30,062	100.0
Portugal	South Portugal[a]	1998	97.5	0.0	2.5	0.0	0.0	31,569	97.5	822	2.5	32,391	100.0
Scotland	Scotland[a]	1963	87.0	4.3	8.7	0.0	0.0	118,397	91.3	11,258	8.7	129,655	100.0
Slovenia	Slovenia	1956	93.2	3.8	2.9	0.1	0.0	33,154	97.0	1,030	3.0	34,184	100.0
Spain	Navarra	1985	91.0	2.7	5.8	0.4	0.1	11,109	93.7	742	6.3	11,851	100.0
	Tarragona	1985	92.4	2.2	5.1	0.2	0.0	11,602	94.7	653	5.3	12,255	100.0
Sweden	Sweden	1959	89.8	6.4	3.6	0.1	0.0	190,154	96.2	7,502	3.8	197,656	100.0
Switzerland	Basel	1981	81.9	6.6	10.4	0.9	0.1	8,583	88.5	1,114	11.5	9,697	100.0
	Geneva	1980	82.6	6.9	9.5	0.9	0.1	8,399	89.5	987	10.5	9,386	100.0
Wales	Wales	1978	86.5	5.1	7.8	0.6	0.0	65,414	91.6	6,008	8.4	71,422	100.0
Total		-	90.7	3.7	5.4	0.2	0.0	2,862,846	94.4	170,006	5.6	3,032,852	100.0

[a]Original sequence number
[a]First of two or more primaries
Reg, Registry; *Y*, starting year; *OPO*, one primary only; *Sub Prim*, subsequent primaries; *N*, number of cases

Table 2.10 Subsequent primary tumors (%) by registry and cancer site (patients age 15–99. Eurocare period 1995–1999)

Country	Reg	B[b]	CR	L	P	S	NH-	Pa	Cancer site K
Austria	Austria	9.2	14.9	10.9	14.4	4.7	3.1	2.5	5.8
	Tyrol	8.6	12.5	14.5	13.4	6.1	2.1	1.8	6.2
Belgium	Flemish	16.1	14.0	13.5	14.7	2.3	2.9	0.6	5.8
Czech Republic	West Bohemia	13.1	21.0	13.1	5.1	2.9	1.9	2.0	9.3
DenmarK	Denmark	10.4	16.7	18.1	8.0	2.9	3.4	3.5	4.0
Finland	Finland	15.2	11.8	10.9	12.9	4.5	4.1	3.3	5.1
FRANCE	Herault	5.6	13.0	9.3	20.9	2.8	4.2	0.9	4.7
	Isere	5.6	16.8	13.9	11.1	2.7	2.8	2.4	2.7
	Manche	3.6	12.0	13.5	13.5	3.1	1.0	0.5	7.3
	Somme	3.8	14.9	13.0	11.4	3.8	2.5	0.3	3.5
	Tarn	6.4	17.0	7.4	13.5	3.9	2.9	2.3	4.2
Germany	Saarland	7.8	17.9	13.9	12.6	4.8	3.7	1.6	4.2
Iceland	Iceland	10.5	14.6	14.4	10.8	4.5	3.1	3.2	7.4
Ireland	Ireland	10.4	21.2	9.9	12.1	3.8	2.6	2.1	3.9
Malta	Malta[a]	11.0	11.0	11.0	9.8	6.1	4.9	0.0	3.7
Netherland	North Neth.	15.1	18.6	15.3	10.2	3.2	2.8	1.6	4.5
Northern ireland	Northern Ireland[a]	4.5	18.3	12.5	6.9	4.0	4.6	2.1	5.5
Norway	norway[a]	13.8	22.3	9.5	10.6	3.8	2.7	2.8	3.9
Poland	warsaw[a]	15.3	12.7	15.7	5.9	3.7	2.6	1.6	5.0
Portugal	South Portugal[a]	11.6	15.7	8.4	12.0	5.2	4.1	1.3	3.0
Scotland	Scotland[a]	12.7	15.4	18.9	6.6	3.6	2.9	2.4	3.5
Slovenia	Slovenia	6.0	14.9	16.8	6.4	5.1	3.2	1.7	3.6
Spain	Navarra	3.4	13.2	13.7	10.6	5.7	3.5	2.8	5.5
	Tarragona	5.1	12.3	15.3	10.1	5.1	3.8	1.5	4.9
Sweden	Sweden	17.1	17.6	5.9	13.0	2.3	3.0	1.7	5.8
Switzerland	Basel	15.6	16.8	12.2	14.1	2.6	3.9	2.5	4.3
	Geneva	12.4	13.2	13.0	9.7	1.9	2.9	2.6	3.5
Wales	Wales	7.0	12.9	13.7	9.9	4.6	4.1	3.0	2.9
Total		10.9	15.2	14.2	10.1	4.1	3.4	2.5	4.1

[a]Original sequence number
[b]Females only
Reg, Registry; *B*, breast; *CR*, colon and rectum; *L*, lung; *P*, prostate; *S*, stomach; *NH*, non-Hodgkin and neck; *Br*, brain; *H*, Hodgkin

Sk	Le	O	U	E	HN	Br	H	Other	All sites
3.1	2.3	2.3	3.9	1.0	2.4	0.7	0.2	18.6	100.0
2.1	2.1	2.8	4.5	1.5	2.2	0.5	0.1	18.9	100.0
1.5	2.1	1.0	2.6	1.5	4.8	0.4	0.4	16.0	100.0
2.7	3.5	2.4	4.0	1.3	1.5	0.3	0.1	16.1	100.0
3.0	4.0	2.7	3.3	2.1	2.5	1.2	0.2	14.1	100.0
2.5	2.5	1.8	3.1	1.0	1.1	1.1	0.3	18.7	100.0
0.9	3.7	1.4	2.3	2.3	9.3	0.0	0.0	18.6	100.0
2.0	2.8	1.1	2.9	2.9	9.0	1.1	0.1	20.1	100.0
1.0	1.0	2.1	1.6	5.2	15.1	1.6	0.0	17.7	100.0
0.6	1.6	1.9	3.2	6.0	13.3	0.0	0.0	20.3	100.0
1.3	4.2	2.3	2.3	2.3	6.8	0.3	0.6	22.5	100.0
1.4	3.7	1.9	3.8	1.9	3.6	0.7	0.3	16.3	100.0
1.4	3.4	2.2	3.1	1.4	1.6	0.7	0.4	17.1	100.0
3.5	3.4	2.3	3.3	1.7	1.7	0.8	0.2	17.2	100.0
1.2	7.3	1.2	2.4	1.2	1.2	1.2	0.0	26.8	100.0
2.0	2.6	1.4	2.6	1.2	3.5	0.6	0.1	14.6	100.0
1.5	2.2	5.0	2.1	3.0	4.4	0.6	0.5	22.3	100.0
4.7	2.1	2.1	2.2	1.1	1.7	1.1	0.2	15.5	100.0
1.7	2.2	4.3	5.1	0.9	1.9	1.0	0.2	20.1	100.0
2.8	3.0	2.9	3.8	2.3	2.9	0.2	0.6	20.0	100.0
2.5	2.7	2.3	2.3	3.0	2.8	0.7	0.3	17.4	100.0
2.0	2.9	2.0	5.2	1.5	9.7	0.3	0.3	18.3	100.0
0.9	3.2	2.2	3.6	1.9	3.1	1.8	0.5	24.3	100.0
1.5	2.3	1.4	4.0	1.2	4.0	0.8	0.3	26.5	100.0
3.9	3.4	1.7	2.7	0.8	1.2	0.5	0.3	19.1	100.0
3.5	2.6	1.1	2.2	1.5	3.3	0.5	0.4	12.8	100.0
4.3	4.3	0.9	2.5	2.3	8.3	1.2	0.4	16.5	100.0
2.1	4.1	2.7	2.9	2.6	2.7	0.8	0.2	23.8	100.0
2.4	3.1	2.3	3.0	2.1	2.5	0.8	0.2	18.9	100.0

s; *K*, kidney; *Sk,* skin (melanoma); *Le*, leukemia; *O*, ovary; *U*, corpus uteri; *E*, esophagus; *HN*, head due to its large size, long follow-up of cancer survivors, and highly representative sample covering more than 10% of the U.S. population [8]. The criteria applied by the SEER Program for MPM are different from those adopted by the IARC; therefore, the SEER data cannot be directly compared with those of AIRTUM and EUROCARE.

In USA, 5-year relative survival rates for all cancers combined increased steadily, from 50% in 1975–1979 to 66% in 1996–2002 among adults, and from 61to 79% among children. It has been estimated that, among those cancer survivors alive as of January 1, 2002, at least 750,000 (nearly 8%) had more than one form of cancer diagnosed between 1975 and 2001 [9].

In SEER, the risks of subsequent cancers are systematically examined by gender, age at diagnosis of the first tumor, and time since diagnosis, as well as the initial treatment and histologic type of certain tumors. Whenever relevant, the differences in subsequent cancer risk are noted by racial group.

Based on the nine original cancer registries comprising the program, SEER provided data on more than 2 million cancer patients who survived at least 2 months (including nearly 390,000 patients surviving at least 10 years and 76,000 patients surviving ≥20 or more years), yielding close to 11 million person-years at risk over the follow-up period from 1973 to 2000. Overall, cancer survivors had a 14% higher risk of developing a new malignancy than would have been expected in the general SEER population (O/E = 1.14, 95% CI = 1.14–1.15) (Table 2.11).

A total of 185,407 new primary cancers were observed compared with 162,602 expected. (The risk of subsequent prostate cancers diagnosed following an initial prostate cancer was excluded from the analysis, since typically these second tumors are not reportable to SEER.) The estimate of the excess absolute risk (EAR) among all patients combined was 21 excess subsequent cancer cases per 10,000 person-years. A very large proportion (93%) of patients with multiple cancers had microscopic confirmation of each malignancy (first, second, and subsequent cancers), reflecting the high reliability of the SEER database and the low likelihood that metastatic spread from the original malignancy would be reported as a new tumor. For most cancer sites, subsequent risk according to age at diagnosis was examined. As shown in Table 2.11, there were striking differences with respect to age, with a more than six-fold relative risk for survivors of childhood cancer (O/E = 6.13).

This finding is consistent with previous studies of childhood tumors, which have implicated initial therapy and genetic susceptibility as major risk factors in the development of new cancers [10, 11]. An age effect was further illustrated by the 2- to 3-fold increased risk for patients diagnosed as young adults (ages 18–39 years), and by the 1.2- to 1.6-fold elevated risks for those ages 40–59 years. By contrast, the observed number of new malignancies was lower than expected for survivors whose first cancer occurred at older ages (ages >80 years, O/E = 0.92), which may be due to underreporting of second cancers among elderly patients who are more likely to have competing risks from comorbid conditions. In the combined analysis of all initial sites, the greatest burden of new

Table 2.11 Risk of subsequent primary tumor after any first cancer, by age at initial diagnosis (SEER 1973–2000)

Age at initial diagnosis	O	Total O/E	EAR	O	Male O/E	EAR	O	Female O/E	EAR
All ages	185,407	1.14*	21	100,428	1.11*	22	84,979	1.17*	21
00–17 years	351	6.13*	15	176	6.44*	15	175	5.84*	15
18–29 years	1,401	2.92*	22	562	3.39*	22	839	2.67*	23
30–39 years	4,909	2.37*	39	1,530	2.88*	40	3,379	2.20*	38
40–49 years	13,537	1.61*	39	4,466	1.83*	52	9,071	1.52*	34
50–59 years	34,159	1.27*	32	15,957	1.33*	46	18,202	1.21*	24
60–69 years	62,286	1.13*	23	35,986	1.11*	25	26,300	1.14*	22
70–79 years	52,321	1.02*	4	32,419	1.00*	0	19,902	1.05*	9
>80 years	16,443	0.92*	-19	9,332	0.92*	-26	7,111	0.93*	-14

*$p < 0.05$

Note: All first primary cancers except for non-melanoma skin cancers are included in the analysis. Subsequent cancers include 2nd. 3rd,. and later primaries and encompass all cancer sites, except non-melanoma skin and subsequent prostate cancers following first primary prostate cancer due to their large impact on subsequent cancer risks for males. O, O/E, and EAR were adjusted by excluding observed and expected numbers of subsequent prostate cancers following an initial prostate cancer (O=44. E=15.185). The population at risk includes 2,036,597 patients who survived 2 or more months after an initial diagnosis during 1973–2000 (1,038,089 males and 998,508 females. 9 SEER registries). Numbers of patients surviving at least 5, 10, and 20 years were 789,221; 387,436; and 75,859 patients, respectively. The age distribution at initial diagnosis was 3.4%, 14.2%, 44.2%, 25.6%, and 12.6% for age groups <30, 30–49, 50–69, 70–79, and >80 years, respectively. The average age at initial cancer diagnosis was 64.6 years for men and 62.5 years for women

O, Observed number of subsequent (2nd. 3rd. etc.) primary cancers; *E*, expected numbers of subsequent cancers; *O/E*, ratio of observed to expected cancers, *EAR*, excess absolute risk (excess cancers per 10,000 person-years)

malignancies was experienced by cancer patients initially diagnosed between the age of 30 and 59 years, with EARs ranging from 32 to 39 per 10,000 person-years. Overall, females had a slightly higher relative risk than males for all subsequent cancers combined (O/E = 1.17 for females vs. 1.11 for males) (Table 2.11). However, the risk for males consistently exceeded that for females among patients whose initial cancer occurred before the age of 60 years.

Tobacco smoking and alcohol intake are major causes of cancer in the general population and also appear to account for a sizable proportion of the new malignancies among cancer survivors [12, 13]. More than 11,000 of the 25,000 subsequent cancers observed following the diagnosis of an initial cancer typically related to tobacco and/or alcohol (e.g., oral cavity/pharynx, esophagus, larynx, and lung) occurred at sites also related to these exposures (Table 2.12). In terms of absolute excess risk, tobacco/alcohol-related cancer sites accounted for about 10,000 excess subsequent cancers, or >35% of the total excess subsequent cancers occurring in this survey (initial cancer sites with O/E >1.0).

Table 2.12 Risk of subsequent primary tumor after any first cancer strongly related to tobacco and/or alcohol exposure (oral cavity and pharynx, esophagus, larynx, lung, and bronchus), by sex (SEER 1973–2000)

Subsequent primary cancer	Total O	Male O/E	EAR	O	Female O/E	EAR	O	O/E	EAR
All sites	24,688	1.64*	114	17,491	1.58*	120	7,197	1.82*	105
Oral/pharynx	2,510	9.04*	26	1,742	7.78*	28	768	14.29*	23
Larynx, lung/bronchus	8,084	2.95*	63	5,704	2.62*	66	2,380	4.26*	59
Esophagus	999	5.49*	10	738	4.74*	11	261	9.94*	8
Bladder, renal pelvis, ureter	1,325	1.42*	5	1,116	1.38*	6	209	1.68*	3
Kidney parenchyma	447	1.48*	2	333	1.40*	2	114	1.78*	2
Pancreas	531	1.36*	2	346	1.28*	1	185	1.55*	2
Cervix uteri	60	1.16	<1	–	–	–	60	1.16	<1
Stomach	474	1.39*	2	395	1.44*	2	79	1.17	<1

*p <0.05
Note: The population at risk includes 410,688 patients who survived 2 or more months after an initial diagnosis of cancer of the oral cavity/pharynx, esophagus, larynx, or lung/bronchus during 1973–2004. Cancers of the oral cavity/pharynx are defined to include cancers of the tongue, tonsil. mouth/floor of mouth, oropharynx, and hypopharynx. All subsequent cancers include 2nd, 3rd, and later primaries and encompass all cancer sites except for non-melanoma skin cancer
O, Observed number of subsequent (2nd. 3rd. etc.) primary cancers; *E*, expected numbers of subsequent cancers; *O/E*, ratio of observed to expected cancers, *EAR*, excess absolute risk (excess cancers per 10,000 person-years)

Conclusions

The majority (>80%) of MPM reported in the AIRTUM, EUROCARE, and SEER databases arose in separate or independent organ systems. While a certain fraction of the subsequent tumors would be expected to develop at the same rate as in the general population, the patterns of excess risk that emerged are sufficiently distinctive to suggest risk factors that may be shared by the primary and subsequent tumors, or an effect of cancer therapies that are potentially carcinogenic. The burden of second-cancer occurrence is not borne equally among all cancer survivors. Instead, there are specific constellations of multiple tumors, so that it is possible to tailor strategies for primary and secondary prevention, including long-term medical surveillance aimed at the early diagnosis and treatment of subsequent tumors [14, 15]. Lowering of the second-cancer risk, as reported among survivors who changed their high-risk behaviors, most notably by cessation of smoking and alcohol intake, indicates the need for behavioral research and educational programs to reinforce the importance of lifestyle changes that curtail exposure to cancer risk factors. Increased diet and physical activity to reduce excess body weight, workplace and environmental improvement, limited exposure to UVA and ionizing radiation should decrease the risk not only of a first primary cancer, but also of subsequent ones for those at risk and the population at large.

Acknowledgement. We thank the working group AIRTUM for providing cancer registry data. We thank for their collaboration and suggestions: Dr. Stefano Rosso (CPO, Piedmont Cancer Registry, Torino, Italy) and Riccardo Capocaccia (Cancer Epidemiology Unit, National Centre for Epidemiology, Surveillance and Health Promotion, Istituto Superiore di Sanità, Rome, Italy). The contribution of Prof. Alberto Cavallo (Dipartimento di Ingegneria dell'Informazione, Seconda Università di Napoli, Aversa, Italy) in producing the SEER tables is acknowledged.

References

1. Curtis RE, Freedman M, Ron E et al (eds) (2006) New malignancies among cancer survivors: SEER Cancer Registries, 1973–2000, NCI, Bethesda pp 1–7
2. IARC/IACR (2004) International rules for multiple primary cancer. ICD-O, 3rd edn. International Agency for Research on Cancer, Lyon, Internal Report 2004/02
3. Crocetti E, Lecker S, Buiatti E, Storm HH (1996) Problems related to coding of multiple primary cancers. Eur J Cancer 32A:1366–1370
4. National Cancer Institutes (2007) SEER program coding and staging manual. Released May 15, 2007. Available at http://seer.cancer.gov/tools/codingmanuals/ (last access July 2008)
5. Banca Dati Airtum. Available at www.registri-tumuri.it/cms/?q=bancadati (last access July 2008)
6. EUROCARE website. Available at http://www.eurocare.it/Scripts/Document.htm (last access July 2008).
7. Rosso S, De Angelis R, Ciccolallo L et al (2008) Survival with multiple tumors. Eur J Cancer (in press)
8. National Cancer Institute (2006) About SEER. NIH publication no. 05-4772. Available at http://seer.cancer.gov/about/ (last access July 2008)
9. Mariotto AB, Yabroff KR, Feuer EJ et al (2006) Projecting the number of patients with colorectal carcinoma by phases of care in the US: 2000–2020. Cancer Causes Control 17(10):1215–1226
10. Neglia JP, Friedman DL, Yasui Y et al (2001) Second malignant neoplasms in five-year survivors of childhood cancer: childhood cancer survivor study. J Natl Cancer Inst 93(8):618–629
11. Bhatia S (2005) What is the risk of second malignant neoplasms after childhood cancer? Nat Clin Pract Oncol 2(4):182–183

12. Boffetta P, Hashibe M, La Vecchia C et al (2006) The burden of cancer attributable to alcohol drinking. Int J Cancer 119(4):884–887
13. Vineis P, Alavanja M, Buffler P et al (2004) Tobacco and cancer: recent epidemiological evidence. J Natl Cancer Inst 96(2):99–106
14. Aziz NM, Rowland JH (2003) Trends and advances in cancer survivorship research: challenge and opportunity. Semin Radiat Oncol 13(3):248–266
15. Bellizzi KM, Rowland JH, Jeffery DD et al (2005) Health behaviors of cancer survivors: examining opportunities for cancer control intervention. J Clin Oncol 23(34):8884–8893

Chapter 3

Bioinformatics in MPM: Using Decision Trees To Predict a Second Tumor Site

Alberto Cavallo, Concetta Dodaro

Introduction

The availability of large databases of medical data has made it possible to apply statistical methodologies designed to deal with large data sets to medical applications. One of the largest databases, comprising data on multiple primary malignancies (MPM), is that of the NCI's Surveillance, Epidemiology and End Results (SEER) program [1]. SEER cases have been collected since 1973, with constant updates and upgrades of the program during the subsequent years. SEER thus provides an appealing source for statistical investigations of MPM.

The so-called data mining approach [2], with its corollary of event forecasting, has been the subject of great interest in recent investigations. Its applications range from weather forecasting to "smart" internet research engines, to fault detection for mechanical and electrical machines. In data mining, information can be extracted directly from the data, without the need for pre-existing knowledge or beliefs that could bias the conclusions. The technique makes use of a "non-invasive approach to knowledge discovery" [3] by using different data mining methodologies, e.g., fuzzy classification [4], rough sets [5], and decision trees [6]. Basically, one property in the database, called the *decision variable* or *consequence*, is assumed to be the result of other information, the *attributes*, or *premises*. The idea is to extract "significant" information from a large mass of data by obtaining only a minimal set of premise variables to describe the consequence datum. This strategy can be used to filter out non-essential information, thus revealing the inner structure of the physical phenomenon subtending the data. In dealing with a large mass of data, some of the apparent relationships among variables turn out to be due to chance, while others show themselves as essential, thus belonging to the "true" structure of the phenomenon. When this operation is completed, a *model* of the phenomenon is obtained, enabling the analyst to predict future values of the decision variable based on the values assumed by a known set of attributes. Different statistical techniques have been developed to discover essential variables, mainly the use of "randomized" [7] approaches. These result in a description of the phenomenon under study that is reasonably free from random effects.

A. Renda (ed.), *Multiple Primary Malignancies.*
©Springer-Verlag Italia 2009

Here, a set of such methodologies is applied to the analysis of the occurrence of a second primary neoplasm after the first one has been diagnosed. Although very recent, the use of decision trees is not new in medical applications [8, 9]; what, to our knowledge, is new is their use in the *prediction* of second primary cancers given the diagnostic data of a first malignancy. This prediction can suggest follow-up strategies focusing on the symptoms of the possible – or, better, of the most probable – subsequent primary tumors so as to allow for early-warning approaches to the future malignancy.

Moreover, also an estimate of *when* the next neoplasm will show itself is of interest. Roughly speaking, the time between the two diseases turns out to be a stochastic variable with an exponential or geometric distribution; this result is not surprising and is confirmed by the current literature. The interesting point is that the choice between the above distributions depends on the premise variable. This aspect is not detailed in this chapter but simply pointed out in the most apparent cases, and it is the subject of further research. The chapter presents an organ-based investigation in which some of the more common sites for the localization of a first tumor are considered. The most frequent second localizations are then sought (i.e., those whose relative frequency exceeds 5%) and associated with premise variables by using a randomized algorithm to exclude unessential premises. The result is compared to the relative risk associated with the first cancer, so as to give a physical interpretation of the results of the algorithm. Mean, variance, and median of the time-to-the-next malignancy are also reported.

Methodology

The problem of predicting the most probable (i.e., most frequent) second tumors based on a set of precursors is addressed herein. Specifically, different primary sites are considered, i.e., anatomic districts where the first primary has made its appearance, and then selected as the most significant according to the current literature and the authors' experience. For each one of these sites, the probability of a second tumor has been computed using the SEER data [10] from 1973 to 2004. Second tumors are associated with different variables and conditions, measured at the time of diagnosis of the first cancer. These variables are considered as *precursors* (or premises) of the following cancer. In particular, the following premise variable is considered:

1. Age at diagnosis
2. Sex
3. Histologic type, with different coding criteria applied over the years, harmonized according to [11] and the SEER documentation
4. Stage A, to be used cautiously, as reported in [12], with values: in situ (non-invasive neoplams), localized (confined to the organ of origin), regional (extended into surrounding organs), distant (extended to remote organs),

localized/regional (only prostate), unstaged (insufficient information). See [13] for further details

5. Grade, with the following values: I, well differentiated, differentiated, NOS; II, moderately differentiated, moderately well differentiated, intermediate differentiation; III, poorly differentiated, differentiated; IV, undifferentiated, anaplastic; T-cell, T-precursor; B-cell, pre-B, B-precursor; null cell, non-T-non B; NK (natural killer) cell
6. Primary organ (in case the primary site consists of different organs, as in the case of the colon, which is divided into ascending colon, transverse colon, etc.)
7. Race (white, black, Hispanic, other)

It must be stressed that, in spite of its impressive volume of data, the SEER database lacks certain important elements, like familiarity of the disease and the administration of chemotherapy. Radiotherapy is present, but a preliminary analysis shows that its isolated presence is not sufficient to assess the influence of the initial treatment on the second-tumor type, as reported also in [14]. Moreover, obviously the treatment has not yet happened at the time of the diagnosis, hence, strictly speaking, this variable is not available at the time of diagnosis. Finally, this piece of information is not uniformly available on the SEER database but instead starts at different years (in some cases from 2003), and thus still must be consolidated to be fully usable. For the above reasons, radiotherapy information has been discarded from the analysis. Moreover, reducing the cardinality (number) of the variables improved the readability of the results.

Based on the above precursors, a decision tree was trained on individual records, such that, for each patient, information regarding the location of the new (second) tumor, the precursors, and the time of the second diagnosis was collected. The resulting tree was used to display the most frequent locations for the second tumor and the significant premise variables (i.e., those appearing in the tree) and their values. Generally speaking, the most influential variables are sex and age at first cancer diagnosis, followed by the primary cancer location, and this confirms common sense. An interesting result is that information about the patient's race is absolutely unessential. Although it is well known that the risk of different neoplasms is influenced by race [15], the effect of racial differences is null on the frequency of the second malignancy.

At this point, a short discussion on the method used is in order. The relative risk of subsequent primary cancer is generally assessed based on the SIR (standardized incidence ratio) index, which is basically the ratio between the number of observed second tumors and the number of expected subsequent cancers (O/E). Starting from a cohort of patients affected by a given malignancy, their clinical history is followed, and the number of patients hit by a second tumor is counted and compared with the number expected in the general case of patients without any previous neoplasm. This approach is interesting, and if the O/E ratio is high (>1) *in both directions*, i.e., when the role of the two tumors (first and second) is reversed, it indicates the presence of common factors predisposing to *both* cancers [16]. However, computing the SIR may be misleading, due to the presence of bias factors [17], e.g., increased diagnostic screening following the first primary cancer. Moreover, the role of the SIR as a "relative risk" index has been criticized by authors showing that the SIR may, in some cases, overestimate the true relative risk [18].

Nonetheless, in some specific cases there is a striking difference between increase in risk and probability of a second tumor. For example, esophageal cancer as a first tumor increases the risk of a second cancer involving the oral cavity and pharynx by more than 900%, although the probability of being hit by this kind of cancer is still <5% for patients diagnosed with esophageal cancer. If the prediction of a second cancer is the goal, a simple frequency computation may yield more reasonable results, with the SIR explaining the discrepancies between the frequencies in the general population and in patients hit by a previous cancer. For this reason, both indices, the SIR, as an index of increased risk, and the frequency, as an index of the more probable second malignancy, have been reported in this study.

The general approach followed in epidemiologic studies is the cohort study, which divides the general population into classes according to prescribed attributes (e.g. sex, age at diagnosis) and follows the clinical history of the classes over the years. However, decision regarding which selection attribute to use to define the cohort is rather arbitrary and is usually based on the researcher's knowledge and experience. An alternative approach, used in the field of dynamic system identification [19], is to obtain partitions directly from the data by using statistical techniques such as the data mining approach.

In this study, a prediction (frequency) is deduced and presented by employing a decision tree computed with the MATLAB software [20] on data extracted from the SEER database and using the SEER*Stat software [21]. However, since a prediction of the second cancer is sought, not a simple classification, the possibility that some apparent associations are due to chance has to be considered. In order to account for this possibility, a randomized method was considered in building the decision tree, splitting the data set into different subsets to be used for training and validation of the tree. Thus, only truly significant associations are retained in the final tree, while rejecting those not significant enough from a statistical point of view. For the same reason, a minimum split parameter of 10% of the size of the group of individuals under study was selected.

Another result of the study is the estimate of the time to second tumor (TST) for the different classes induced by the tree. For each anatomic district, the values of mean (μ), standard deviation (σ), and median (m) are reported below the "leaves" of the tree. Further studies are needed to determine the best stochastic model fitting the TST, although at first glance both the exponential and the geometric distributions give good results.

Case Study

As mentioned in the previous section, specific tumor sites must first be selected. This is done by computing the most frequent cancer sites (whatever the order of occurrence of the cancer) and the researchers' experience, and selecting the first anatomic districts.

A SEER-Stat frequency session gives the results, sorted by frequency (Table 3.1).

Moreover, based on literature reports and experience, some anatomic districts have to be specified, thus obtaining the following primary sites: (1) colon, (2) rectum, (3) stomach, (4) esophagus, (5) lung and bronchus, (6) breast , (7) prostate, (8) Hodgkin lymphoma, (9) urinary bladder, (10) kidney and renal pelvis, (11) uterus, and (12) ovary.

Related to the frequency of the tumor is the concept of incidence, i.e., the number of *new* cancers appearing each year. The incidence of the above malignancies as first tumor is computed and shown in Table 3.2. The incidence is obtained by computing only the first or only tumor in the SEER database. Incidence rates are per 100,000 and age-adjusted to the 2000 USA Std Population (19 age groups, Census P25-1130) standard.

Table 3.1 Frequency of tumor sites by broad anatomic districts, ordered

Sites (broad)	Count	Frequency (%)
Digestive system	898,088	19.97
Respiratory system	673,141	14.97
Breast	669,083	14.88
Male genital system	661,673	14.71
All lymphatic and hematopoietic diseases	380,260	8.46
Urinary system	313,122	6.96
Female genital system	290,635	6.46
Skin, excluding basal and squamous cell carcinomas	165,962	3.69
Miscellaneous	115,330	2.56
Oral cavity and pharynx	114,862	2.55
Endocrine system	74,974	1.67
Brain and other nervous system	66,007	1.47
Soft tissue, including heart	27,524	0.61
Kaposi sarcoma	18,764	0.42
Mesothelioma	9,808	0.22
Bones and joints	9,384	0.21
Eye and orbit	8,400	0.19
Total	4,497,017	100.00

Table 3.2 Age-adjusted incidence rates (per 100,000) for broad groupings of malignancies as first cancer

Broad districts	Male and female	Male	Female
Breast	58.7	0.9	106.9
Prostate	55.9	133.9	0
Lung and bronchus	53.9	77.8	36.1
Colon excluding rectum	34.7	39.2	31.3
Urinary bladder	17.1	30.1	7.6
Non-Hodgkin lymphoma	14.7	17.8	12.1
Rectum and rectosigmoid junction	14.1	18.2	10.9
Corpus and uterus, nos	13.1	0	23.9
Melanoma of the skin	12.2	14.4	10.8
Kidney and renal pelvis	8.5	11.8	5.8
Stomach	8.4	12.2	5.6
Ovary	7.2	0	13.2
Esophagus	3.8	6.4	1.8
Hodgkin lymphoma	2.8	3.2	2.4

Now it is possible to begin our detailed analysis of different anatomic districts. For each one, a prediction tree is computed showing only the second tumors with a probability of occurrence >5%. SIR tables are derived in which stratification is based on the first (the most important) subdivision defined by the root node of the tree. This enables the comparison between results from the tree analysis and the increase in risk suggested by the SIR.

Colon

With the primary site being the colon, the following anatomic districts are highlighted: cecum, appendix, ascending colon, hepatic flexure, transverse colon, splenic flexure, descending colon, sigmoid colon, and large intestine.

By training a decision tree on the data obtained from the SEER database, the tree for the most probable second tumors is shown (Fig. 3.1). As the main split in the tree is based on the sex of the patient, the SIR is computed according to the stratification of sex. Table 3.3 shows the SIR results for the main anatomic districts. A further refinement can be made by using the SEER Stats software to show that the influence of the colon (O/E = 1.57) alone within the digestive system (O/E = 1.37) is rather high.

Female breast cancer, although very frequent, does not show significantly increased risk.

Only three interesting variables have to be noted, according to the above tree: sex, age at diagnosis, and sub-location of the first (colon) cancer. The strong impact of an initial colon cancer on a second colon neoplasm is evidenced by

3 Bioinformatics in MPM: Using Decision Trees To Predict a Second Tumor Site

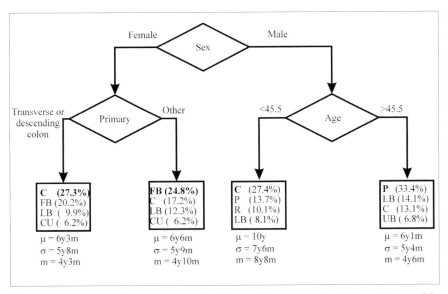

Fig. 3.1 Frequency tree for colon cancer. *C*, Colon; *CU*, corpus uteri; *FB*, female breast; *LB*, lung and bronchus; *P*, prostate; *R*, rectum; *UB*, urinary bladder. μ, Mean; σ, standard deviation; m, median

Table 3.3 Standard incidence rate (SIR) for colon cancer (*p <0.05)

Broad districts	Male and female	Male	Female
Oral cavity and pharynx	0.98	1.01	0.92
Digestive system	1.37*	1.34*	1.42*
Respiratory system	0.93*	0.89*	1.01
Bones and joints	0.8	0.6	1.04
Soft tissue, including heart	1.07	1.12	1
Skin, excluding basal and squamous carcinomas	0.97	0.98	0.95
Breast	1.02	0.8	1.02
Female genital system	1.12*	0	1.12*
Male genital system	1	1	0
Urinary system	1.04	1.05	1.02
Eye and orbit	1.14	1.23	1.03
Brain and other nervous system	0.82*	0.73*	0.94
Endocrine system	1.14	1.02	1.22
All lymphatic and hematopoietic diseases	0.93*	0.91*	0.96
Mesothelioma	0.73*	0.74	0.62
Kaposi sarcoma	0.92	0.99	0.73

both the 57% increase in the SIR and the high frequency (for females with a first cancer at the descending or transverse colon, or males under age 45 another colon cancer is the event with highest probability). Generally, a second cancer is expected after about 6 years. After about 4.5 years, half of the patients affected by a colon tumor are struck by a second malignancy. However, male patients under age 45 at first diagnosis are more likely to have a second colon tumor; also the number of years between the two cancers is higher, perhaps due to the younger age of these patients. Moreover, further investigation showed that the importance of patients <45 years is much lower than that of patients above 45, as the former represent only about 300 cases vs. more than 12,000.

Rectum

If the primary site is the rectum, the rectum and rectosigmoid junction are the relevant anatomic districts. Figure 3.2 shows the prediction tree. The O/E ratio is globally between 0.98 and 1.01, hence, no final consideration can be drawn about the

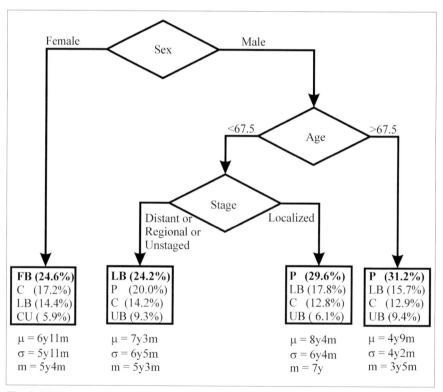

Fig. 3.2 Frequency tree for rectal cancer. *C*, Colon; *CU*, corpus uteri; *FB*, female breast; *LB*, lung and bronchus; *P*, prostate; *R*, rectum; *UB*, urinary bladder. μ, Mean; σ, standard deviation; *m*, median

increase in risk. However, in some specific cases, the risk increases: digestive system (O/E = 1.17), respiratory system (O/E = 1.07), urinary system (O/E = 1.14); and for some anatomic districts the risk decreases: oral cavity and pharynx (O/E = 0.86), male genital system (O/E = 0.81), all lymphatic tumors (O/E = 0.90).

The complete data including male/female distinct SIR are reported in Table 3.4, where some differences between the sexes are apparent.

For women, breast cancer, although not correlated to rectal cancer, is still the most frequent cancer. However, there is a high occurrence of colon malignancy, as measured by the increased SIR for the digestive system; indeed, it is the second most probable tumor for females. For males the analysis is more complex in that, even if there is a reduced incidence of cancers of the genital system, in two out of three subdivisions (elderly and younger men with stage-localized disease) prostate cancer is the most probable malignancy. In the remaining case, age under 67 and stage-distant, regional, or unstaged disease, Lung cancer is the most probable, even if the O/E does not show any increased risk. Hence, for men hit by rectal cancer the second most frequent malignancy is not defined by an increased risk. Moreover, elderly men (over 67) are subject to a second cancer in about half the time span than other patients, with a mean below 5 years and 50% of new cases occurring within 3 years and 5 months from the first diagnosis.

Stomach

For the stomach as primary site, no sub-districts are defined. The prediction tree is reported in Fig. 3.3, which shows that the only interesting variable is sex. The O/E ratio is globally 0.94, at p <0.05, with excess risk -11.17 (i.e., about 11 people less than what is expected) per 10,000. Only for the male endocrine system does the risk increase (O/E = 2.14), while for the male genital system it decreases (O/E = 0.83). All the remaining anatomic districts have confidence levels <95%.

It has to be stressed that for females there is no significant risk increase; hence, the most frequent second cancers are the ones that could be expected without a first cancer (see Table 3.1). For males, the reduction in prostate cancer is not strong enough to remove this cancer as the predominant second malignancy, and the risk increase for low-frequency endocrine cancers is not high enough to include the latter among the most frequent (>5%) second cancers. Thus, the distribution of the second tumor follows the general pattern shown in Table 3.1.

Esophagus

For esophageal tumors, no sub-districts are defined. The O/E ratio is globally 1.34, at p <0.05, with an excess risk of 63.6 per 10,000. In some specific cases, the risk increases: oral cavity and pharynx, endocrine system, respiratory sys-

Table 3.4 SIR for rectal cancer (*p <0.05)

Broad districts	Male and female	Male	Female
Oral cavity and pharynx	0.86*	0.92	0.68*
Digestive system	1.17*	1.11*	1.26*
Respiratory system	1.07*	1.02	1.18*
Bones and joints	1.01	0.83	1.3
Soft tissue, including heart	0.86	0.99	0.62
Skin, excluding basal and squamous carcinomas	0.99	0.99	1
Breast	1	1.28	1
Female genital system	0.96	0	0.96
Male genital system	0.81*	0.81*	0
Urinary system	1.14*	1.12*	1.20*
Eye and orbit	0.79	0.67	1.01
Brain and other nervous system	0.8	0.65*	1.06
Endocrine system	1.14	1.06	1.21
All lymphatic and hematopoietic diseases	0.90*	0.87*	0.95
Mesothelioma	0.79	0.8	0.76
Kaposi sarcoma	1.21	1.08	1.78

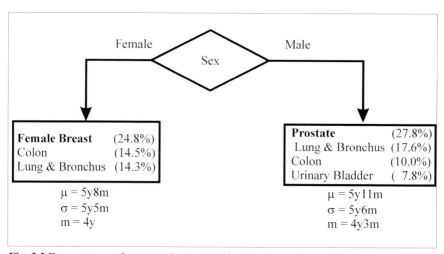

Fig. 3.3 Frequency tree for stomach cancer. μ, Mean; σ, standard deviation; m, median

tem, digestive system, while for two, male genital system and lymphatic diseases, the risk decreases. The global SIR is reported in Table 3.5.

There is no tree, since the only predictive conclusion that can be drawn, independently of the precursors, is that, after an esophageal cancer, the frequency of cancers of the lung and bronchus may reach 20.2%, followed by prostate cancer (15.0%) and colon cancer (9.1%). The increased frequency of cancers of the lung and bronchus with respect to the standard values of prostate and digestive system cancers (see Table 3.1) is easily explained by the increased risk of a second cancer involving the respiratory system, as shown in Table 3.5.

Table 3.5 SIR for esophageal cancer ($*p <0.05$)

Broad districts	Global
Oral cavity and pharynx	9.07*
Digestive system	1.33*
Respiratory system	1.83*
Bones and joints	0
Soft tissue, including heart	0
Skin, excluding basal and squamous carcinomas	1.23
Breast	0.83
Female genital system	0.6
Male genital system	0.78*
Urinary system	1.04
Eye and orbit	0
Brain and other nervous system	1.05
Endocrine system	2.78*
All lymphatic and hematopoietic diseases	0.64*
Mesothelioma	0.53
Kaposi sarcoma	0

Lung and Bronchus

For lung (and bronchus) as first primary site, no sub-districts are defined. The prediction tree is rather complex, as seen in Fig. 3.4. Note that many precursors are important in the prediction of a second neoplasm resulting from this type of cancer, namely sex (the most important), age, stage, and grade. The O/E ratio is globally 1.38 at $p <0.05$, with an excess risk 67.95 per 10,000. The risk increases for oral cavity and pharynx and for the respiratory, endocrine, urinary, and digestive systems, while decreasing for the genital system (male and female), skin, brain and nervous system, and mesothelioma. For other anatomic districts, the risk increase or decrease cannot be assessed by the 95% confidence level. The most important variable for prediction is sex. The SIR, with partitioning by sex, is shown in Table 3.6.

Also in this case, the behavior for females is far easier understood than that for males. Indeed, both the SIR and the frequency tree show that a first cancer at the lung or bronchus region is strongly correlated with a second cancer at the respiratory system. For males, another tumor at the respiratory system can be

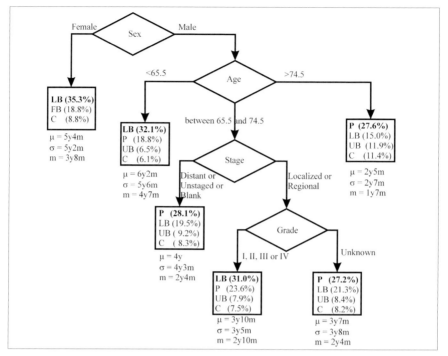

Fig. 3.4 Frequency tree for cancers of the lung and bronchus. *C*, Colon; *CU*, corpus uteri; *FB*, female breast; *LB*, lung and bronchus; *P*, prostate; *R*, rectum; *UB*, urinary bladder. μ, Mean; σ, standard deviation; m, median

roughly foreseen if the first tumor appeared before the age of 65. After age 74, a prostate tumor has to be expected, otherwise the most frequent second cancer involves either the prostate or the respiratory system, depending on the stage and grade of the first malignancy. The increase in risk of a second tumor to the respiratory system is confirmed by the SIR (Table 3.6).

Breast

No sub-districts are defined when the breast is the primary site. Breast cancer is mainly present in females, as apparent from the male:female ratio (M/F) of 1.02, i.e. male breast cancers are less than 1% of all cancer cases. For this reason, the main decision variable in defining the most frequent cancer is not sex, but age, as shown by the prediction tree in Fig. 3.5. The O/E ratio is globally 1.17, at $p < 0.05$, with an excess risk of 21.39 per 10,000. In some specific cases the risk increases: breast, soft tissues, female genital system, skin, excluding squamous and basal carcinomas, and endocrine system, while for the respiratory and brain and nervous systems the risk decreases.

3 Bioinformatics in MPM: Using Decision Trees To Predict a Second Tumor Site

Table 3.6 SIR for cancers of the lung and bronchus (*p <0.05)

Broad districts	Male and female	Male	Female
Oral cavity and pharynx	2.33*	2.24*	2.65*
Digestive system	1.28*	1.27*	1.31*
Respiratory system	2.54*	2.09*	3.77*
Bones and joints	1.07	0.92	1.36
Soft tissue, including heart	1.14	1.09	1.23
Skin, excluding basal and squamous carcinomas	0.85*	0.81*	0.93
Breast	1	1.39	1
Female genital system	0.74*	0	0.74*
Male genital system	0.91*	0.91*	0
Urinary system	1.59*	1.52*	1.88*
Eye and orbit	0.55	0.62	0.41
Brain and other nervous system	0.73*	0.68*	0.83
Endocrine system	1.94*	2.07*	1.84*
All lymphatic and hematopoietic diseases	0.98	0.95	1.04
Mesothelioma	0.55*	0.59*	0.27
Kaposi sarcoma	0.84	0.96	0

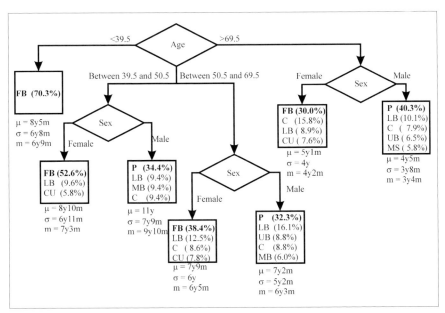

Fig. 3.5 Frequency tree for breast cancer. *C*, Colon; *CU*, corpus uteri; *FB*, female breast; *LB*, lung and bronchus; *MB*, male breast; *MS*, melanoma of the skin; *P*, prostate; *R*, rectum; *UB*, urinary bladder. μ, Mean; σ, standard deviation; m, median

The SIR, partitioned according to age at diagnosis is given in Table 3.7.

The SIR and the frequency analysis are in agreement, showing that in patients under the age of 39 a subsequent breast cancer has to be expected after the first (confirmed by the high SIR of 4.64). It has to be pointed out that the statistics for this situation apply almost exclusively to women, as the number of males affected by a breast cancer before the age of 39 and subsequently hit by a second cancer is very low (only 5 cases observed vs. 2,591 for women). For females, after the age of 40 a second breast cancer is the most frequent malignancy, although other the occurrence of other types is also significant, while for males prostate cancer is the most frequent, as confirmed by the SIR in patients until age 50. After 50, the probability of getting a prostate cancer is naturally high for males, hence the SIR reduces to 1.12, with a further reduction after the age of 70. This figure is not high enough to assess an increase in the risk of prostate cancer, as the 95% confidence interval is [0.94, 1.32]. By contrast, there is an increase in breast cancer in men 50–69, as confirmed by the SIR (not reported here) for males only, which is very high (35.8) and reflects the relatively high frequency (6.0%) of second breast cancer. For females, the constant risk increase in cancers of the genital system following a first breast cancer it noteworthy and is confirmed by the high frequency of second tumors occurring in the corpus uteri.

Table 3.7 SIR for breast cancer (*p <0.05)

Broad districts	Age at diagnosis (years)				
	0–39	40–49	50–69	70+	All ages
Oral cavity and pharynx	1.46	1.19	1.1	0.95	1.07
Digestive system	1.19	1.05	1.02	0.95*	0.99
Respiratory system	1.87*	1.23*	0.99	0.76*	0.96*
Bones and joints	2.43	2.34*	1.31	0.62	1.29
Soft tissue, including heart	3.34*	1.32	1.48*	1.07	1.38*
Skin, excluding basal and squamous carcinomas	1.11	1.29*	1.12*	1.20*	1.17*
Breast	4.64*	1.99*	1.43*	1.20*	1.56*
Female genital system	2.29*	1.29*	1.17*	1.26*	1.24*
Male genital system	4.07	2.00*	1.12	1.11	1.16
Urinary system	1.22	1.13	1.08*	0.93	1.03
Eye and orbit	2.12	1.73	0.82	1.21	1.08
Brain and other nervous system	1.62	1.24	0.84*	0.65*	0.86*
Endocrine system	1.19	1.2	1.16*	1.1	1.16*
All lymphatic and hematopoietic diseases	1.87*	1.16*	0.99	0.87*	0.97
Mesothelioma	0	0.76	0.87	0.91	0.86
Kaposi sarcoma	3.59	0	0.82	0.85	0.86

Prostate

No sub-districts are defined for the prostate as primary site. As prostate cancers subsequent to a prostate cancer are not reported to the SEER, this disease has been excluded from the analysis. The global O/E ratio is 0.91. Figure 3.6 shows the prediction tree.

The risk of second cancer involving the endocrine or urinary systems or the soft tissues increases, whilst for Kaposi sarcoma, all lymphatic cancers, cancers of the oral cavity, digestive and respiratory systems decreases. Other anatomic districts have a confidence level <95%. The only variable of interest in computing the prediction tree is the age at the first malignancy. For this reason, a SIR with the same age divisions was computed (Table 3.8).

Interpretation of the results is rather straightforward. For patients below 80 years of age, cancers of the respiratory system are highly frequent, although there is a 20% reduction from the standard incidence. Over the age of 80, the increase in the SIR for cancers of the digestive system, along with the decrease in the SIR for those of the respiratory system, makes colon cancer the most frequent. Note that for patients over age 80, due to the low number of cases, only three anatomic districts have SIR values with 95% confidence.

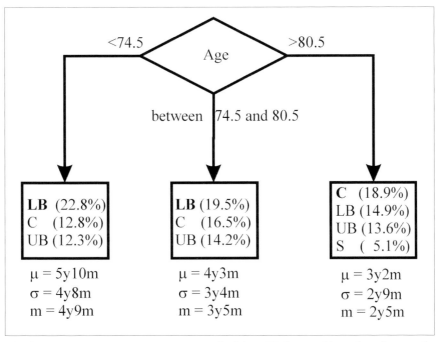

Fig. 3.6 Frequency tree for prostate cancer. *C*, Colon; *LB*, lung and bronchus; *S*, stomach; *UB*, urinary bladder. μ, Mean; σ, standard deviation; *m*, median

Table 3.8 SIR for prostate cancer (*p <0.05)

Broad districts	Age at diagnosis (years)			
	0–74	75–79	>80	All ages
Oral cavity and pharynx	0.80*	0.90	0.77*	0.81*
Digestive system	0.90*	0.97	0.95*	0.92*
Respiratory system	0.80*	0.80*	0.72*	0.79*
Bones and joints	1.15	1.38	0.88	1.16
Soft tissue, including heart squamous carcinomas	1.20*	1.04	1.26	1.18*
Skin excluding basal and	1.12*	1.12*	0.96	1.10*
Breast	1.02	0.91	1.07	1.01
Urinary system	1.05*	1.08*	0.99	1.05*
Eye and orbit	1.02	0.79	1.06	0.98
Brain and other nervous system	1.00	1.01	1.05	1.01
Endocrine system	1.22*	1.25	1.27	1.23*
All lymphatic and hematopoietic diseases	0.99	0.92*	0.94	0.97*
Mesothelioma	1.07	1.10	0.85	1.05
Kaposi sarcoma	0.78	0.84	0.46	0.73*

Hodgkin Lymphoma

In the case of Hodgkin lymphoma two sub-districts are defined, nodal and extra-nodal. The prediction tree is presented in Fig. 3.7. It shows a broad division based on the sex attribute only. Accordingly, the SIR, shown in Table 3.9, is also stratified by sex. The O/E ratio is globally 2.20, at p <0.05, with an excess risk of 50.63 per 10,000. The risk increases for all lymphatic and hematopoietic diseases, cancers of the oral cavity and pharynx, endocrine system, bones and joints, soft tissues, respiratory, digestive and urinary systems, as well as for breast cancer, Kaposi sarcoma, cancers of the female genital system, and skin cancer; it decreases for cancers of the male genital system.

A comparison of the prediction tree with the SIR table leads to the following considerations. For women, the high incidence of breast cancer together with the increased risk due to a lymphoma as a first cancer makes the probability of being hit by a breast cancer as a second tumor very high. For men, the increased risk and the high incidence of lung cancer makes this cancer the most probable second malignancy, while the very high frequency of prostate cancer is somewhat counteracted by the reduced risk probability, apparent from Table 3.8. This reduces the total probability of getting a second prostate cancer to 11.3%.

3 Bioinformatics in MPM: Using Decision Trees To Predict a Second Tumor Site

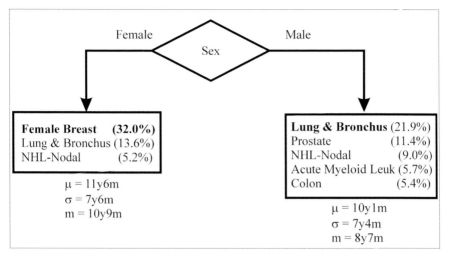

Fig. 3.7 Frequency tree for Hodgkin lymphoma. μ, Mean; σ, standard deviation; m, median

Table 3.9 SIR for Hodgkin lymphoma (*p <0.05)

Broad districts	Male and female	Male	Female
Oral cavity and pharynx	3.36*	2.73*	5.47*
Digestive system	1.58*	1.63*	1.47*
Respiratory system	2.97*	2.75*	3.50*
Bones and joints	6.94*	2.83	13.41*
Soft tissue, including heart	6.91*	5.94*	8.57*
Skin, excluding basal and squamous carcinomas	1.56*	1.63*	1.46
Breast	2.49*	3.88*	2.48*
Female genital system	1.69*	0	1.69*
Male genital system	0.83*	0.83*	0
Urinary system	1.29*	1.23	1.51
Eye and orbit	0	0	0
Brain and other nervous system	1.11	1.27	0.82
Endocrine system	3.30*	3.43*	3.25*
All lymphatic and hematopoietic diseases	4.95*	4.64*	5.53*
Mesothelioma	2.08	2.49	0
Kaposi sarcoma	2.16*	1.92*	18.09*

Urinary Bladder

No sub-districts are defined with the urinary bladder as primary site. Figure 3.8 shows the prediction tree. The O/E ratio is globally 1.21, at $p < 0.05$, with the excess risk of 45.21 per 10,000. The risk increases for cancers of the urinary, respiratory, and male genital systems and decreases for skin cancers, excluding basal and squamous carcinomas, and for Kaposi sarcoma. The detailed table, divided by sex, is reported in Table 3.10.

In this case, the large SIR for cancers of the female respiratory system is responsible for the high frequency of cancers of the lung and bronchus for women, while for men the high underlying frequency of prostate cancer, although associated with a relatively moderate increase in risk of 15%, makes prostate cancer the second tumor in about one third of the cases considered. The second most frequent cancer is breast cancer for women, basically due to its own high frequency, and cancers of the lung and bronchus for men.

Kidney and Renal Pelvis

In the case the primary site is the kidney or the renal pelvis, only "kidney" and "renal pelvis" sub-districts are considered. The prediction tree is in Fig. 3.9. The O/E ratio is globally 1.33, at $p < 0.05$, with an excess risk of 53.42 per 10,000. In some specific cases, the risk increases, i.e., for skin cancers, excluding basal and squamous carcinomas, and for cancers of the urinary, endocrine, respiratory, and male genital systems; it decreases for cancers of the oral cavity.

In this case the main branch variable is histologic type ICD-O-3, which is not

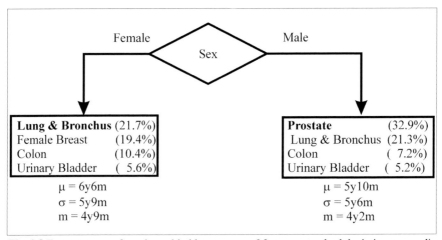

Fig. 3.8 Frequency tree for urinary bladder cancer. μ, Mean; σ, standard deviation; m, median

3 Bioinformatics in MPM: Using Decision Trees To Predict a Second Tumor Site

Table 3.10 SIR for urinary bladder cancer (*p <0.05)

Broad districts	Male and female	Male	Female
Oral cavity and pharynx	0.92	0.91	0.98
Digestive system	1.02	1.01	1.07*
Respiratory system	1.62*	1.54*	2.15*
Bones and joints	1.55	1.45	1.92
Soft tissue, including heart	1.16	1.18	1.06
Skin; excluding basal and squamous carcinomas	0.90*	0.86*	1.1
Breast	0.96	1.03	0.96
Female genital system	1	0	1
Male genital system	1.15*	1.15*	0
Urinary system	1.66*	1.48*	3.28*
Eye and orbit	0.95	1	0.7
Brain and other nervous system	0.89	0.91	0.8
Endocrine system	1.01	1.04	0.96
All lymphatic and hematopoietic diseases	0.96	0.93*	1.08
Mesothelioma	1.04	1	1.78
Kaposi sarcoma	0.54*	0.47*	1.39

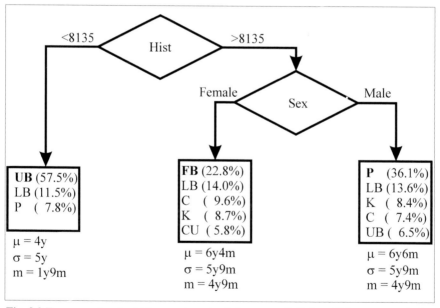

Fig. 3.9 Frequency tree for kidney and renal pelvis cancer. *C*, Colon; *CU*, corpus uteri; *FB*, female breast; *K*, kidney; *LB*, lung and bronchus; *P*, prostate; *UB*, urinary bladder. μ, Mean; σ, standard deviation; *m*, median

a very intuitive variable. Roughly speaking, and considering only the most frequent values comprising the data, histologic types below 8,135 are related to urothelial/transitional cell tumors, while values above 8,135 refer to renal cancers. In order to gain deeper insight into the importance of this variable, a SIR table was computed with the same histologic partitioning (Table 3.11).

The table clearly shows that the risk of a second cancer to the urinary system for histologic types below 8,135 is so high that this variable assumes the role of an almost certain indicator of second malignancy. Indeed in more than half of patients with histologic type less than 8,135, the second cancer involved the urinary bladder (see Fig. 3.9). The SIR exhibits the usual behavior for histologic types above 8,135. This explains why the second branch of the tree is the classic variable "sex", with the classic sex-based second malignancies (prostate cancer for males and breast cancer for females).

Table 3.11 SIR for urinary kidney and renal pelvis cancer (*p <0.05)

Broad districts	Total	8000–8135	8136–9989
Oral cavity and pharynx	0.75*	0.96	0.72*
Digestive system	1.03	1.02	1.03
Respiratory system	1.12*	1.78*	1
Bones and joints	0.98	0	1.14
Soft tissue, including heart	1.39	1.01	1.46
Skin excluding basal and squamous carcinomas	1.24*	1.41	1.22*
Breast	0.97	1.01	0.96
Female genital system	0.94	1.15	0.91
Male genital system	1.18*	1.03	1.20*
Urinary system	3.93*	14.39*	1.99*
Eye and orbit	1.02	1.94	0.86
Brain and other nervous system	1.06	1.03	1.07
Endocrine system	2.90*	1.35	3.11*
All lymphatic and hematopoietic diseases	1.07	0.75	1.12*
Mesothelioma	1.26	1.72	1.18
Kaposi sarcoma	0.7	0	0.81

Uterus

In the case of the uterus, tumor data for three anatomic sub-districts are defined: cervix uteri, corpus uteri and uterus, NOS (not otherwise specified). The prediction tree is given in Fig. 3.10. The O/E ratio is globally 0.96 at p <0.05, with a negative excess risk of -4.39 per 10,000. This is due in large part to the selection of both kinds of tumors together. If only cervix uteri cancer is considered, the O/E ratio increases to 1.25, with an excess risk of 19.41 per 10,000. Even when

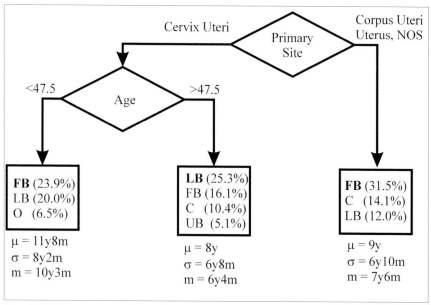

Fig. 3.10 Frequency tree for uterine cancer. *C*, Colon; *FB*, female breast; *LB*, lung and bronchus; *O*, ovary; *UB*, urinary bladder. μ, Mean; σ, standard deviation; *m*, median

both sites are considered together, in some specific cases the risk increases, i.e., for bones and joints, soft tissues, urinary, and digestive systems, whilst it decreases for breast, eye and orbit, and female genital system. According to the frequency tree (Fig. 3.10), a division between primary cancer of the cervix uteri and other forms involving the uterus has to be made. The SIR table has been computed accordingly (Table 3.12).

The results in Table 3.12 and in Fig. 3.10 can be explained by noting that the increased risk in the case of corpus uteri and uterus NOS is not enough to justify a true risk from different sites. Therefore, the most frequent second cancer is the high-frequency breast cancer, while if the primary site is the cervix uteri there is an increase in the risk of cancer at the respiratory system, as shown by the high frequency of cancers of the lung and bronchus in the elderly (see also [22]).

Ovary

In the case of ovary tumor data, no sub-districts are defined. There is no tree, since the only predictive conclusion that can be drawn, independently of the precursors, is that after an ovarian cancer the frequency of breast cancer reaches 31.4%, followed by colon cancer (11.5%), and cancers of the lung and bronchus (11.4%). The time between the occurrence of the first and second tumors is a

Table 3.12 SIR for uterine cancer (*p <0.05)

Broad districts	Cervix uteri	Corpus and uterus, NOS
Oral cavity and pharynx	1.78*	0.71*
Digestive system	1.32*	1.06*
Respiratory system	2.36*	0.79*
Bones and joints	2.95*	1.66
Soft tissue, including heart	1.59	1.54*
Skin, excluding basal and squamous carcinomas	0.70*	0.98
Breast	0.74*	1.02
Female genital system	1.16*	0.33*
Male genital system	0	0
Urinary system	2.02*	1.27*
Eye and orbit	0.29	0.55
Brain and other nervous system	0.67	0.93
Endocrine system	0.92	0.9
All lymphatic and hematopoietic diseases	1.1	0.93*
Mesothelioma	1.25	0.92
Kaposi sarcoma	2.74	1.29

mean 10 years and 2 months, with a standard deviation of 7 years and 10 months and a median 8 years and 5 months. The O/E ratio is globally 1.05 at $p<0.05$, with an excess risk of 4.62 per 10,000. In some specific cases the risk increases: eye and orbit (O/E = 2.71), all lymphatic and hematopoietic diseases (O/E = 1.46), urinary (O/E = 1.37) and digestive systems. For breast cancer and cancers of the female genital system, the risk decreases (O/E = 0.44).

The frequency results are clearly in accordance with the general incidence data (female breast first) and with the increased: whenever a cancer has a high frequency and the SIR does not show a strongly reduced risk, this cancer has a good probability to appear as a second tumor.

Conclusions

In this chapter; the occurrence of a second tumor after a possible cure from the first one has been considered. Our approach is not based on an increase in risk due to the primary, but on the most frequently appearing second cancer. Several factors contribute to this type of analysis, including sex, race, age at diagnosis, location of the first cancer, histology, grade and stage. Globally, the most important elements are sex and age at diagnosis, followed by location and stage of the first tumor. In the case of the first malignancy at the respiratory system, tumor grade is important, while tumor histology is important in the case of a first tumor involving the kidney and renal pelvis. Interestingly, the patient's race does not affect the location of the second neoplasm. The SIR, which is based on a partition induced by the prediction trees for each district, was used as a measure of relative risk in order to explain the differences between cancer frequencies before and after being hit by a malignancy. Determination of the time-to-second-tumor provided a stochastic variable of which the mean, standard deviation, and median were presented. At a first approach this variable can be modeled only as an exponential stochastic variable; however, it deserves further, specific investigation since it can offer clues about the need for a time-varying description of the classes defined by the trees, especially when the constant rate hypothesis of the exponential distribution cannot be assumed to hold.

References

1. Overview of the SEER Program, available at http://seer.cancer.gov/about/
2. Larose DT (2005) Discovering knowledge in data: an introduction to data mining. Wiley-Interscience, Hoboken, NJ
3. Daüntsch I, Gediga G (2000) Rough set data analysis: road to non-invasive knowledge discovery. Methoδos Publishers, Bangor, UK
4. Zhang H, Liu D (2006) Fuzzy modeling and fuzzy control. Birkhäuser, Boston Basel Berlin
5. Polkowski L (2001) Rough sets. Physica-Verlag, Heidelberg, New York
6. Breiman L, Friedman JH, Olshen R, Stone CJ (1993) Classification and regression trees. Chapman & Hall, Boca Raton
7. Motwani R, Raghavan P (1995) Randomized algorithms. Cambridge University Press, New York
8. Tsumoto S (2004) Mining diagnostic rules from clinical databases using rough sets and medical diagnostic model. Inf Sci (Ny) 162:65–80
9. Mugambi EM, Hunter A, Oatley G, Kennedy L (2004) Polynomial-fuzzy decision tree structures for classifying medical data. Knowledge-based Systems 17:81–87
10. Incidence - SEER 9 Regs Limited-Use, Nov 2006 Sub (1973–2004) - Linked To County Attributes - Total U.S., 1969-2004 Counties, National Cancer Institute, DCCPS, Surveillance Research Program, Cancer Statistics Branch, released April 2007, based on the November 2006 submission
11. Multiple Primary and Histology Coding Rules, January 01, 2007, National Cancer Institute Surveillance Epidemiology and End Results Program, Bethesda, MD. Available at http://seer.cancer.gov/tools/mphrules/2007_mphrules_manual_04302008.pdf
12. Localized/Regional/Distant Stage Adjustments, documentation available on the web at http://seer.cancer.gov/seerstat/variables/seer/yr1973_2004/lrd_stage/
13. Young JL Jr, Roffers SD, Ries LAG et al (eds) (2001) SEER Summary Staging Manual - 2000: Codes and Coding Instructions. National Cancer Institute, Bethesda, NIH Pub 01-4969
14. Adjadj E, Rubino C, Shamsaldim A et al (2003) The risk of multiple primary breast and thyroid carcinomas: role of radiation dose. Cancer 98:1309–1317
15. Curtis RE, Freedman DM, Ron E et al (eds) (2006) New malignancies among cancer survivors: SEER cancer registries, 1973–2000. National Cancer Institute, Bethesda, NIH Pub 05-5302
16. Curtis RE, Ries LAG (2006) Methods. In: Curtis RE, Freedman DM, Ron E et al (eds) New malignancies among cancer survivors: SEER cancer registries, 1973–2000. National Cancer Institute, Bethesda, NIH Pub 05-5302, pp 9-14

17. Neugut AI, Meadows AT, Robinson E (eds) (1999) Multiple primary cancers. Lippincott Williams & Wilkins, Philadelphia
18. Begg CB (1999) Methodological and statistical considerations in the study of multiple primary cancers. In: Neugut AI, Meadows AT, Robinson E (eds) Multiple primary cancers. Lippincott Williams & Wilkins, Philadelphia, pp 13–26
19. Nelles O (2001) Nonlinear system identification. Springer-Verlag, Berlin Heidelberg
20. MATLAB with Statistic Toolbox, ver. 2007a, The Mathworks. Available at http://www.mathworks.com/products/statistics/
21. Surveillance Research Program, National Cancer Institute SEER*Stat, version 6.3.6, available at: www.seer.cancer.gov/seerstat
22. Kleinerman RA, Kosary C, Hildesheim A (2006) New malignancies following cancer of the cervix uteri, vagina, and vulva. In: Curtis RE, Freedman DM, Ron et al (Eds) New malignancies among cancer survivors: SEER cancer registries, 1973–2000. National Cancer Institute, Bethesda, NIH Pub 05-5302, pp 207-229

Chapter 4
Carcinogenesis

Nicola Carlomagno, Francesca Duraturo, Gennaro Rizzo, Cristiano Cremone, Paola Izzo, Andrea Renda

Introduction

Carcinogenesis is the process that determines the evolution of cancer and it is triggered from mutations in the DNA of normal cells. The resulting alteration in the equilibrium between proliferation and programmed cell death leads to uncontrolled cell division and, therefore, tumor formation. Before the arrival of biomolecular techniques, which revealed that cancer is a pathology with genetic origins, there were various hypotheses regarding the etiology of this complex disease.

Historical Notes

The discovery of cancer has very deep roots in the history of humanity. The first hypothesis, valid until the Modern Era, was inherent in the Galenic-Hippocratic theory, which established that human health depends on an equilibrium of the four "humors" (blood, mucus, and yellow and black bile). The tumor was thus a tangible expression of a grave humoral disturbance (provoked, for example, by a local concentration of black bile), and its excision would eliminate any consequences of the illness but would not completely resolve the disease. Surgical removal of the tumour was merely symptomatic. Instead, the aim of treatment was to restore the internal humoral equilibrium, as indicated by Galeno. This view was confirmed by the observation of the disease course, as tumor-related illness was often fatal and not influenced by surgical interventions. In the 16th–17th century, the humoral theory was still very much accepted. Fabricius Hildanus (1560–1634) [1], one of the Fathers of German surgery and author of the six-volume work, *"Observationum et curationum chirurgicarum centuriae"*, (Fig. 4.1), analyzed the causes of unsuccessful surgery, above all in the treatment of tumours. In addition to pointing out insufficient technique, he stigmatized the lack of general cognition of medicine among surgeons: *"poorly educated and reckless as they are, they do not take into consideration and do not treat the humoral problem, the fundamentals of the growth of tumours!"*

A. Renda (ed.), *Multiple Primary Malignancies.*
©Springer-Verlag Italia 2009

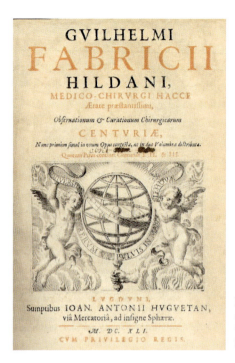

Fig. 4.1 *Observationum et curationum chirurgicarum centuriae,* a six-volume work by Fabricius Hildanus (1560–1634), father of German surgery

Signs of change developed in the 18th century, when the famous English surgeon Percival Pott (1714–1788) posed the question: How does cancer arise? Almost 100 years later, A.W. Volmann was able to correlate environmental factors (skin contact with asphalt and black smoke) with the occurrence of tumors. This was followed in the 19th century by the insights of Muller and Virchow into carcinogenesis. Rudolph Virchow, in his *"Die Cellular pathologie"*, (1858), translated into English in 1860, first observed that new cells always come from pre-existent ones *'omnis cellula e cellula'* (every cell from cell). He demonstrated that cancerous cells do not exist in and of themselves, regardless of how large or widespread the tumor may be; rather, it arises from a normal cell. The cancerous cell is not strange to our organism; it is a mutated, degenerate cell and therefore, can originate, at any time, from a very small cellular alteration.

In 1915, the Japanese researchers K. Yamagiwa and K. Ichigawa were able to experimentally reproduce tumors in laboratory animals. H.A. Gaylord (1906) hypothesized that tumors were of autoimmune origin. He observed that mice, infected with tumor cells, healed spontaneously, rejecting the carcinogenic cells upon subsequent inoculation, or became resistant. Further progress was made based on the work of the biologist T. Boveri, who demonstrated that in tumor cells, alongside the usual diploid configuration, abnormal mitotic figures, often tetraploid, at times even polyploid and irregularly distorted, could be seen during cell division. These observations gave rise to "the hypothesis of chromosome mutations." In 1920, R.C. Whitman and K.H. Bauer proposed the "theory of somatic mutations," in which tumor proliferation was suggested to originate from genetic lesions of somatic cells. In 1928, Karl Heinrich Bauer [2] was one of the first to propose a genetic basis for the development of cancer, which was confirmed many years later by molecular biology. Today, the genetic features of tumor cells are the focal point of oncological research [3–5].

It has now been shown conclusively that cancer results from the accumulation of DNA damage. Substances that cause mutations are known as mutagens, and mutagens that cause cancer are referred to as carcinogens. Already in 1955, E. Bonser identified carcinogenic substances in metabolic products. Since then many substances and behaviors have been associated with specific types of cancer, e.g., cigarette smoking, prolonged exposure to radiation, in particular to UVA, the inhalation of asbestos fibers). In more general terms, a carcinogen is the chemical, physical or biological agent that causes, promotes, or spreads cancer, either by acting directly action on DNA or by interfering with metabolic processes regulating programmed cell death. Carcinogens are classified according to international guidelines. In 1971, Ryser [6] summarized the main properties of carcinogenic agents and their effects: irreversibility, additive action, long latency period, transmission of the provoked lesion with cell replication.

The Molecular Basis of Cancer

As a genetic disease, or one that is determined by a genomic mutation, cancer can be viewed on a cellular level as the development of clones that differentiate in a diverse manner with respect to the parent cell. Therefore, all tumor cells originate from a single cell in which the regulation of proliferate has been altered. Currently, hundreds of genetic alterations have been linked to neoplastic pathologies.

Accordingly, the education of a surgeon must be enriched by an understanding of the basic principles of molecular biology, and thus the pathogenesis and clinical implications of genetic mutations. The surgeon must be familiar with the terms and concepts formerly used only by the laboratory physician, such as gene, genome, protein, transcription, mRNA, mutation, codons, exons, etc.

Cells are the fundamental unit of life. They are capable of maintaining chemical and physical conditions that differ from those of the surrounding environment and which are necessary to carry out vital metabolism. The numerous cells that constitute multicellular organisms derive from continuous divisions but originate from a single original cell.

The progression from normal tissue to cancer is marked by defects in cellular processes. Such "hits" are determined by the presence of mutations, or other alterations, of genes involved in cellular proliferation and interactions. The fundamental mechanisms can involve DNA synthesis and thus cellular replication, due, for example, to exposure to carcinogenic factors, including ionizing or UV radiations, viruses, and chemical substances, (drugs, pesticides, conserving agents, etc.), or, in hereditary forms of cancer, to defective germinal cells.

Different genes can be implicated in carcinogenesis, such as those responsible for mutations in what will thus become tumor cells. These oncogenic, oncosuppressor, and DNA repair genes can bring mutations either in the germinal or in the somatic line.

Normal cellular proliferation is the result of an equilibrium between the genes that promote and those that suppress growth. If the first type of gene is activated by an amplification or mutation in a hyperfunctional sense, the effect on cellular growth will be positive. These genes are known as oncogenes. They encode proteins that regulate the cell cycle and are often targets of mutations during neoplastic transformations. Oncogenes generally stimulate cell proliferation and/or inhibit programmed cell death (apoptosis). So-called proto-oncogenes are typically involved in the transmission of stimulating signals from the receptors of growth factors [7] whereas onco-suppressor genes have opposing actions, encoding anti-proliferation proteins (i.e., pRb, p15 and p16) that negatively control cell division. Onco-suppressors are inactivated in some tumors, leading to the loss of proliferation control. However, in contrast to proto-oncogene, both copies of an oncosuppressor gene must be lost or inactivated to produce a malignant transformation.

DNA-repair genes maintain the integrity of genetic information and scan for eventual DNA mismatches; therefore, they are responsible for correct DNA synthesis during replication. Replication errors are recognized by hMSH2, hMSH6, and hMSH3 proteins, homologous to yeast mutS. Formation of a complex consisting of hMLH1 and hPMS2, homologous to yeast mutL proteins, is necessary for detecting and repairing mismatches.

The oncogene, oncosuppressor and DNA repair genes responsible for hereditary colorectal cancer (CRC) can be divided into two categories: caretaker and gatekeeper. Caretakers maintain the integrity of the genetic information contained in each cell. They arrest proliferation in cells with chromosomal damage. The loss of these genes does not cause uncontrollable cell growth but accelerates carcinogenesis, facilitating the accumulation of mutations in gatekeeper genes. These codify proteins that stimulate or inhibit cellular proliferation, differentiation, or apoptosis.

The relationship between the somatic and germinal mutations that cause some tumors was clarified in the 1970s. In observations of sporadic and inherited cases of retinoblastoma, Knudson 8, 9] noted that hereditary neoplasms were more frequently bilateral, multicentric, and occurred earlier than neoplasms that arose sporadically. He hypothesized a model in which two mutational events ("hits") were required for tumor development. In the inherited form of retinoblastoma, the first hit occurred in the germ line (and therefore in all cells of the individual) and the second, later hit in the somatic line. An important implication of this model is that the gene affected in the familiar form is the same one that is subsequently affected by a somatic mutation, i.e., both alleles are altered. The analysis of such tumors has provided important information that has furthered our understanding of the biological basis of the most common cancers provoked by somatic mutations, and thus of carcinoma progression.

4 Carcinogenesis

The hypothesis formulated by Fearon and Vogelstein [3] described carcinogenesis as a multi-step process in which a series of sequential genetic mutations specified the biological nature of the tumors. For example, a series of steps was needed in the malignant transformation of a normal epithelial cell to a cancerous cell. In each step a specific proto-oncogene and/or onco-suppressor gene (APC, K-ras, DCC, MCC, p53) was mutated (Fig. 4.2). Such alterations could be caused by casual errors of replication, by exposure to environmental carcinogens, by ionizing radiation, and/or by viral or hormonal factors. Consistent with the two-hit hypothesis, people who were carriers of genetic mutations in the above-mentioned genes would be particularly vulnerable to these agents.

Currently, this model has been irrefutable, but it is likely that other mechanisms, still unknown, intervene in the malignant transformation process. The multiple characteristics of a metastatic cell make it highly likely that more than the inactivation of a single gene is required for the spectrum of events that result in cancer.

Carcinogenesis is the result of DNA damage in a normal cell that confers a growth and survival advantage [9–13]. DNA damage is the result of gene-environment interactions on multiple levels, including the susceptibility for genetic alterations, inherited from parental genes [14, 15]. Along with this inherited genetic background, cells are assaulted by a variety of gene-damaging environmental agents, including radiation, viruses and other microbes, and chemical carcinogens, as well as the free radicals that are products of normal cellular processes and which accumulate with age. These DNA-damaging agents are modulated by host defenses and intrinsic cellular and extrinsic noncellular risk modulators. Host defenses include the state of the patient's immune system, nutritional status, and comorbid conditions. Intrinsic risk modulators are inherited traits that do not contribute directly to DNA damage but modulate the cellular environment; for example, how well hepatic metabolic enzymes such as

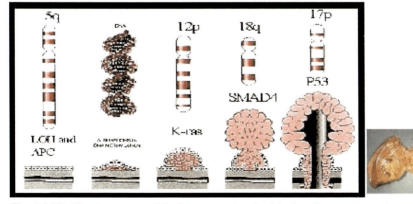

Fig. 4.2 The Vogelgram, a model of the genes involved in the adenoma to carcinoma progression of colorectal cancer (*bottom right*)

CYP3A modulate drug and hormonal activities [16]. Extrinsic risk modulators are best characterized by chemopreventative agents, including antioxidants such as selenium and vitamin E, which remove damaging oxygen radicals from the intracellular space by facilitating their breakdown to water [17].

Regardless of how damage to the genome originates, cancers arise from mutations that result in a group of common characteristics, or "hallmarks," that define the minimum set of survival traits that a cancerous cell must acquire to flourish. The common characteristics of malignant cells include: genetic instability, limitless replicative potential (immortality), anchorage-independent growth, stimulation of angiogenesis, evasion of programmed cell death (apoptosis), and ability to grow independently of stimulation by growth factors.

The physiological, programmed cell death is known as apoptosis, from the Greek term that indicates the falling of leaves and petals. It is the process by which cell proliferation is balanced by an appropriate cellular death thereby maintaining tissue homeostasis [7, 18–21]. Since the early 1990s, apoptosis research has yielded spectacular results. Apart from its importance as a biological phenomenon, apoptosis is of enormous medical importance, since defective apoptosis plays a role in numerous diseases, such as the loss of cells in Parkinson's disease, while the absence of apoptosis may contribute to the underlying uncontrolled growth of tumors.

In contrast to apoptosis, which is a physiological, genetically programmed process that is highly regulated and requires energy (in the form of ATP), necrosis is passive, energy-independent, and provoked by acute physiological damage (e.g., ischemia, mechanical damage, and toxins). During necrosis there is destruction of cytoplasmic membrane resulting in the swelling and, ultimately, lysis of cells. As a result, the contents of the cytoplasm are freed into the extracellular space, causing inflammation with necrosis and destruction of neighboring tissues.

Angiogenesis is the development of new blood vessels from the existing vasculature. It occurs in a highly regulated manner in normal physiological processes such as wound healing and is closely bound to the hemostatic system in the presence of vascular damage. Following injury, hemostasis regulates platelet adherence and fibrin formation, thereby stopping the bleeding; while angiogenesis governs the formation of new blood vessels, a vital step in wound healing. Once clot stabilization is achieved, angiogenesis is modulated by proteins and peptide fragments generated from the coagulation and fibrinolytic systems [21–23]. Angiogenesis consists of several steps: endothelial cell (EC) proliferation and migration, basement membrane degradation, and new lumen organization [24, 25]. This multi-step process is determined by a net balance between circulating pro- and anti-angiogenesis regulators that are released from activated ECs, monocytes, smooth muscle cells, and platelets [24, 25]. The regulation of cellular and molecular mediators by autocrine and paracrine mechanisms results in a coherent interplay between angiostimulators and angioinhibitors (Table 4.1) [26].

Tumor survival depends on new blood vessel growth, which consists of three

Table 4.1 Factors influencing neoangiogenesis (adapted from [26])

Angiostimulators	Vascular endothelial growth factor (VEGF)
	Basic and acidic fibroblast growth factors (bFGF, aFGF)
	Platelet-derived endothelial cell growth factor
	Matrix metalloproteinases (MMPs)
	Insulin-like growth factor (IGF)
	Epidermal growth factor (EGF)
	Interleukins: IL-1, IL-4, IL-6, IL-8, IL-15
	Angiogenin
	Integrins ?v1?3 and ?v1?5
	Endotoxin
	Endothelin-1
	Angiopoietin-1 (Ang-1)
	Tumor necrosis factor (TNF)-α (in vivo))
Angioinhibitors	Thrombospondins-1, -2
	Endostatin
	Angiostatin
	Interferons: IFN-α, IFN-β
	Interleukin-12
	Drugs: Tamoxifen, thalidomide, captopril, dexamethasone, indomethacin, diclofenac
	Angiopoietin-2 (Ang-2)
	TNF-α (in vitro)

steps: angiogenesis, vasculogenesis, and intussusception [27]. In 1971, Folkman described the crucial role of angiogenesis in cancer growth [28]. Tumors need oxygen and essential nutrients to grow. Angiogenesis is fundamental to tumor growth, invasion, and metastasis. For a cancer to grow more than 2–3 mm, it requires its own blood supply to meet the demands of cell metabolism [28]. When tumors are very small, oxygen and nutrients can diffuse into the cells, whereas tumor growth and metastasis require the development of an adequate vasculature. In addition, the rich vascular network typical of solid tumors allows the entry of malignant cells into the circulation, facilitating the metastatic process. By activating the haemostatic system, tumor cells induce the production of proangiogenic factors. The newly formed blood vessels allow the tumor to enlarge more rapidly and increase the surface area through which tumor cells can escape and metastasize [29–33].

Once the angiogenic switch has occurred, the tumor cells can grow exponentially, due in part to the their symbiotic relation with endothelial cells: angiogenic factors secreted by malignant cells increase the number of local blood vessels, which in turn secrete paracrine factors that promote tumor growth [34].

Angiogenesis also has an important prognostic role, determining resistance to chemotherapy (poor penetration of drugs) and to radiotherapy (due to the distortion of the vascular architecture of the tumor and the increased interstitial pressure); furthermore, the inhibition of specialized cells decreases the efficacy of immune surveillance, and thus facilitates tumor formation.

Metastasis results from a very complex series of events involving many different molecules. Recently, progress has been made in elucidating these events. Genes encoding proteins that are directly or indirectly involved in adhesion, invasion, survival, and cell growth have been linked to mechanisms of liver metastasis, such occurs in colorectal cancer (Table 4.2) [35]. Moreover, the expression of some of these genes are indicative of a poor prognosis (SNRPF, EIF4EL3, HNRPAB, DHPS, PTTG1, COL1A1, COL1A2, LMNB1) whereas others correlate with a low risk of metastases (ACTG2, MYLK, MYH11, CNN1, HLA-DPB1, RUNX1, RBM5). Several cellular factors (chemokines, cytokines, proteases, coagulation cascade) involved in metastasis have been further identifies as determinants of a lethal phenotype [10].

Table 4.2 Genes encoding proteins that are directly or indirectly involved in liver metastasis (adapted from [35])

Function	Protein
Adhesion	E-Cadherin,
	Epithelial cell adhesion molecule
	P-and L-selectin
	Carcinoembryonic antigen (CEA)
	Integrin $\alpha v \beta 5$
	sLex and sLea
	Osteopontin (OPN)
	Intracellular adhesion molecule (ICAM-1)
	Vascular cell adhesion molecule (VCAM-1)
	CD44v6
Invasion	Cathepsin B
	MMP-7, MMP-2, MMP-9
Angiogenesis	Angiopoietin
	Vascular endothelial growth factor (VEGF)
	Thrombospondin-1 (TSP-1)
	Angiostatin
	Endostatin
	Thymidine phosphorylase (dThdPase) or platelet-derived endothelial cell growth factor (PDECGF)
	Survival FAS receptor (CD95)
	TRAIL receptors (-R1, -R2, -R3, -R4)
Cell growth	Epidermal growth factor receptor
	c-erb-2
	c-Src/β-arrestin 1

Multiple Cancerogenesis

Multiple cancerogenesis is an interesting, complex, and fascinating phenomenon, an understanding of which draws upon much of the above discussion. Drugs, radiations, and a genetic predisposition are among the many factors/carcinogens that, acting alone or together and at the same or different time, lead to the development of multiple primary malignancies (MPM). Nonetheless, further biomolecular and epidemiological studies are needed to shed light on their exact associations with MPM. For example, it remains to be determined which factors are predominantly or exclusively hereditary. The effects of the simultaneous or metachronous occurrence of single or multiple external factors and their relationship to each other also remains poorly understood.

The prolonged exposure to carcinogens acting at multiple anatomic sites must be taken in account. It is well known that some substances or behaviors provoke cancer in more than one organ, with different latencies (cigarette smoking, chemical agents, viruses). Thus, a person who has recovered from a tumor generated by one of these causes must change his or her lifestyle with respect to exposure to avoid developing MPM.

Iatrogenic MPM is extensively discussed elsewhere in this volume. Many types of antiblastic and radiotherapies, especially at particular doses, can act as carcinogens. This is evidenced by the high percentage of MPM in some oncology patients, with the later onset of leukemia, lymphoma, or other solid tumors years after therapy. Some immunologic disorders predispose patients to MPM. They are also extensively reviewed in this volume.

In an attempt to explain from a biological point of view the increased frequency of MPM, several hypotheses from a recent paper by Anisimov [36] on aging and cancer of interest. The author cited three major concepts to explain the well-documented association between cancer and age. First, the association is a consequence of the duration of carcinogenesis, i.e., longer life implies a more prolonged exposure to carcinogens. Second, age-related progressive changes in the internal milieu of the organism may provide an increasingly favorable environment for the induction of neoplasms and the growth of otherwise latent malignant cells. Third, the cancer-prone phenotype of older humans may reflect the combined effects of cumulative mutational load, increased epigenetic gene silencing, telomere dysfunction, and altered stromal milieu.

An enhancement of our knowledge regarding the origins of MPM will no doubt derive from genetic insights. Just as identification of the genes responsible for hereditary syndromes (FAP, MEN, HNPCC, HBOC) has clarified the onset of these malignancies, so new genes or association of cofactors may someday be recognized as being responsible for what are now referred to as "sporadic" associations with MPM.

The recent discoveries made by molecular biology have opened the door to new possibilities, such as the mapping of the sequence of the entire human genome. Between 1985 and 1987, the goal to obtain a complete map of the genes comprising the human genome, to be achieved by the year 2005, was established a series of international scientific congresses. In 1988, two American governmental institutions, the National Institutes of Health (NIH) and the Department of Energy (DOE), allocated the necessary funds and formalized coordination of the research and technical procedure needed for this study. In 1991 the Human Genome Project began. Aided by the work of the private research company of Craig Venter, the sequence was completed earlier than expected (February 2, 2001). In addition to the intrinsic importance of this newfound knowledge, there are many other relevant implications. In addition to new sequencing strategies that could be applied in other applications of molecular biology and genetic engineering; it has stimulated the development of an integrated information system, including the creation of a database to organize the immense quantity of information collected [37–41].

By identifying people who are at high risk for the development of cancer, surgeons will play an increasingly important role in genetic evaluation and therapy. Prophylactic surgery could soon become a first-line treatment in the fight against cancer. Especially regarding MPM and hereditary syndromes (MEN, FAP, HNPCC, HBOC), interesting changes, dictated by biomolecular information, have begun to influence the clinical approach, as discussed in detail in the following chapters.

References

1. Jones E (1960) The life and works of Guilhelmus Fabricius Hildanus (1560–1634) Part I Med Hist 4(2):112–134
2. Bauer KH (1928) Mutationstheorie der Geschwulst-Entstehung. Übergang von Körperzellen in Geschwulstzellen durch GenÄnderung. Springer, Berlin
3. Fearon ER, Vogelstein B (1990) A genetic model for colorectal tumorigenesis. Cell 61:759–767
4. Kinzler KW, Vogelstein B (1996) Lessons from hereditary colorectal cancer. Cell 87:159–170
5. Hahn M, Saeger HD, Schackert HK (1999) Hereditary colorectal cancer: clinical consequences of predictive molecular testing Int J Colorectal Dis 14:184–193
6. Ryser HJ (1971) Chemical carcinogenesis. N Engl J Med 23 285(13):721–734
7. Ko TC, Evers BM (2003) Biologia molecolare e cellulare. In: Sabiston (ed) Trattato di chirurgia. Le basi biologiche della moderna pratica chirurgica, prima edizione italiana sulla sedicesima americana. Antonio Delfino Editore, Rome, pp 13–27
8. Knudson A (2001) Alfred Knudson and his two-hit hypothesis (Interview by Ezzie Hutchinson). Lancet Oncol 2(10):642–645
9. Devilee P, Cleton-Jansen AM, Cornelisse CJ (2001) Ever since Knudson. Trends Genet 17(10):569–573
10. Loberg RD (2007) The lethal phenotype of cancer: the molecular basis of death due to malignancy. CA Cancer J Clin 57:225–241
11. Radman M, Matic I, Taddei F (1999) Evolution of evolvability. Ann NY Acad Sci 870:146–155
12. Greaves M (2002) Cancer causation: the Darwinian downside of past success? Lancet Oncol 3:244–251
13. Nowell PC (1976) The clonal evolution of tumor cell populations. Science 194:23–28
14. Hanahan D, Weinberg RA (2000) The hallmarks of cancer. Cell 100:57–70

15. Nesse RM, Williams GC (1998) Evolution and the origins of disease. Sci Am 279:86–93
16. Coffey DS (2001) Similarities of prostate and breast cancer: Evolution, diet, and estrogens. Urology 57:31–38
17. Farinati F, Cardin R, Della Libera G et al (1994) The role of anti-oxidants in the chemoprevention of gastric cancer. Eur J Cancer Prev 3(suppl):93–97
18. Abastado JP (1996) Apoptosis: function and regulation of cell death. Res Immunol 147:443–456
19. Raff M (1998) Cell suicide for beginners. Nature 396:119–122
20. Wang J, Han W, Zborowska E et al (1998) Reduced expression of transforming growth factor beta type 1 receptor contributes to malignancies of human colon carcinoma cells. Science 280:1077–1082
21. Staton CA, Lewis CE (2005) Angiogenesis inhibitors found within the haemostasis pathway J Cell Mol Med 9:286–302
22. Browder T, Folkman J, Pirie-Shephered S (2000) The hemostatic system as a regulator of angiogenesis. J Biol Chem 275:1521–1524
23. Dardik R, Loscalzo J, Inbal A (2006) Factor XIII (FXIII) and angiogenesis. J Thromb Haemost 4:19–25
24. Liu CC, Shen Z, Kung HF, Lin MCM (2006) Cancer gene therapy targeting angiogenesis: an updated review. World J Gastroenterol 12(43):6941–6948
25. Tandle A, Blazer DG 3rd, Libutti SK (2004) Antiangiogenic gene therapy of cancer: recent developments. J Transl Med 2:22
26. Atkin GK, Chopada A (2006) Tumour angiogenesis: the relevance to surgeons. Ann R Coll Surg Engl 88:525–529
27. Cao Y (2005) Tumor angiogenesis and therapy. Biomed Pharmacother 59(Suppl 2):S340-S343
28. Folkman J (1971) Tumor angiogenesis: therapeutic implications. N Engl J Med 285:1182–1186
29. Nijziel MR (2006) From Trousseau to angiogenesis: the link between the haemostatic system and cancer. Netherlands J Med 64 (11):403–410
30. Ellis LM, Liu W, Ahmad SA et al (2001) Overview of angiogenesis: biologic implications for antiangiogenic therapy. Semin Oncol 28(Suppl 16):94–104
31. Folkman J (1990) What is the evidence that tumors are angiogenesis dependent? J Natl Cancer Inst 82:4–6
32. Hanahan D, Folkman J (1996) Patterns and emerging mechanisms of the angiogenic switch during tumorigenesis. Cell 86:353–364
33. Poon RT, Fan ST, Wong J (2003) Clinical significance of angiogenesis in gastrointestinal cancers: a target for novel prognostic and therapeutic approaches. Ann Surg 238:9–28
34. Rak J, Filmus J, Kerbel RS (1996) Reciprocal paracrine interactions between tumour cells and endothelial cells: the "angiogenesis progression" hypothesis. Eur J Cancer 32A:2438–2450
35. Nadal CP, Garcea G, Doucas H et al (2006) Molecular prognostic markers in resectable colorectal liver metastases: a systematic review. Eur J Cancer 42:1728–1743
36. Anisimov VN (2007) Biology of aging and cancer. Cancer Control 14 (1):23–31
37. Brown I, Heys SD, Schofield AC (2003) From peas to "chips" – the new millennium of molecular biology: a primer for the surgeon. World J Surg Oncol 21:1–6
38. Dulbecco R (1986) A turning point in cancer research: sequencing the human genome. Science 231(4742):1055–1056
39. Hood LE, Smith LM, Sanders JZ et al (1986) Fluorescence detection in automated DNA sequence analysis. Nature 321(6071):674–679
40. International Human Genome Sequencing Consortium (2001) Initial sequencing and analysis of the human genome. Nature 409(6822):860–921
41. The Human Genome Project (2001) In their own words. Science 291(5507):1196

Chapter 5
Iatrogenic Second Tumors

Pietro Lombari, Loredana Vecchione, Antonio Farella, Sebastiano Grassia, Fernando De Vita, Giuseppe Catalano, Marco Salvatore, Andrea Renda

Introduction

The recent introduction of new chemotherapeutic and radiotherapeutic schemes into clinical practice has led to the improvement in the overall survival of cancer patients. Hodgkin's disease, testicular cancer, and pediatric malignancies are the pathologies with the highest survival rate; improved cure rates have also been achieved for breast cancer, ovarian cancer, and non-Hodgkin's lymphoma. However, the long-term survival and/or recovery conferred by these treatments paradoxically expose cancer patients to a higher risk of important long-term complications, the most serious of which is the development of a second tumor.

Even if several international studies reported in the medical literature have well-documented the oncologic risk related to cytotoxic agents and ionizing radiation, it is necessary to underline that not all second primary malignancies are due to oncologic therapies; rather, multiple factors play important roles in the development of iatrogenic tumors, including patient age, genetic predisposition, immunodeficiency, concomitant use of drugs with possible pharmacological interactions, and continuous environmental and occupational exposure to oncogenic agents.

Role of Chemotherapy in the Genesis of Second Tumors

In 1948, A. Haddow experimentally demonstrated the oncogenic potential of antineoplastic drugs, after the discovery of the carcinogenic effects of ionizing radiation. Since then, numerous in vitro and in vivo studies have tested the carcinogenic potential of every single cytotoxic drug. Those that show high oncogenic activity are: alkylating agents, nitrosoureas, dacarbazine, procarbazine, topoisomerase II inhibitors, and hormones (Table 5.1). The platinum compounds cisplatin and carboplatin are carcinogenic both in vitro and in laboratory animals; but it is still not clear whether cisplatin has leukemogenic activity, either alone or in association with other chemotherapic agents, in vivo [1]. The antimetabolites do not seem to be carcinogenic [2], although there are reports in

Table 5.1 Potentially carcinogenic chemotherapeutics

Alkylating agents	Mechlorethamine, chlorambucil, melphalan, busulfan, carmustine, prednimustine, lomustine, semustine, dacarbazine, procarbazine
Topoisomerase II inhibitors	Non-intercalating: Etoposide, teniposide Intercalating: Adriamycin, epirubicin
Hormone therapy	Tamoxifen

the medical literature of second brain tumors in children with acute lymphatic leukemia (ALL) with wild-type thiopurine methyltransferase who were treated with panencephalic prophylactic radiotherapy and high-dose 6-mercaptopurine-based chemotherapy [3].

Generally, chemotherapic drugs are responsible for the appearance of acute myeloid leukemia (whereas radiotherapy causes second solid tumors). Exceptions are bladder cancer and urinary tract carcinoma following cyclophosphamide-based chemotherapy [4] and endometrial carcinoma after hormone therapy with tamoxifen.

Mechanism of Action

The mechanisms by which chemotherapeutic drugs lead to the development of second tumors have not been fully elucidated. There is no direct correlation between antineoplastic drugs and the appearance of iatrogenic tumors. Not all second malignancies are induced by oncologic therapies; rather, multiple factors seem to play important roles in the development of these neoplasms, such as age, genetic predisposition, immunodeficiency, concomitant use of drugs, and continuous environmental and occupational exposure to oncogenic agents. Nevertheless, the most reliable and widely studied mechanisms are: gene polymorphism in drug-metabolizing enzymes [5], alterations in the mechanisms of DNA repair [6], germline mutations in tumor-suppressor genes [7], concomitant administration of other cytostatics/cytotoxics and/or chemo-protective drugs, inter-patient variation in hepatic and renal function, and interindividual differences in drug absorption, distribution, metabolism, and excretion (Fig. 5.1).

Alkylating agents transfer and/or replace alkylating groups by the formation of covalent bonds with DNA, either on a single strand or on both strands, thereby interfering with cell replication. Generally, cellular repair enzymes are able to repair damaged DNA. The most frequent repair mechanism is excision. Specific endonucleases recognize the damaged nitrogenous base and cut the DNA at this site; the cut area is degraded by exonucleases and a DNA polymerase re-synthesizes the missing DNA stretch, thus guaranteeing the continu-

5 Iatrogenic Second Tumors

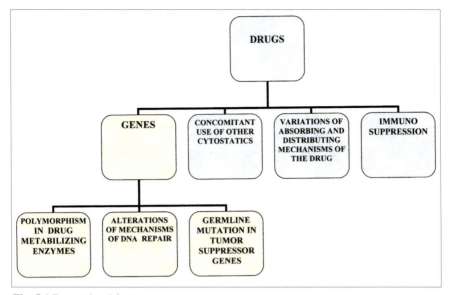

Fig. 5.1 Drug-related factors

ity of the DNA itself. O^6-alkyl guanine transferase repairs damage at the O^6-guanine position by transferring the alkylated group from the guanine residue on the nitrogenous base of the DNA to its own cytosine residue. As a result, the repair enzyme inactivates and progressively consumes itself. Cytoplasmic levels of the enzyme are therefore faithful indicators of the cell's ability to repair damage caused by alkylating agents. Hematopoietic precursors of the bone marrow lack enzymes with alkyltransferase activity, instead reacting to damage suffered by a rapid increase in proliferation. This explains why second tumors arising from alkylating agents are hematological.

Topoisomerase I and II inhibitors bind to the complex DNA topoisomerase, thereby inhibiting the enzymatic reaction such that DNA fragments consisting of strands of the double helix bound to proteins accumulate. The persistence of this lesion during DNA duplication or mRNA transcription prevents proper closure of the strands with subsequent translocations and cell death due to apoptosis or necrosis [8].

Clinical Aspects

Antineoplastic Drugs and Second Acute Myeloid Leukemia

In 1970, Kyle described the occurrence of second acute myeloid leukemia (AML) in patients treated with chemotherapy. Currently, 10–20% of all AMLs are correlated with antineoplastic treatments [7]. The drugs with greatest leukemogenic activity are alkylating agents and topoisomerase II inhibitors; therefore, AML secondary to chemotherapy is classified AML induced by alkylating agents and AML induced by topoisomerase II inhibitors [9, 10] (Table 5.2).

The median latency of AML induced by alkylating agents and nitrosourea is 4–5 years. Such cases are usually preceded by a pre-leukemic phase (myelodysplastic syndromes) lasting about 11 months and subdivided into M1 and M2 forms in according to the French-American-British (FAB) classification [11] (Table 5.3). The most frequent chromosomal abnormality consists of loss of either part or the entire chromosome 5 and/or 7 [12]. Chromosomal damage induced by alkylating agents involves intra-strand bonds in the double helix of DNA. These defects may lead to a delay in anaphase, cause difficulties in correct chromosomal segregation in daughter cells, and induce a loss of chromosomal material. The latter can be considered the first but not the only step in leukemogenic evolution. This would explain why AML secondary to alkylating agents is preceded by a pre-leukemic phase [13].

Table 5.2 Acute myeloid leukemia (AML) resulting from antineoplastic drugs

	Alkylating	Topoisomerase II inhibitors
Latency	4–5 years	2–3 years
Myelodysplastic syndromes	Yes	No
Type of mutation	Deletions: 7q e/o 5q (not balanced)	Translocations: 11q23, 21q22 3q32 (balanced)
FAB classification	M1, M2	M4, M5
Therapeutic response	Poor	Good

FAB, French-American-British Cooperative Group classification

Table 5.3 Acute myeloid leukemias: FAB classification

M0	Minimally differentiated
M1	Myeloblastic with no maturation
M2	Myeloblastic with maturation
M3	Hypergranular promyelocytic
M4Eo	Increase of anomalous medullary eosinophils
M4	Myelomonocytic
M5	Monolithic
M6	Erythroleukemic
M7	Megaloblastic

Moreover, AML secondary to alkylating agents is refractory to treatment, so the prognosis is inauspicious. Alkylating agents with high leukemogenic acivity are: mechlorethamine, chlorambucil, melphalan, carmustine, busulfan, prednimustine, lomustine, semustine, dacarbazine, and procarbazine. Cyclophosphamide has a lower leukemogenic activity; probably due to the presence of an aldehyde deydrogenase in hematopoietic stem cells. This enzyme degrades cyclophosphamide into inactive compounds, i.e., that lack cytotoxic and cancerogenic activity. The risk of the AML secondary to alkylating agents increases with increasing the cumulative dose, the intensity of the dose, and the duration of therapy.

The AML induced by non-intercalating topoisomerase II inhibitors (epipodophyllotoxins, etoposide, and teniposide) appears in younger patients and is not preceded by a pre-leukemic phase. The latency period is less than 2–3 years. Morphologically, the AML is classified as M4 or M5, according to the FAB classification; there is a balanced translocation of chromosomes 11q23, 21q22, 3q32. These patients have a better prognosis because they respond to chemotherapy [12, 14, 15].

The leukemogenic activity of intercalating topoisomerase II inhibitors (anthracyclines) is not well-understood. However, some studies have found a very high risk of AML in women treated with mitoxantrone compared to patients treated with adriamycin and epirubicin.

Tumors with a Higher Risk of Second Malignancies

Hodgkin's Disease

Patients who survive Hodgkin's disease are at higher risk of second tumors than the general population. In these patients, there is a 22-fold relative higher risk for AML, followed by a 6-to14-fold increased risk for non-Hodgkin's lymphomas, a 4- to 11-fold higher risk for mesenchymal tumors of the bone and the thyroid, a 2- to 4-fold higher risk for lung cancer, esophageal cancer, and breast and colon cancers.

The risk of leukemia and non-Hodgkin's lymphoma secondary to chemotherapy is especially high 3–9 years after treatment. The probability of developing second leukemias is greater for patients who were treated with alkylating agents. In fact, it has been estimated that the 15-year cumulative risk of developing an AML after MOPP chemotherapy (mechlorethamine, procarbazine, vincristine, and prednisone) is 9.5% compared to 0.7% for patients treated with the ABVD scheme (doxorubicin, bleomyicina, vinblastine, and dacarbazine) [16].

The combination of chemotherapy and radiotherapy exposes the patient to a higher risk of AML. Actually, for each radiotherapy dose range (<10 GY, 10–20 GY, >20 Gy) the risk of leukemia is significantly higher with increasing number chemotherapeutic cycles [17]. By contrast, for patients receiving a standard number of chemotherapeutic cycles, the risk is not higher with increasing of radiotherapy dose.

The risk of second AML is possible even in patients treated with rescue therapy. The literature reports that patients who received MOPP rescue therapy after radiotherapy had a higher risk of acute leukemia than patients who received initial combined treatment. Finally, there are data indicating the risk of iatrogenic leukemia in patients treated with high-dose chemotherapy associated with autologous bone marrow transplant or hematopoietic progenitor reinfusion [18, 19].

Immunosuppression related to the same disease and immunosuppression secondary to antineoplastic therapies seem to be the cause of the development of post-Hodgkin iatrogenic non-Hodgkin's lymphomas. Unlike the acute leukemias, iatrogenic non-Hodgkin's lymphoma is curable in 50% of cases. These seem correlated with predominantly lymphocytic Hodgkin's lymphomas, compared to those variants featuring nodular sclerosis [20].

Patients with Hodgkin's disease who received radiotherapy have a high risk of developing solid tumors. Specifically, patients who receive radiotherapy and an alkylating-agent-based chemotherapy are at higher risk to develop lung cancer than patients treated with radiotherapy only. Conversely, the risk of developing breast cancer is higher in patients treated only with "mantle" radiotherapy than in patients treated with a combination of chemotherapy and radiotherapy. The reason is that chemotherapy is responsible for premature estro-progestrogenic deprivation (pharmacological menopause), which plays a protective role in the development of breast cancer [21].

Non-Hodgkin's Lymphoma

The risk of developing a second tumor in patients treated for non-Hodgkin's lymphoma is lower than in patients treated for Hodgkin's disease. This can be explained by the quite recent introduction of effective therapies that increase survival and by the older age of these patients at the time of diagnosis, which limits long term observation. The most frequent iatrogenic tumors affecting this cancer patient population are leukemias and bladder carcinomas. Acute leukemias are correlated with the administration of cyclophosphamide-based chemotherapeutic schemes; their incidence does not increase with cumulative dose or with duration of treatment. A very high risk of iatrogenic tumors has been observed in patients treated with prolonged maintenance therapy and/or with simultaneous total body irradiation. As is the case with some patients treated for Hodgkin's disease, the risk of acute leukemia seems to be related to the administration of high-dose therapy in association with autologous bone marrow transplant.

The incidence of bladder carcinoma correlates with the cumulative dose of cyclophosphamide. For a cumulative dose <20 g, no statistically relevant correlation was noted between cyclophosphamide-based treatment and bladder cancer. However, at a cumulative cyclophosphamide dose of 20–50 g or >50 g, the increased risk of bladder carcinoma is 6- and 14.5-fold, respectively, which is statistically significant. Moreover, the risk is higher in patients who were treated concomitantly with radiotherapy and cyclophosphamide-based chemotherapy [22].

Breast Cancer

The risk of a second tumor developing in a woman who has recovered from breast cancer is only in part related to the treatment she received. Breast cancer patients have a higher predisposition to develop a second, contralateral breast tumor or a second breast cancer on the previously operated breast; the risk of uterine, ovarian, colon, esophageal, and lung cancer is also higher. Thus it is difficult, in the absence of knowledge regarding individual risk factors, to determine whether the development of a second tumor is the result of radiotherapy, chemotherapy, hormone therapy, or a combination thereof, or whether there is no correlation at all.

The use of tamoxifen for 2 years is associated with two-fold increased risk of of endometrial carcinoma whereas the risk is 4- to 8-fold higher for those patients taking the drug for 5 years. Moreover, this risk is higher in women pretreated with estrogen hormone therapy before tamoxifen [23]. Nevertheless, due to its protective effects, i.e., lower risk of loco-regional recurrence, distance recurrence, and a second, contralateral breast tumor, and improved disease-free survival (DFS) and overall survival (OS), tamoxifen still represents one of the most important drugs for breast cancer patients in the adjuvant and advanced settings.

Chemotherapy increases the risk of second acute leukemia, and the risk is higher for alkylating-agent-based regimens and for concomitant administration of radiotherapy once chemotherapeutic regimens have reached the cumulative leukemogenic dose. Currently, the leukemogenic activity of antineoplastic drugs used in adjuvant therapy for breast cancer is more closely correlated with dose intensity than with cumulative dose. It may well be that the intensified schedules increase the rate of DNA deletions and/or translocations beyond that allowing repair.

Role of Radiotherapy in the Genesis of Second Tumors

Radiotherapy administered for curative and palliative purposes is, for many patients, the therapy of choice. The biological assumption is that radiotherapy yields the "inactivation" of malignant cells, by irradiation of a specific tumor volume, with the least damage to healthy tissues, through the choice of optimized therapy schemes such as TCP (tumor control probability) and NTCP (normal tissue complication probability) models. However, beyond the well-known beneficial effects, there is a wide range of complications, the most fearsome of which is the oncologic potential of ionizing radiation, as widely analyzed in nuclear catastrophes survivors [24, 25].

The risk of tumor induced by high-dose radiotherapy was clearly established as early as 1956, J.P. Palmer [26, 27]. Indeed, the development of a second primary tumor represents the most fearsome complication of this form of therapy. A neoplasm is defined as "radio-induced" based on the following parameters: (a) it must appear in the irradiated area after a defined latency; (b) it must be absent prior to irradiation; (c) it must be histologically different from the original tumor treated with radiotherapy; (d) its incidence must be higher in irradiated patients; (e) a genetic diathesis or familial relationship to the development of the neoplasm must be excluded [28]. The time of onset of an iatrogenic, radiation-induced tumor ranges from 2–3 years for hematological malignancies to 5–10 years for solid ones.

Ionizing Radiation

In order to understand the mechanisms through which ionizing radiation damages cells, the fundamental concept in radiobiology of linear energy transfer (LET), that is the ability of radiation to determine ionization in penetrating irradiated tissues, must be understood. LET is a function of the charge and the speed of the ionizing particle; thus, there is high LET (particle α, neutrons and protons) and low LET (X rays and γ rays) radiation (Fig. 5.2).

Since the biological effect of radiation depends on the quantity of energy released as the radiation source passes through the tissues, it is clear that high LET radiation produces greater damage to DNA (Fig. 5.3) as the density of ionization, expressed as the relative biological effectiveness (RBE), is higher than that of low LET radiation [20].

The degree of radiation-induced damage at the molecular level is a function of physical, biological, and chemical factors. Specifically, physical factors include whether the dose is single or fractional, the irradiated volume, and the intensity and type of radiation used. Biological factors are related to: cellular kinetics (i.e., cell cycle phase at the moment of irradiation), the radiosensitivity

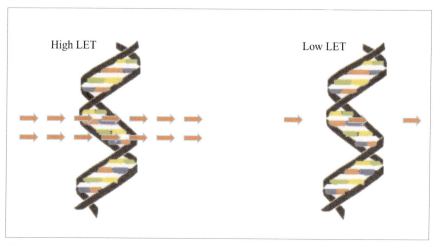

Fig. 5.2 Radiation with different linear energy transfers (LETs)

5 Iatrogenic Second Tumors

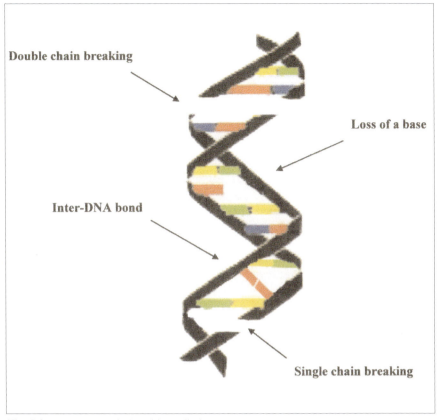

Fig. 5.3 DNA Damage induced by radiation

of the cellular population, and the repair capacity of the cells or tissues. Chemical factors include the action of agents that can enhance (sensitizers) or diminish (protective action) the efficacy of the radiation dose.

Ionizing radiation effects can also be divided into those that are stochastic (probabilistic) vs. those that are graduated (deterministic) (Table 5.4). Stochastic effects are manifested by the appearance of leukemia or a solid neoplasm, as a result of alterations in the genetic inheritance of somatic cells, and by the appearance of malformations in the patient's progeny, if the alterations involve the germinal cells. For stochastic effects it is difficult to establish a causal connection, since other factors (not related to radiation exposure) influence the degree of cell damage. They become evident when the incidence of a leukemia or solid tumor is higher than the spontaneous one, as discussed in the next section.

Graduated effects usually reveal themselves in patients who are treated with radiotherapy or who were accidentally exposed to important radiation doses (contamination) [29]. In either case, it is possible to make a connection between

Table 5.4 Biological effects of irradiation

Effects	Threshold to dose	Proportional to dose	Level-size damage	Cause-effect relationship
Deterministic	Yes	Damage	Specific	Certain
Stochastic	No	Probability	Aspecific	Uncertain

the radiation dose, which exceeds the threshold dose, and the biological damage. The timing with which these effects reveal themselves can vary from a minimum of hours or days to a maximum of several years. Other relevant factors influencing the time in which graduated effects become apparent include the delivery modality of the dose (single or fractional dose), the irradiated organ or tissue type, and the ability of the affected cell population to repair the damage. *Acute* effects occur generally within 6 months of exposure, *subacute* effects between 6 and 12 months of exposure, *chronic* effects within 2–5 years, and *late* effects after 5 years (Table 5.5).

It is particularly important to establish the radiosensitivity of a biological system since it as indicator of whether graduated (deterministic) effects are likely. This may prove difficult because of the contribution of several cell- and tissue-specific variables; however, it is possible to define a relative radiosensitivity scale for different cell populations [30] (Table 5.6).

Table 5.5 Late-type tiered effects

Organ	Possible damages within 5 years from irradiation
Skin	Ulceration, serious fibrosis
Esophagus, stomach, small intestine, colon, rectum	Ulceration, stenosis
Salivary glands	Xerostomia
Liver	Hepatitis, ascites
Kidney	Sclerosis
Testicle	Sterility
Lung	Pneumonia, fibrosis
Heart	Pericarditis
Bone	Necrosis, fracture
Encephalus	Necrosis
Spinal marrow	Necrosis, myelitis

5 Iatrogenic Second Tumors

Table 5.6 Scale of relative radiosensitivity

Cell population	Radiosensitivity
Spermatogonia	High
Lymphocytes, erythroblasts	High
Intestine, stomach, colon basal cells	Medium
Cutaneous and endothelial cells	Medium
Nerve cells	Low
Muscle cells	Low

Stochastic (Probabilistic) Effects and Second Tumor Formation

Stochastic effects arise from ionizing-radiation-induced alterations in the cell's genetic material. In somatic cells, they are responsible for the possible onset of second tumor following radiotherapy, whereas in gonadal cells they explain the occurrence of genetic defects that cause mutations transmittable to the patient's progeny. Tumor induction is accidental and ensues after a long latency period, i.e., from the exposure to and action of a potential oncogenic agent to the clinical onset of illness. After entering the tissue, the radiation must interact with that tissue by delivering energy (giving rise to ionization) such that there is irreparable damage to the DNA giving rise to a neoblastic mutation, and ultimately a clinically evident tumor, rather than destruction of the cell by the body's defense mechanisms (Table 5.7). Based on the follow-up of a sufficiently large series of patients, the onset of a tumor can be statistically correlated with exposure to low-dose ionizing radiation, although not with a specific dose.

Our knowledge of the effects of irradiation on the human body comes from studies of individuals who have survived of nuclear disasters (Hiroshima, Chernobyl) as well as those working in professions in which there is exposure to a very fractionated but cumulative irradiation dose, such as radiologists, radiographers, surgeons, etc.), and uranium-mine workers. Radio-induced skin cancers in the former group are "typical" malignancies, while in the latter the extended exposure to radon is associated with a 3- to 3- to 4-fold higher incidence of lung tumors compared to control groups. In such patients, it is often difficult to precisely calculate the absorbed dose, or the contribution of different forms of radiation (low or high LET). Moreover, since the radiation exposure is sometimes only partial (involving only certain organs and tissues), the estimates have a high margin of error. Nonetheless, the findings are conclusive enough to allow us to state that even a minimum dose exposure confers effects, and there is no threshold dose below which an exposure-related risk can be excluded [30].

Table 5.7 Sequence of irradiation effects

Time (latency)	Event	Effect
0	Irradiation	
10^{-15} seconds	Physical	Ionization-excitation
Minutes	Biochemical (macromolecules)	Enzymatic and DNA damage
Hours-Days	Genetic mutations, mitotic inhibition, activation of polymerase	Phenotypic and genotypic alterations, cell death, damage repair
Weeks-months	Biological system changes	Alterations in organ function, death
Years	Expression of somatic and genetic mutations	Radio-induced tumors, hereditary diseases

Clinical Aspects

Colorectal Cancer Following Radiotherapy

The radio-induced neoplasm has a latency time of 5–15 years after exposure and an onset site inside the irradiated field. Prostate cancer is associated with a 10-year survival of over 80%; treatment consists of radiotherapy or surgical resection. In the former group of patients, a link to the development of rectal cancer is suspected since, during pelvic prostate irradiation (Fig. 5.4), the rectum receives high-dose radiation, with smaller doses to other areas of the colon (particularly the rectosigmoid, the sigmoid, and the cecum). However, the literature is inconsistent and contradictory, with the exception of a US study that uses SEER data (Surveillance, Epidemiology and End Results) from the period between 1973 and 1994 [31].

The selection criteria of were patients with non-metastatic, histologically confirmed disease. Only patients who had survived at least 5 years from the follow-up for prostate cancer were included, while patients with a previous diagnosis of colorectal tumor as well those who had developed the tumor within the first 5 years post-therapy or who did not undergo any type of therapy were excluded. The series thus consisted of 85,815 men, age about 67 years, and a period of observation >9 years. These patients were divided in two groups: (I) 55,263 only-surgery patients and (II) 30,552 radiotherapy (with or without surgery) patients. The colorectal cancers that developed were also subdivided according to site: (a) located in a definite irradiated field (rectum), (b) located in a potential irradiated field (rectosigmoid, sigmoid, cecum), and (c) located in a non-irradiated field (ascending colon, hepatic flexure, transverse colon, splenic flexure, descending colon) (Fig. 5.5).

5 Iatrogenic Second Tumors

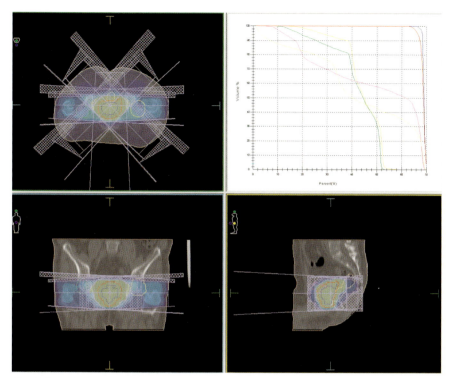

Fig. 5.4 Irradiation fields "3D Conformational Therapy" for prostate cancer

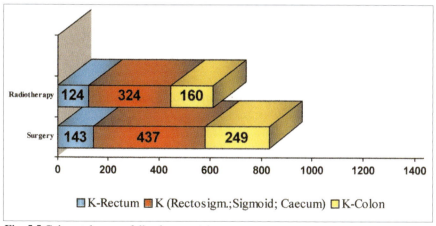

Fig. 5.5 Colorectal cancer following prostate cancer

The number of colorectal neoplasms observed after at least 5 years was 1,437, divided as follows: 267 rectal tumors; 686 rectosigmoid, sigmoid, and caecum; and 484 other sites in the colon (Table 5.8).

Table 5.8 Summary data

Neoplasm site (n)	Surgery only	Radiotherapy only
Radiotherapy field: rectum (267)	143 (15.8%)	124 (23.2%)
Bordering area: rectosigmoid colon, sigmoid colon, cecum (686)	437 (48.4%)	249 (46.8%)
No radiotherapy: other sites of the colon (484)	324 (35.8%)	160 (30%)
Total number of neoplasms: 1,437	904	533

The percentage of patients who developed rectal cancer was higher in the group that had undergone radiotherapy, with a hazard ratio of 1.7 (95% CI: 1.4–2.2). Regarding the development of tumors in potentially irradiated or non irradiated sites, the data of the two groups were essentially superimposable. Radiation and older age at diagnosis were identified as the main factors responsible for radio-induced second tumors.

The increased risk of iatrogenic second tumor in the rectum can be explained by the fact that the rectum is so close to the prostate that the two structures receive almost the same dose of radiation. This association has important implications for the screening of colorectal cancer; prostate irradiation must be included among the risk factors for rectal cancer and such patients should undergo endoscopic examination starting from the fifth year after radiotherapy.

Moreover, a possible reverse correlation was established by the Swedish Cancer Registry, in a report published by Birgisson [32]. In 115 patients treated with radiotherapy for rectal cancer who subsequently developed a second neoplasm, prostate (21), colon (17), and bladder (12) were the most common sites of second tumor development.

Carcinogenic Effects of Radiotherapy for Seminoma

Seminoma is a highly curable neoplasm; its radio-chemo sensitivity results in a 10-year survival of 90–95%, despite the fact that nearly 15% of seminomas at first stage present with occult lymph node involvement. In such patients, postoperative radiotherapy has been shown to provide excellent adjuvant treatment (Fig. 5.6). In most cases, treatment concerns the radiation of lymph nodes of the lumbo-aortic tract with extension to the homo or bilateral iliac station. The total dose of radiation is low (25–30 Gy). Radioprotection of the patient includes screening of the other testicle, even if only lumbo-aortic fields are irradiated, and the use of "multi leaf" or lead screens.

Nonetheless, the possibility of a radio-induced second neoplasm is high since most patients are young and have a long life expectancy. The Netherlands Cancer Institute reported a global actuarial risk of 9.8% at 15 years post-treat-

5 Iatrogenic Second Tumors

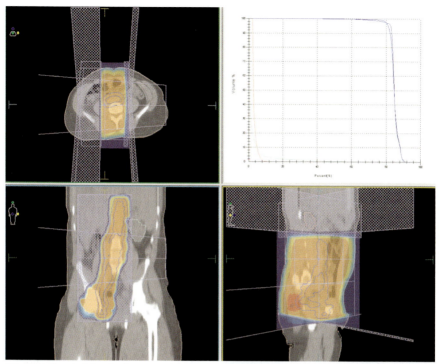

Fig. 5.6 Classic "dog-leg" approach encompasses para-aortic and ipsilateral pelvic nodes

ment. A risk of 3.4% for gastrointestinal tumors and 2.4% for contralateral testicular tumors was estimated based on the case histories of 1909 patients followed on average for 7.7 years. A recent update of the same case histories (median 10.8 years) confirmed an increased relative risk of tumors of the stomach (6.5), pancreas (6.0), kidney (5.1), and bladder (4.4) [33].

The risk of a contralateral testicular tumor was ascribed to predisposing factors, such as cryptorchidism or the presence of an atrophic testicle. However, the increased risk of a gastrointestinal tract tumor (in particular, stomach and pancreas) seemed to be closely connected to previous radiotherapy and to represent a dose-effect response, since the risk increased three-fold after 30–35 Gy and of 27-fold after 40–45 Gy. Today, the tendency is to use a lower radiation dose; nevertheless the possibility of a second radio-induced neoplasm must be taken into consideration in follow-up protocols.

Radiotherapy for Hodgkin's disease and the Development of Second Tumors

Current therapies for Hodgkin's disease have resulted in a very high percentage of recoveries (80–90%) in some subgroups, and therefore an increase in long-time survival. Consequently, over time, side effects linked to different therapeutic strategies are likely to occur. With the wider use of sequential treatment of low-dose chemotherapy and radiotherapy, the incidence of post-irradiation sequelae is lower than in the past. However, radiotherapy for Hodgkin's disease often requires high-energy radiation (between 32 and 36 Gy) and the treatment of a large number of lymph nodes at different sites involving large "mantle" fields (for example, cervical, axillary, mediastinal, and hilar) (Fig. 5.7) while protecting critical organs and tissues with lead and multi-leaf screens. Given the high percentage of recovery of Hodgkin's disease patients and thus the longer observation time, the onset of a second tumor, especially in patients who received radiotherapy, is not surprising. Almost 80% of these tumors appear in previously irradiated sites, or at the edge of them, and the risk is about 13% at 15 years post-treatment, increasing with increasing number of years of follow-up [34].

Recently, an international retrospective study was carried out on over 32,000 Hodgkin's lymphoma patients. This study, by the National Cancer Institute, evaluated the risk of developing a second neoplasm among Hodgkin's disease

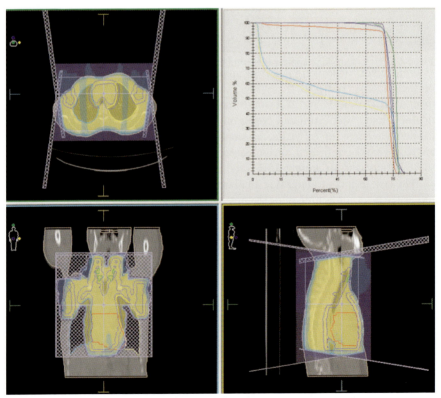

Fig. 5.7 "Mantle" radiotherapy for Hodgkin's lymphoma

survivors, as determined using the database of 16 tumor registries in the USA, Canada, and several European countries. Patients in the series had the longest follow-up of any study thus far; 1,111 patients had been followed for 25 years. The study concluded that survivors had double the probability to develop a second tumor compared to the general population, and this probability remained significantly high for 25 years, after which the relative risk declined [35]. Previous studies had demonstrated that the risk of a second neoplasm remained high 20 years after the initial diagnosis. In particular, we have seen that "mantle radiation" or radiation of cervical sites is associated with a 2.4- to 14-fold higher risk of inducing thyroid tumors, depending on the age of the patient. Children have a considerably higher risk (60- to 65-fold) than adult patients (about 15-fold). There is also a 1.5- to 2.1-fold higher risk of a breast tumor [20]. Recent research from Stanford University pointed out that the risk of developing a breast neoplasm is four times higher in Hodgkin's disease patients who underwent "mantle therapy" than in the same age-matched population.

The increased risk of breast carcinoma is most prominent 15 years after the initial exposure, and in almost all the published case histories the carcinoma developed within or at the edge of the radiotherapy field, mostly involving internal quadrants of the breast. Another important aspect connected to previous radiotherapy treatments is the frequent bilateralism of breast neoplasms, the same histological characteristics, in both locations, and the premature age of onset. Finally, there is an increased risk of developing a lung tumor after treatment for Hodgkin's disease, particularly in patients who were irradiated with "mantle fields" who were smokers, and middle-aged (40–42 years) at the time of the diagnosis [22].

Conclusions

The benefits of current therapies exceed by far the possible side effects of such treatments. Maintenance of these high recovery and survival rates and a reduction of the occurrence of second neoplasms to a minimum require that patients at high risk are identified. This can be achieved by the use of targeted screening programs and therapies with both documented effectiveness and a low rate of carcinogenicity.

References

1. Greene MH (1992) Is cisplatin a human carcinogen? J Natl Cancer Inst 84:306
2. IARC (1987) Overall evaluations of carcinogenicity: an updating of IARC monographs volumes 1 to 42. IARC Monogr Eval Carcinog Risks Hum Suppl 7:1
3. Cheson BD, Vena DA, Barrett J, Freidlin B (1999) Second malignancies as a consequence of nucleoside analog therapy for chronic lymphoid leukemia. J Clin Oncol 17(8):2454
4. Travis LB, Curtis RE, Grimelius B et al (1995) Bladder and kidney cancer following cyclophosphamide therapy for non-Hodgkin's lymphoma. J Natl Cancer Inst 87:524

5. Felix CA (1999) Chemotherapy-related second cancers. In: Neugut AI, Meadows AT, Robinson E (eds) Multiple primary cancers. Lippincott Williams & Wilkins, Philadelphia, p 137
6. Ben-Yehuda D, Krichevsky S, Caspi O et al (1996) Microsatellite instability and p53 mutations in therapy-related leukemia suggest mutator phenotype. Blood 88(11):4296
7. Smith MA, McCaffrey RP, Karp JE (1996) The secondary leukemia: challenges and research directions". J Natl Cancer Inst 88(7):407
8. Davies Stella M (1995) Mechanisms of cytotoxicity and leukemogenesis: topoisomerase II inhibitors and alkylating agents. In ASCO Educational Book, American Society of Clinical Oncology Educational Symposia. 31st annual meeting; May 20-23, 1995, Los Angeles, p 204
9. Pedersen-Bjergaard J, Rowley JD (1994) The balanced and the unbalanced chromosome aberrations of acute myeloid leukemia may develop in different ways and may contribute differently to malignant transformation. Blood 83:2780
10. Smith MA, Rubinstein L, Ungerleider RS (1994) Therapy-related acute myeloid leukemia following treatment with epipodophyllotoxins: estimating the risks. Med Pediatric Oncol 23:86
11. Levine EG, Bloomfield CD (1992) Leukemias and myelodysplastic syndromes secondary to drug, radiation, and environmental exposure. Semin Oncol 19:47
12. Pedersen-Bjergaard J, Philip P, Larsen G, Byrsting K (1990) Chromosome aberrations and prognostic factors in therapy-related myelodysplasia and acute nonlymphocytic leukemia. Blood 76:1083
13. Van Leeuwen FE, Chorus AM, van der Belt-Dusebout AW et al (1994) Leukemia risk following Hodgkin's disease: relation to cumulative dose of alkylating agents, treatment with teniposide combinations, number of episodes of chemotherapy, and bone marrow damage. J Clin Oncol 12:1063
14. Pedersen- Bjergaard J, Pedersen M, Roulston D, Philip P (1995) Different genetic pathways in leukemogenesis for patients presenting with therapy-related myelodysplasia and therapy-related acute myeloid leukemia. Blood 86(9):3542
15. Pedersen- Bjergaard J, Philip P (1991) Balanced translocations involving chromosome bands 11q23 and 21q22 and highly characteristic of myelodisplasia and leukemia following therapy with cytotatic agents targeting at DNA-topoisomerase II (Letter). Blood 78:1147
16. Valagussa PA, Bonadonna G (1995) Carcinogenic effects of cancer treatment. In: Peckham M, Pinedo H, Veronesi U (eds) Oxford textbook of oncology. Oxford University Press, Oxford, p 2348
17. Kaldor JM, Day NE, Klarke EA et al (1990) Leukemia following Hodgkin's disease (see comments). N Engl J Med 322:7
18. Park S, Brice P, Noguerra ME et al (2000) Myelodysplasias and leukemias after autologous stem cell transplantation for lymphoid malignancies. Bone Marrow Transplant 26(3):321
19. Metayer C, Curtis RE, Vose J et al (2003) Myelodisplastic syndrome and acute myeloid leucemia after autotransplantation for lymphoma: a multicenter case control study. Blood 101(5):2015
20. Bonadonna G, Valagussa G (2003) Tumori iatrogeni. In: Bonadonna G, Valagussa G, Robustelli della Cuna G (eds) Medicina Oncologica, VII edizione. Elsevier Masson, Bologna, pp 1663-1680
21. Van Leeuwen FE, Klokman WJ, Stovall M et al (2003) Roles of radiation dose, chemotherapy and hormonal factors in breast cancer following Hodgkin's disease. J Natl Cancer Inst 95(13):971
22. van Leeuwen FE, Travis LB (2005) Second cancers. In: De Vita VT, Hellman S, Rosenberg SA (eds) Cancer: principles and practice of oncology, 7th edn. Lippincott Williams & Wilkins, Philadelphia, pp 2575-2600
23. Bernstein L, Deapen D, Cerhan JR et al (1999) Tamoxifen therapy for breast cancer and endometrial cancer risk. J Natl Cancer Inst 91(19):1654
24. Lend CE, Tokunaga M, Koyama K et al (2003) Incidence of female breast cancer among atom-

ic bomb survivors, Hiroshima-Nagasaki 1950–1990. Radiat Res 160:707–717
25. Thompson DE, Mabuchi K, Ron E et al (1994) Cancer incidence in atomic bomb survivors. Part II: Solid tumors, 1958-1987. Radiat Res 137(2 Suppl):S17-S67
26. Sachs RK et al (2005) Solid tumor risks after high doses of ionizing radiation. Proc Natl Acad Sci USA 102(37):13040–13045
27. Palmer JP et al (1956) Pelvic carcinoma following irradiation for benign gynecological diseases. Am J Obstet Gynecol 72:497–505
28. Bernstein M et al (1991) Radiation-induced tumors of the nervous system In: Gutin Ph et al (eds) Radiation injury to the nervous system. Raven, New York, pp 455–472
29. Perez CA, Brady LW (1998) Principles and practice of radiation oncology. JB Lippincott, Philadelphia
30. Orecchia R, Lucignani G, Tosi G (2001) Elementi di radiobiologia clinica e radioprotezione. Archimedica, Turin
31. Baxter NN et al (2005) Increased risk of rectal cancer after prostate radiation: a population-based study. Gastroenterology 128:819–824
32. Birgisson H et al (2005) Occurrence of second cancers in patients treated with radiotherapy for rectal cancer. J Clin Oncol 23:25
33. Travis LB et al (1997) Risk of second malignant neoplasm among long-term survivors of testicular cancer. J Natl Cancer 89:1429–1439
34. Valagussa P (1993) Second neoplasm following treatment of H.D. Current Opinion Oncol 5:805–811
35. Kennedy BJ (1998) The National Cancer data base report on Hodgkin's disease. Cancer 83 (5):1041–1047

Chapter 6

Immunodeficiency and Multiple Primary Malignancies

Michele Santangelo, Sergio Spiezia, Marco Clemente, Andrea Renda,
Arturo Genovese, Giuseppe Spadaro, Concetta D'Orio, Gianni Marone,
Stefano Federico, Massimo Sabbatini, Eliana Rotaia,
Pierluca Piselli, Claudia Cimaglia, Diego Serraino

Immunology and Cancer

The relationship between cancer onset and the immune response became a subject of great interest in the early 1900s, and led Ehrlich [1] to establish what came to be known as the theory of immunological surveillance. This theory is based on three principles: (1) cancer cells are antigenic, (2) these cells can be destroyed by the immune response of the organism (by a mechanism similar to that observed in transplanted tissue or organ rejection), and (3) immune depression is related to a higher incidence of neoplastic disease [2]. The theory is based on the concept that the immune system is able to recognize cancer cells as non-self and consequently to destroy them. Furthermore, this response involves both branches of the immune system. However, this defensive system is not as perfect as it may seem at first sight, because more often than not a certain number of cancer cells do avoid surveillance and subsequent destruction by immune-competent cells and thus continue to proliferate, until they give rise to the various forms of malignancies. The mechanisms by which cancer cells elude immunological surveillance may be explained by some intrinsic characteristics of these cells and/or the patient's condition, including an immune deficiency.

Immune Deficiencies

The immune response is the result of complex interactions between the various mechanisms that make up the defensive system of the organism. Specifically, it is the result of a cooperation between surface barriers (mucous membranes and skin), innate immunity (including the monocyte/macrophage system and complement), and the adaptive or specific immune system (antibodies and cell-mediated immunity). Defects in one or more of these systems compromise the immune response, leading to the development of an immune deficiency (ID).

The IDs are classified as primary and secondary. The primary immune deficiencies (PIDs) make up a large group of genetically determined pathological conditions. While these apparently differ from a pathogenetic point of view, all are caused by an intrinsic dysfunction of the cells of the immune system. Therefore, it is possible to schematically classify PIDs according to the mechanisms involved (Table 6.1). By contrast, secondary immune deficiencies (SIDs) represent a group of diseases in which the immune system is compromised by a pathological process, such as infections (human immunodeficiency virus, cytomegalovirus, Epstein-Barr virus), cancer, or therapeutic interventions (drug therapy, radiotherapy, surgery, etc.) (Tables 6.2, 6.3). The fundamental feature of a primary or secondary immune deficiency is obviously an increased susceptibility to infections, but there is also evidence that immune system defects can, in turn, determine the development of a neoplastic disease. In this context, of particular interest are multiple primary malignancies (MPM); that is, the presence in the same subject of two or more malignancies that show specific characteristics, such as time of appearance, histology and site of onset, that allow each lesion to be considered as a new cancer and not simply as secondary or recurrent tumors.

For practical purposes, the relationship between MPM and primary or secondary immune deficiencies are considered separately, in this latter case based on observations of transplanted patients (the vast majority of patients with iatrogenic immune suppression) and patients with acquired immumodeficiency syndrome (AIDS) (the largest group of patients with acquired immune suppression).

Table 6.1 Classification of primary immune deficiencies (modified from the WHO classification)

Deficiencies affecting antibody production
– Agammaglobulinemia X-linked (Bruton's disease)
– Common variable immune deficiencies
– IgA selective deficit
– Transient hypogammaglobulinemia of infancy
Combined immunodeficiency
– Hyper-IgM disease
– Adenosine deaminase (ADA) disease
– Severe combined immunodeficiency disease (SCID)
– Reticular dysgenesis

Defects in phagocyte function
– Chronic granulomatous disease
– Neutropenia
– Chediak-Higashi syndrome

Immunodeficiency-syndrome-associated
– Ataxia-telangiectasia
– DiGeorge syndrome
– Wiskott-Aldrich syndrome
– Hyper-IgE syndrome

Table 6.2 Secondary immunodeficiencies

Physiologic causes	Prematurity, prenatally, pregnancy, senescence
Pathologic causes	Lost protein enteropathy, nephrotic syndrome, alcoholic cirrhosis, diabetes, malnutrition, scald, diarrhea, Cushing syndrome, splenectomy
Iatrogenic causes	Drugs, surgery, radiotherapy
Cancer	Leukemia, lymphoma B cell, cancer, Good's syndrome
Infection	HIV, congenital rubella virus, measles virus, mononucleosis, CMV, toxoplasmosis

Table 6.3 Pharmacological immunodepression

Cytostatic	Azathioprine, methotrexate
Immunosuppressants	Cyclosporine A, FK-506
Steroids	
Biologicals	Infliximab, etanercept
Others	Barbiturates, carbamazepine, phenytoin, penicillin, sulfasalazine, captopril

Primary Immune Deficiencies, Cancer, and Multiple Primary Malignancies

It has been observed that cancer-related mortality in patients with PID may be 10–200 times higher as than in the age-matched general population. Several mechanisms have been hypothesized as possible causes of the increased susceptibility of PID patients to neoplastic disease [3], including: (a) suppressed immune response to oncogenic viruses, (b) loss of immune surveillance, (c) chronic stimulation and proliferation of lymphocytes that respond to specific antigens, and (d) possible disorders with independent effects on oncogenesis and on the immune system.

As already mentioned, the incidence of tumors appears to be higher in PID patients [4], but this increase seems to be particularly significant in those with ataxia-telangiectasia or Wiskott-Aldrich syndrome and in those with a defective humoral immune response, such as recently described in individuals with common variable immune deficiency (CVID), Bruton's disease, and selective IgA deficit [5].

Ataxia-telangiectasia (A-T) is an autosomal recessive syndrome characterized by progressive immune deficiency, progressive cerebellar ataxia, oculocutaneous telangiectasia, radiosensitivity and increased levels of α-fetoprotein. Neoplastic disease is a frequent complication and a principal cause of mortality in approximately one-third of these patients. The tumors more frequently associated with A-T are those of the lymphoreticular system, mainly in patients under 15 years of age. In this context, over 40% of the tumors are non-Hodgkin's lymphomas, approximately 20% acute lymphocytic leukemias, and 5% Hodgkin's lymphomas.

The Wiskott-Aldrich syndrome is an X-linked recessive disorder with a symptomatological triad of microthrombocytopenia, eczema, and recurrent infections. In this group of patients, approximately 13% develop neoplastic lesions, mainly non-Hodgkin's lymphomas, all of which occur in early age, with average survival rates of approximately 6 years [6].

Furthermore, controlled study results showed that neoplastic disease develops in approximately 10% of patients with CVID, a heterogeneous disorder in which serum immunoglobulin levels are reduced. In this group, the most frequent neoplasias are gastrointestinal cancer (adenocarcinoma of the stomach and colon), especially in case of co-existing IgA deficiency, and lymphoreticular cancer (Hodgkin's and non-Hodgkin's lymphomas) [7, 8]. Moreover, CVID patients often show evidence of a lymphoproliferative disease but without signs of malignancy, at least at the time of diagnosis, such as lymphonodal involvement with follicular hyperplasia and intestinal nodular lymphoid hyperplasia; the clinical evolution of the latter is poorly defined and therefore necessitates careful patient monitoring. It has also been hypothesized that certain microorganisms, such as Epstein-Barr virus (EBV), human herpesvirus 8 (HHV-8) and *Helicobacter pylori* are involved in carcinogenesis in CVID patients [8–12].

The small number of cases reported in the literature do not allow for a reliable evaluation of the incidence of MPM in PID patients,, as there are no meaningful clinical statistics [3, 12]. The absence of MPM in PID may well be due to the decreased survival of such patients. In fact, the clinical picture is rather severe throughout the course of their disease, and often features infections, which are most likely responsible for the overall reduction of survival. Fortunately, today, a diagnosis of PID can be established very early and, more importantly, appropriate strategic therapies can be implemented that prolong the life expectancy of ID patients. The results of these therapeutic approaches are that patients live longer despite the persistence of a compromised immune response. However, this increases the possibility of developing complications related to immunodeficiency, including MPM.

Besides the recent description of multiple malignancies of the colon in patients with Bruton's disease [13], we reported two cases of MPM in CVID patients. More precisely, MPMs (metachronous) were detected in two patients, one with gastric and gallbladder adenocarcinoma and the other with non-Hodgkin's lymphoma and cervical carcinoma. Furthermore, antineoplastic surveillance implemented in CVID patients admitted to our clinic showed that 15% had gastric metaplasia.

In conclusion, since the number of patients with PID and MPM probably is likely to increase in the next few years, antineoplastic surveillance appears to be more than necessary in this patient population, especially those individuals who have already had a neoplastic disease.

Secondary Immune Deficiencies, Cancer, and Multiple Primary Malignancies: Transplants

Today, the high standards in the surgical, anesthesiological, and clinical management of transplant patients have resulted in extremely positive results regarding short and medium-term survival, of both the transplanted organs and the patients. However, these results have been partially nullified by the long-term complications reported in these subjects, especially the development of cancer. In fact, the incidence and aggressiveness of neoplastic diseases appear to be remarkably increased in this group of patients compared to the age-matched general population (Fig. 6.1). Moreover, within the population of renal transplant patients, mortality over the long term due to cancer is higher than that due to cardiovascular diseases. It has been calculated that the prevalence of neoplastic disease at 10 years post-renal transplant is 20–30%, with peaks of 40% at 20 years

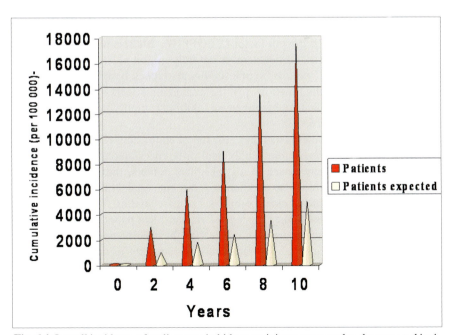

Fig. 6.1 Overall incidence of malignancy in kidney recipients compared to the expected incidence in general population

[14]. Observing this same problem from a different point of view, we can say that approximately 75% of subjects undergoing renal transplant will develop a skin cancer during their post-transplant life [15]. However, it must also be noted that in the population of patients undergoing an organ transplant, the main factor among those facilitating the development of a neoplastic lesion (age, male sex, genetic predisposition, cigarette smoking, the baseline disease responsible for organ failure and determining the need for transplant, UV exposure, use/abuse of drugs) is undoubtedly immune-suppressive treatment. This conclusion is supported by the following observations: (1) subjects undergoing immune-suppressive treatment for reasons other than transplant also have an increased risk of developing neoplastic lesions, even in the absence of other pro-carcinogenic factors [16]; (2) some types of tumors that develop in transplanted patients regress if the immune-suppressive therapy is suspended or substituted [17]. The association between pharmacological immune suppression and an increased risk of cancer is a very widely discussed topic in clinical medicine, and much attention has been given to, among others, the duration of immune suppression therapy, the intensity of treatment, and the drugs or combination of drugs used. Regarding the carcinogenic potential of the various immune-suppressive agents administered to transplant patients, the prevailing hypotheses are that anti-lymphocyte antibodies increase the risk of viral infections and, consequently, facilitate the development of virus-induced neoplastic lesions [17]; azathioprine (a purine analogue) induces chromosomal aberrations and makes cells particularly susceptible to the carcinogenic effect of UVA [18, 19]; calcineurin inhibitors (cyclosporine and tacrolimus) interfere with the synthesis of cytokines, leading to an over-expression of transforming growth factor (TGF)-β and vascular endothelial growth factor (VEGF) [16, 20, 21]; with chronic treatment and at higher doses, corticosteroids not only inhibit macrophage functions and pro-inflammatory cytokines synthesis, but also block lymphocyte proliferation and reduce NK cells functions [3]; the mutagenic effects of mycophenolate (an inosine monophosphate dehydrogenase inhibitor) amplify the aggressiveness of neoplastic lesions [16, 22].

Nonetheless, the numerous studies still report contrasting results due to, e.g., the fragmentation of case studies, individual differences among patients, different therapeutic approaches used in all transplant centers, the switch from one immune-suppressive protocol to another, and, last but certainly not least, the pressure exercised by pharmaceutical companies in case studies. Thus, perhaps the truth is that, globally, the higher cancer risk in transplant patients is more generically related to immune suppression rather than the specific compound(s) used.

Malignant tumors are an important cause of mortality in the United States, second only to cardiovascular diseases [17]. Nonetheless, it has been calculated that if malignant tumors carried a lower mortality rate and were more uniformly distributed in the general population, we could still expect to find that one out nine cancer patients would develop a second neoplasia during the course of his life and that within this latter group 1 out 27 would probably have a third primary cancer [23]. This type of statistical projection obviously refers to the general population. Accordingly, it would be logical to conclude that, from a merely theoretical and statistical point of view, immune-suppressed patients are at potentially higher risk of developing MPM. However, this conclusion is not substantiated by clinical findings, perhaps because these patients die of cancer before the appearance of a "second primary malignancy" but also because of the difficulty in finding transplant patients who survive a first cancer and continue immune-suppressive treatment long enough to develop a second primary cancer related to the iatrogenic immune deficiency state. Nonetheless, a few observations have been made regarding the correlation between iatrogenic immune suppression and MPM.

The possibility that a transplant patient undergoing immune-suppressive treatment develops a second cancer should be examined in particular situations:
1. The patient recovers from a cancer, undergoes transplantation, and then has a new cancer at follow-up
2. The patient recovers from a cancer, undergoes transplantation, and develops a new cancer transmitted by the organ donor
3. The patient develops MPM after transplantation
These three situations are discussed in detail below.

Detection of a New, Second Cancer in Transplant Patients Who Previously Recovered from Cancer

In 1997, Penn [24] studied 1297 subjects such patients and reported a cancer recurrence rate of approximately 21%; but in these cases it was only recurrence of the disease, not MPM. Regarding MPM, theoretically, all patients who had a virus-linked cancer before transplant have a higher chance than a control population of developing MPM induced by the same virus during the post-transplant period. Similarly, patients with chronic renal failure who developed cancer of the kidney or bladder prior to renal transplantation are at higher risk for a new urogenital cancer because of the underlying urinary or renal pathology or because of the deleterious effects of the loss of renal function on the urogenital system. In 2005, Kauffman [25, 26] studied 1,358 renal transplant patients and 561 heart transplant patients, all with a previous history of cancer, and 50291 renal transplant patients and 16,160 heart transplant patients without a previous history of cancer. The incidence of new, post-transplants malignancies was 7.8 and 15.3%, respectively, in the first group vs. 2.8 and 8.8% in the latter group.

Our workgroup has no experience regarding this class of patients but has studied the incidence of neoplasms, including MPM, in transplant patients (Tables 6.4–6.6). The results of the only Italian study that considered this scenario from a statistical point of view [27] do not seem to confirm Kauffman's findings, nor does the data of other case studies (Tables 6.7, 6.8).

Table 6.4 Overall incidence of neoplasm among 968 kidney transplant patients followed at Federico II University Medical School between 1975 and 2005

Type of neoplasm	Number of patients
Skin single cancer (included melanoma)	17
Multiple skin cancer (included melanoma)	19
No skin single cancer	31
Multiple primary malignancies	3
Precancerous skin lesion	19
No benign skin lesion[a]	3
Total	92

[a]Two more benign skin lesions were associated with other cancers

Table 6.5 Incidence of primary and multiple primary malignancies among 968 kidney transplanted patients followed at Federico II University Medical School between 1975 and 2005

Kidney transplant patients ($n = 968$)	Number of patients with cancer ($n = 70$, 7.2%)[a]	Number of cancer patients with MPM ($n = 3$, 4.3%)
Males ($n = 610$)	53 (8.7%)	3 (5.7%)
Females ($n = 358$)	17 (4.7%)	0

[a]Not considered: 3 benign and 19 precancerous lesions

Table 6.6 Characteristics of the three male patients who developed multiple primary malignancies, among 968 kidney transplanted patients followed at Federico II University Medical School between 1975 and 2007

Patient	Type of first cancer	Type of second cancer	Characteristics
1	Prostate	Kidney	Synchronous, treated surgically, disease-free for 2 years
2	Kaposi's sarcoma	MALToma	Metachronous, medical and surgical treatment disease-free for 1 year, exitus at 18 months
3	Lung	Squamous carcinoma	Metachronous, surgical treatment, disease-free at 8 months, exitus at 12 months

Table 6.7 Incidence of primary and multiple primary malignancies among 8,047 transplanted patients[a]

	Number	With a cancer (%)	With MPM (%)
Kidney transplant	7,001	411 (5.9)	19 (4.6)
Heart, lung, liver transplant	1,046	122 (11.7)	4 (3.3)
Overall	8,047	533 (6.6)	23 (4.3)
Male	5,415	141 (5.4)	5 (3.5)
Female	2,632	141 (5.49	5 (3.5)

[a] Patients transplanted at: S.Raffaele Hospital, Milan; Policlinico Hospital, Milan; Policlinico Hospital, Verona; Policlinico Hospital, Padua; Ca Foncello Hospital, Treviso; S.Maria della Misericordia Hospital, Udine; Riuniti Hospitals, Bergamo; Civic Hospital, Brescia; S.Bartolo Hospital, Vicenza; Niguarda Hospital, Milan; Policlinico "Gemelli" Hospital, Rome; Policlinico "S.Matteo" Hospital, Pavia. (Data: courtesy of Dr. P. Piselli, MD)

Table 6.8 Characteristics of the 23 patients who developed multiple primary malignancies among 8,047 transplanted patients[a]

Patient number	Sex	Transplanted organ	Type of first cancer	Type of second cancer
1	F	Kidney	Breast	Skin (squamous cell)
2	F	Kidney	Cervix	Breast
3	F	Kidney	Gastric	Liver
4	F	Kidney	Kaposi's sarcoma	Nasal mucosa
5	F	Kidney	Thyroid	Breast
6	M	Kidney	Burkitt lymphoma	Skin (squamous cell)
7	M	Kidney	Colon	Melanoma
8	M	Kidney	Hodgkin lymphoma	Non-Hodgkin lymphoma (NHL)
9	M	Kidney	Kaposi's sarcoma	Kidney
10	M	Kidney	Kaposi's sarcoma	Skin (squamous cell)
11	M	Kidney	Kaposi's sarcoma	Skin (squamous cell)
12	M	Kidney	Kidney	Skin (basal cell)
13	M	Kidney	Kidney	Skin (squamous cell)
14	M	Kidney	Kidney	Skin (squamous cell)
15	M	Kidney	Larynx	Lung
16	M	Kidney	Melanoma	Anus
17	M	Kidney	NHL	Kaposi's sarcoma
18	M	Kidney	Prostate	Skin (squamous cell)
19	M	Kidney	Rectum	Skin (squamous cell)
20	M	Heart	Bladder	Skin (basal cell)
21	M	Heart	Colon	Skin (basal cell)
22	M	Heart	NHL	Kidney
23	M	Liver	Kaposi's sarcoma	Liver

[a] Patients transplanted at: S.Raffaele Hospital, Milan; Policlinico Hospital, Milan; Policlinico Hospital, Verona; Policlinico Hospital, Padua; Ca Foncello Hospital, Treviso; S.Maria della Misericordia Hospital, Udine; Riuniti Hospitals, Bergamo; Civic Hospital, Brescia; S.Bartolo Hospital, Vicenza; Niguarda Hospital, Milan; Policlinico "Gemelli"Hospital, Rome; Policlinico "S.Matteo" Hospital, Pavia. (Data: courtesy of Dr. P. Piselli, MD).

Detection of a New, Second Donor-Related Cancers in Transplant Patients

In this scenario any discussion would be purely theoretical, as it is highly improbable that a cancer will be transmitted from one subject to another across the transplanted organ. Such cases reported in the literature generally refer to isolated events [28]. Furthermore, the likelihood that a neoplastic lesion is transmitted to a recipient who previously had a tumor and, subsequently, deemed free of cancer, was considered eligible for transplantation is next to zero.

The Development of MPM After Transplantation

Among the predisposing factors for the development of cancer in transplanted patients, besides the already-mentioned immune-suppressive treatment, are the life span of the transplanted patient (and thus the period of time he or she is exposed to immune-suppressive treatment, oncogenic factors, and viral infections) and the age of the population of transplanted patients. Such patients have been shown to have a longer life expectancy, and thus may reach an age at which the neoplastic risk is naturally higher; moreover, transplant is also done directly in older patients, who already have a higher risk for cancer [15]. Certain types of tumors (i.e. cancer of the kidney, liver, lips, skin, vulva and perineum, non-Hodgkin's lymphomas, Kaposi's sarcoma) are more frequent in the transplanted population and in the majority of cases they are caused by a virus. For the other, non-viral types of malignancies that occur in transplanted patients, except for neoplastic lesions of the urinary tract, there is no evidence of a higher incidence than is present in the general control population [26–29]. It is in this context that the problem of MPM in transplanted patients should be considered. The data provided in Tables 6.6 and 6.8 show how often, in the presence of more than one neoplastic disease, the malignancies detected in transplant patients are caused by either the same or by two different oncoviruses. In other patients, a viral etiology is generally recognized in at one least cancer. Viruses are responsible for the majority of MPM, implying that this condition is often characterized by the presence of two or more lesions having similar histologies but localized in different tissues or even different regions of the same organ, e.g., multifocal hepatocarcinoma or multiple cutaneous malignancies. We have also underlined that if two tumors having the same viral etiology are localized in two different sites, they may theoretically appear at different times (metachronous tumors), but clinical experience indicates that very often these malignancies manifest synchronously [30]. These conclusions are confirmed by the clinical experience described in Tables 6.3–6.7.

Secondary Immune Deficiency, Cancer and Multiple Primary Malignancies: AIDS

Interactions between the immune system and viruses are bidirectional. In fact, while in some patients an immune deficiency state can determine an increased susceptibility to viral infections, in others viral infections are responsible for the immune deficiency. In these cases, the viruses themselves become the immune-suppressive agents after their penetration into immune-competent cells (Table 6.9). Among all known viral infections, the most severe and protracted immune suppression is caused by the human immunodeficiency virus (HIV). HIV patients have the highest incidence of neoplastic disease (30–40% of infected patients), i.e. Kaposi's sarcoma (KS) (period-standardized incidence ratio SIR = 192), non-Hodgkin's lymphoma (NHL) (SIR = 76.4) and carcinoma of the cervix (SIR = 8). These lesions are universally considered to be AIDS-defining cancers [31–39]. These neoplastic diseases are, in turn, variably correlated with viral infections (KS/HHV-8; lymphoma/EBV; cervical carcinoma/human papilloma virus) [40]. Therefore, HIV patients have an increased risk of cancer both because of the HIV-induced immune suppression and because of the consequent increased susceptibility to oncoviral infections. Supporting this role of HIV is clinical evidence of a marked reduction in the risk of developing KS or NHL in

Table 6.9 Example of viral infection that cause immunodeficiencies

DNA viruses	Hepatitis B virus (HBV)
	Papova virus
	Herpes simplex virus (HSV)
	Adenovirus
	Epstein-Barr virus (EBV)
	Cytomegalovirus (CMV)
RNA viruses	Hepatitis C virus (HCV)
	Poliovirus
	Rubella virus
	Measles virus
	Respiratory syncytial virus
	Parotid gland virus
	Human parainfluenza virus
	Human influenza virus
Retroviruses	Human immunodeficiency virus (HIV)

HIV patients treated with highly active antiretroviral therapy (HAART) [32]. However, the increased survival of HAART patients has radically modified the spectrum of neoplastic diseases associated with HIV infection. Thus, instead there is a higher incidence of squamocellular skin cancer; non-melanomatous neoplasms of the mucous membranes of the oral cavity, pharynx, and lips; cancer of the anogenital tract; seminomas; cancers of the lungs, bronchi, and trachea; hepatocellular cancer; Hodgkin's lymphoma [41]. These tumors, which make up a pathogenetically heterogeneous group of neoplastic diseases, may occasionally present contemporarily or shortly one after each other in a HAART patient, thus creating the condition known as MPM [42–44]. This has been observed for virus-induced tumors as well as for those neoplasias presumably caused by environmental factors, such as the abuse of certain substances (drugs, cigarettes, alcohol, etc.) [45, 46]. However, there are as yet no studies showing a higher incidence of MPM in HIV patients, even if HAART is expected to facilitate the onset of tumors as a consequence of the patient's longer life expectancy, notwithstanding the persistence of immune suppression [34].

Conclusions

Many observations on the different types of tumors/pre-cancerous lesions and their increased incidence in ID patients have been made. While immune suppression, at least theoretically, is surely a predisposing factor in multicancer syndrome, there are no significant statistical data favoring a correlation between ID and MPM. The lack of evidence for the development of a second cancer in ID patients may be due to the shorter life expectancy of this population. From the few literature reports and our own clinical experience, we can only generally conclude that MPM in immune-suppressed patients are usually synchronous, involve the same organ or tissue but at different sites, have a viral etiology, and at least one lesion is easily explorable (e.g., skin cancer), thereby allowing early diagnosis and treatment. It is our opinion that immune-suppressed patients with MPM should be treated as intensively as possible, so as to completely eradicate the lesion. Moreover, it might be advantageous to suspend immune suppression or to switch to other drugs; this approach has yielded good results in the treatment of some neoplastic diseases. In conclusion, while current clinical and epidemiological data support a primary or secondary ID state as a risk factor for the development of neoplastic disease, they do not furnish sufficient convincing evidence that an ID facilitates the onset of MPM. While a rare problem today, MPM may become an important issue in the future, as new forms of treatment and stricter follow-ups will assure a longer life expectancy in immune-suppressed patients with previous cancers. Thus, in potentially immune suppressed patients (i.e. transplant candidates), greater relevance must be given to measures aimed at preventing oncoviral infections (as is already done for hepatitis B virus infections) and to the measures that reduce exposure to environmental oncogenic factors (drugs, cigarette smoking, alcohol, etc.).

References

1. Piro A, Tagarelli A, Tagarelli G et al (2008) Paul Ehrlich. The nobel prize in phisiology or medicine 1908. Int Rev Immunol 27(1):1–17
2. Totaro G, Ciardiello F, Bianco R (2003) Richiami di biologia dei tumori. In: Manuale di Oncologia Clinica. Mc Growe-Hill, Milan
3. Harrison A, Braunwald KD, Fauci E et al (2004) Harrison's principles of internal medicine. Mc Grow-Hill, Milano Italia
4. Chinen J, Anmuth D, Franklin AR, Shearer WT (2007) Long-term follow-up of patients with primary immunodeficiencies. J Allergy Clin Immunol 120:795–797
5. Ballow M (2002) Primary immunodeficiency disorders: antibody deficiency. J Allergy Clin Immunol 109:581–591
6. Meyn MS (1999) Ataxia-teleangiectasia, cancer and the pathobiology of the ATM gene. Clin Genet 55:289–304
7. Cunningham-Rundles C, Bodian C (1999) Common Variable Immunodeficiency. Clinical and immunological features of 248 patients. Clin Immunol 92:34–48
8. Mellemkjaer GP, Hammarstrom L, Andersen V et al (2002) Cancer risk among patients with IgA deficiency or common variable immunodeficiency and their relatives: a combined Danish and Swedish study. Clin Exp Immunol 130:495–500
9. World Health Organization, International Agency for Research on Cancer (1997) Epstein-Barr virus and Kaposi's sarcoma herpesvirus/human herpesvirus 8. ARC, Lyon
10. Wheat WH, Cool CC, Morimoto Y et al (2005) Possible role of human herpesvirus 8 in the lymphoproliferative disorders in common 999333variable immunodeficiency. J Exper Med 202(4):479–484
11. Bogstedt AK, Nava S, Wadstrom T, Hammarstrom L (1996) Helicobacter pylori infections in IgA deficiency: lack of role for the secretory immune system. Clin Exp Immunol 105:202–204
12. Zullo A, Romiti A, Rinaldi V et al (1999) Gastric pathology in patients with common variable immunodeficiency. Gut 45(1):77–81
13. Brosens LA, Tytgat KM, Morsink FH et al (2008) Multiple colorectal neoplasm in X- linked agammaglobulinemia. Clin Gastroenterol Hepatol 6(1):115–119
14. Berthoux F, Abramowicz D, Bradley B et al (2002) Best practice guidelines for renal transplantation (part 2). Nephrol Dial Transplant 17(suppl 4):1–67
15. Sheil AG (2002) Organ transplantation and malignancy: inevitable linkage. Transplant Proc 34:2436–2437
16. Gutierrez-Dalmau A, Campistol JM (2007) Immunosuppressive therapy and malignancy in organ transplant recipients: a systematic review. Drugs 67(8):1167–1198
17. Dantal J, Pohanka E (2007) Malignancies in renal transplantation: an unmet medical need. Nephrol Dial Transplant 22(Suppl 1):i4-i10
18. Jensen MK, Soborg M (1966) Chromosome aberrations in human cells following treatment with imuran. Preliminary report. Acta Med Scand 179(2):249–250
19. O'Donovan P, Perrett CM, Zhang X et al (2005) Azathioprine and UVA light generate mutagenic oxidative DNA damage. Science 309(5742):1871–1874
20. Hojo M, Morimoto T, Maluccio M et al (1999) Cyclosporine induces cancer progression by a cell-autonomous mechanism. Nature 397(6719):471–472
21. Guba M, von Breitenbuch P, Steinbauer M et al (2002) Rapamycin inhibits primary and metastatic tumor growth by antiangiogenesis: involvement of vascular endothelial growth factor. Nat Med 8(2):128–135
22. Robson R, Cecka JM, Opelz G et al (2005) Prospective registry-based observational cohort study of the long-term risk of malignancies in renal transplant patients treated with mycophenolate mofetil. Am J Transplant 5(12):2954–2960
23. Rheingold SR, Neugut AI, Meadows AT (2000) Secondary cancer: incidence, risk factors and management. In: Holland JF, Frey E (eds) Cancer medicine. Decker, Hamilton

24. Penn I (1997) Overview of the problem of cancer in organ transplant recipients. Ann Transplant 2(4):5–6
25. Kauffman HM, Wida SC, Maureen A et al (2005) Transplant recipient with a history of a malignancy: risk of recurrent and de novo cancers. Transpl Rev 19:55–64
26. Ponticelli C (2007) Medical complications of kidney transplantation. Informa Healtcare, London
27. Taioli E, Piselli P, Arbustini E et al (2006) Incidence of second primary cancer in transplanted patients. Transplantation 81(7):982–985
28. Gandhi MJ, Strong DM (2007) Donor derived malignancy following transplantation: a review. Cell Tissue Bank 8(4):267–286
29. Serraino D, Piselli P, Busnach G et al (2007) Risk of cancer following immunosuppression in organ transplant recipients and in HIV-positive individuals in southern Europe. Eur J Cancer 43(14):2117–2123
30. Neugut AI, Meadows AT, Robinson E (1999) Multiple primary cancer. Lippincott Williams & Wilkins, Philadelphia
31. Hessol NA, Pipkin S, Schwarcz S et al (2007) The impact of highly active antiretroviral therapy on non-AIDS-defining cancers among adults with AIDS. Am J Epidemiol 165(10):1143–1153
32. Biggar RJ, Chaturvedi AK, Goedert JJ, Engels EA (2007) AIDS-related cancer and severity of immunosuppression in persons with AIDS. J Natl Cancer Inst 99:962–972
33. Akanmu AS (2006) AIDS-associated malignancies. Afr J Med Med Sci 35:57–70
34. Clifford GM, Polesel J, Rickenbach M et al (2005) Cancer risk in the Swiss HIV cohort study: associations with immunodeficiency, smoking and highly active antiretroviral therapy. J Natl Cancer Inst 97:425–432
35. Frisc M, Biggar RJ, Engels EA, Goedert JJ (2001) Association of cancer with AIDS-related immunosuppression in adults. JAMA 285:1736–1745
36. Grulich AE, Li Y, McDonald A (2002) Rates of non-AIDS-defining cancers in people with HIV infection before and after AIDS diagnosis. AIDS 16:1155–1161
37. Allardice GM, Hole DJ, Brewster DH et al (2003) Incidence of malignant neoplasm among HIV-infected persons in Scotland. Br J Cancer 89:505–507
38. Dalmaso L, Franceschi S, Polesel J et al (2003) Risk of cancer in persons with AIDS in Italy, 1985–1998. Br J Cancer 89:94–100
39. International collaboration on HIV and Cancer (2000) Highly active antirectroviral therapy and incidence of cancer in human immunodeficiency virus-infected adults. J Natl Cancer Inst 92:1823–1830
40. Arora A, Chiao E, Tyring SK (2007) AIDS malignancies. Cancer Treat Res 133:21–67
41. Grulich AE, Leeuwen M, Falster M, Vajdic CM (2007) Incidence of cancers in people with HIV/AIDS compared with immunosuppressed transplant recipients: a meta-analysis. Lancet 370:59–67
42. Grulich AE, Wan X, Law MG et al (1999) Risk of cancer in people with AIDS. AIDS 13:839–843
43. Antinori A, Larocca LM, Fassone L et al (1999) HHV-8/KSHV is not associated with AIDS-related primary central nervous system lymphoma. Brain Pathol 9(2):199–208
44. Manfredi R, Calza L, Chiodo F (2003) Multiple AIDS-related malignancies just in the era of potent antiretroviral therapy. A rare but intriguing finding. Infez Med 11(3):153–156
45. Aviram G, Fishman JE, Schwartz DS (2001) Metachronous primary carcinomas of the lung in an HIV-infected patient. AIDS Patient Care STDS 15(6):297–300
46. Mussi MG, Correa AR, Moraes DR et al (1996) Astrocytoma and squamous cell lung carcinoma association in AIDS patients. Int Conf AIDS 11:448

Chapter 7
Multiple Primary Malignancies and Human Papilloma Virus Infections

Stefania Staibano, Massimo Mascolo, Lorenzo Lo Muzio, Gennaro Ilardi, Loredana Nugnes, Concetta Dodaro, Andrea Renda, Gaetano De Rosa

Introduction

Patients may develop multiple primary malignancies (MPM) due to the occurrence of many known predisposing factors (i.e. genetic background, environmental factors, hormonal unbalance, and acquired immunosuppression); however, in most cases, no obvious cause of has been found [1–3]. During the last few decades, accumulating evidence has pointed to the involvement of human papillomavirus (HPV) in the development of several neoplastic and preneoplastic lesions of anatomic sites beyond the uterine cervix. In particular, HPV has been associated with squamous cell carcinomas and related precursors in the oral cavity, esophagus, skin, larynx, conjunctiva, paranasal sinuses and bronchus, but even in non-Malpighian-derived tumors, such as urinary bladder carcinoma. At least for a subset of these cases, it has been suggested that exposure to HPV can precede the appearance of cancer by 10 or more years [4, 5]; nonetheless, the true prevalence of HPV DNA in pre-cancerous lesions remains uncertain.

As is well-known, HPV is the most common sexually transmitted infection in the USA and western European countries. Infection with the virus usually regresses without treatment, but in some cases there is malignant transformation.

Infection with high-risk HPV is a prerequisite for virtually all cervical cancers [6] such that HPV DNA testing is currently included in guidelines for cervical cancer screening beyond cytology [7]. It should be noted, however, that only a few women infected with HPV develop cervical cancer, as most women experience only a transient HPV infection [8]. It is thought that high-risk HPV types infection represents the first step in the complex multistep process of cervical carcinogenesis, which requires many concurrent co-factors, including older age, high parity, acquired immunosuppression, and the use of oral steroids [9, 10]. In any case, it can be stated that all the cancers of the uterine cervix are by definition virally derived, thus conferring to these tumors a common "biological background." The differences in clinical behavior between individual cases of cervical carcinoma are probably the result of different genetic mutations accumulated in infected cells during persistent high-risk HPV infection.

A. Renda (ed.), *Multiple Primary Malignancies*.
©Springer-Verlag Italia 2009

Whereas HPV infection in some extragenital human tumors has been extensively described in the literature, there are only limited data addressing the consequences of this infection on the biological behavior of these cancers. In particular, nothing is known about the presence and relevance of HPV infection in patients with MPM.

The aim of the study described here was to partially fill this gap by testing whether HPV played a role in the development of MPM. Clearly, the detection of HPV DNA in tumor tissue alone is neither sufficient evidence of causation nor predictive of the evolution of neoplastic and/or preneoplastic human lesions [11]. For this reason, besides the classical morphological signs of viral infection and positive molecular biological testing for the presence of high-risk HPV types, the same series of cases was examined for co-expression of a 60-kDa protein belonging to the heterotrimeric complex, chromatin assembly factor-1 (CAF-1). CAF-1/p60 has a pivotal role in the epigenetic regulation of cell proliferation and associated DNA-repair process. Recently, this protein has been proposed as a new and sensitive marker of the biological aggressiveness of some human malignancies [12–16]. The study concludes with a discussion of the possible significance of these two parameters in terms of screening options, most common prognosis, progression rates of preneoplastic lesions, and potential alternative therapeutic regimens for a subgroup of MPM patients.

Materials and Methods

Selection of Patients

Files from the Department of Biomorphological and Functional Sciences, Pathology Section, University "Federico II" of Naples, dating from January 2006 to December 2007 were retrieved and used to establish the patient series. Archival paraffin-embedded, formalin-fixed tumoral tissues relevant to MPM of 131 patients who underwent surgery for a second tumor in the same University Hospital was obtained. For each patient, a complete clinical and pathological data set was available.

From the paraffin-blocks representative of MPM, 5-μm-thick serial sections were cut for each patient. One section for each case was stained with hematoxylin and eosin to confirm the original diagnosis and to record the presence of morphological evidence of viral infection; the remaining sections were mounted on slides pre-treated with poly-L-lysine for in situ hybridization (ISH) detection with INFORM HPV (Ventana Medical System, Tucson, Arizona) probes and for immunohistochemical staining.

In Situ Hybridization

To avoid cross-contamination, the microtome was fitted with a new blade for each case. The INFORM HPV probes are analytic specific reagents for the detection of HPV DNA by in situ hybridization (ISH). Two different INFORM HPV probes are able to detect high-risk (16, 18, 31, 33, 35, 39, 45, 51, 52, 56, 58, 68, and 70) and low-risk (6 and 11) HPV types. ISH was carried out according to the manufacturer's guidelines, using the BenchMark Automated Slide Staining System (Ventana Medical System). As a control, CaSki and HeLa (containing, respectively, integrated HPV 16 and HPV 18 genomes), fixed cultured cervical cells, and the HPV-negative cell line C-33A were analyzed. The results of the INFORM HPV slides were evaluated separately by two observers. The pathologists agreed on the results of ISH in all evaluated cases. A positive signal for HPV DNA was defined as the presence of dark blue or black dots in the cell nuclei.

Immunohistochemistry

A section prepared from each block was heated in a microwave oven for antigen retrieval. Antibody detection was carried out using the conventional streptavidin-biotin-peroxidase procedure, as previously reported [17]. Negative and specific positive control slides were added to each run for all antibodies tested. As positive controls, sections of a non-neoplastic, hyperplastic palatine tonsil for PCNA, normal breast tissue, and infiltrating breast carcinoma for CAF-1/p60 were used. Negative controls were performed by substituting primary antibodies with antibodies with irrelevant specificity but of the same isotypes as the primary antibodies.

Immunostaining for PCNA and CAF-1/p60 was evaluated semiquantitatively; the results were graded according to an arbitrary scale as follows: 0 (<5% positive cells), 1 (weak: 5 to ≤15%), 2 (mild: ≥15 to ≤30%), 3 (intense: >30%).

The presence of HPV was investigated by nested PCR; viral genotype was assessed by direct sequencing. Samples were tested in duplicate, with three control slides included in each run (blank, HPV-negative, and HPV-18-positive controls).

HPV-DNA was amplified through a PCR assay using a DNA thermal cycler. This was followed by HPV genotyping.

Data obtained from the study were analyzed using the one-way analysis of variance (ANOVA) and Student-Newman-Keuls multiple comparisons test (SPSS statistical software, version 6.1 for Windows). For the categorical parameters the chi-square test was used; continuous variables were analyzed with the nonparametric Mann-Whitney U-test. P <0.05 was considered significant.

Results

The study population was composed of 131 patients with MPM. All of the lesions were metachronous tumors (time to occurrence of the secondary primitive tumor: ≥6 months). The patients were diagnosed as having at least two primary cancer sites.

Histologically, the tumors were of epithelial origin, either squamous (skin, esophagus, uterine cervix, lung) or glandular (colon, endometrium, lung, breast, prostate, pancreas, ovary, stomach, thyroid); urothelial tumors (urinary bladder), mesothelial tumors (pleura), renal cell carcinomas, liver carcinomas, malignant melanoma (skin and iris melanomas), and testicular and brain tumors.

Among the MPM of our series, 13 squamous cell carcinomas (skin, esophagus, uterine cervix) and three urothelial tumors (urinary bladder cancers) showed morphological features of viral infection and positive results for high-risk HPV DNA. Immunostaining showed a marked overexpression (+++) of CAF-1/p60 in all of the HPV+ tumors (Figs. 7.1, 7.2). By contrast, in the remaining 115 malignancies of our series, CAF-1/p60 expression ranged from low (+) to mild (++), with the highest level of immunoreactivity in malignant melanomas and prostate cancers. Statistical evaluation of these results showed a significant correlation ($p < 0.05$) between CAF-1/p60 overexpression (+++) and HPV infection.

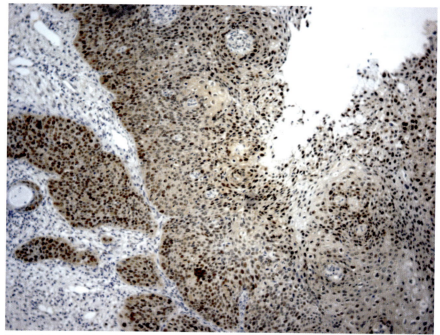

Fig. 7.1 A case of invasive squamous cell carcinoma of the uterine cervix, positive for high-risk human papilloma virus (HPV) DNA, as seen by the extensive immunoreactivity for CAF-1/P60 protein. Streptavidin-biotin peroxidase immunostaining, 150×

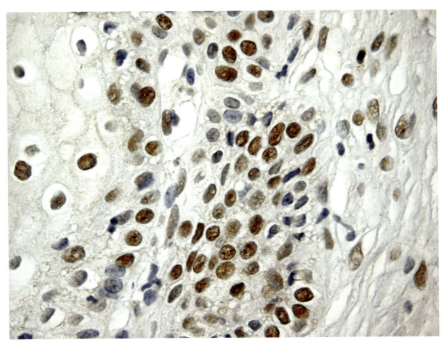

Fig. 7.2 A case of invasive squamous cell carcinoma of the skin, positive for high-risk HPV DNA, as seen by the strong immunoreactivity for CAF-1/P60 protein. Streptavidin-biotin peroxidase immunostaining, 250×

Discussion

Cancer is the result of multiple genetic abnormalities and epigenetic events, most of which are able to influence tumor behavior. The scientific community has devoted significant effort to investigating tumor genetics and to identifying markers that may assist in the diagnosis, prognostic evaluation, and treatment of patients. Unfortunately, the genomic complexity of most solid human malignancies precludes simple molecular screening methods of prognostic and therapeutic relevance.

In MPM, the identification of the molecular events involved in tumorigenesis is greatly hampered by the high variability of possible combinations of a large amount of predisposing factors. However, the recognition of a common pathogenesis, in at least some of these cases, could represent a *fil rouge* that can be followed in a comprehensive evaluation of the patient's "neoplastic background," which, in turn, may provide additional prognostic information.

Progression to invasive cancer requires the concurrent and sequential accumulation of genetic and epigenetic events. Epigenetic instability leads to chromosomal instability, which then favors carcinogenic progression [18]. The molecular events linked to HPV cancerogenesis remain speculative.

Nonetheless, it is well-known that high-risk HPV types induce high-grade epithelial dysplasia and invasive carcinoma of the uterine cervix [19], mainly through interactions between up-regulated E6 viral oncoprotein and p53 tsg (tumor suppressor gene) protein, and between up-regulated viral E7 oncoprotein and pRb tsg protein [20]. These interactions require a shift from productive viral replication (episomal HPV DNA) to integration of the viral genome into the host chromosomes.

High-risk HPV types have the ability to activate the cellular DNA methylation machinery; therefore, they can epigenetically regulate both viral and cellular genes [21–25]. This phenomenon has been observed also in many human malignancies linked to a viral pathogenesis, such as gastric carcinomas positive for Epstein-Barr virus [26, 27], hepatocellular carcinomas in hepatitis-virus-infected patients [28, 29], squamous cell carcinoma and precancerous lesions of the cervix uteri in Epstein-Barr-virus infected women, [30] malignant mesotheliomas in SV40-infected patients [31], and HPV-positive oral carcinoma and head and neck cancers [32, 33]. These observations emphasize the fundamental role of epigenetic changes in virus-associated human cancers [18] and provide a new point of view to better understand the molecular events involved in cancerogenesis.

HPV 16 integration in cervical tumors frequently occurs in common fragile sites (CFS) [34, 35]. These are specific chromosomal loci that, under numerous conditions, tend to form chromosomal abnormalities and represent a target for both estroprogestins and tobacco smoke [34]. The ensuing molecular events probably constitute the basis of the strict interrelationship between epigenetic inactivation of soluble frizzled receptor protein (SFRP) genes, drinking, smoking, and HPV infection, as reported for head and neck squamous cell carcinomas [36]. Clinically speaking, tracking down the epigenetic events linked to cancerogenesis has proved to be a very promising approach to the identification of new therapeutic targets.

Alterations in DNA methylation, histone modification, and the regulation of chromatin assembly are regarded as common hallmarks of human cancer and can be reversed, either spontaneously or by the removal of the pathogenetic event that caused them. This is the case, for example, in *Helicobacter pylori* (HP)-related gastric pathologies, in which eradication of the bacterial infection reversed E-cadherin promoter hypermethylation [37]. This result showed that effective treatment of an infectious agent can reverse the hypermethylation of a tumor suppressor gene.

Besides methylation, epigenetics has identified a new generation of oncogenes and tumor suppressor genes [38]. Recent experimental evidence together with studies on human epithelial tumors [12, 13] have shown that altered expression of CAF-1 proteins may be regarded as a marker of both deregulated cell proliferation and a high risk of malignant progression.

We found marked overexpression of the CAF-1/p60 protein in HPV-positive cases comprising a series of MPM patients. This result is consistent with reports in the literature and may be of considerable utility in the evaluation of a particular subgroup of MPM patients.

As is well known, cytohistological examination and the detection of HPV DNA cannot reliably distinguish those patients who will progress to invasive cancer from the vast majority of those whose abnormalities will spontaneously regress [39]. Thus, it is premature both in terms of the cost and the prognostic consequences to test for HPV infection in MPM patients. The frequent transient nature of HPV infections is such that, as in most females with a positive test for high-risk HPV, MPM patients may not go on to develop cervical cancer or a preneoplastic lesion [39, 40]. Moreover, the biological behavior of well-established HPV cancers presents other, confounding aspects. For example, a subset of patients with HPV-16-positive tonsillar carcinoma was found to have a better overall and disease-specific survival than patients who were HPV-negative [41]. It is therefore mandatory to define the differences in clinical behavior between HPV- and HPV+ MPM, in terms of statistical relevance, on a significant series of cases. In addition, there is a need for more reliable markers of disease progression than those provided by morphological examination or by testing for the presence of high-risk HPV types.

A further goal of this investigation was to provide clinicians with useful information about the biological and molecular characteristics of a subgroup of patients with MPM in which some or all of the primary malignancies were positive for HPV infection. The main questions arising from the identification of this subset of patients: "What is the proper treatment of these HPV-positive lesions? Should be they treated in the same way of their negative counterparts? Can they be ultimately prevented?"

The co-expression of high levels of p60 CAF-1 protein in the HPV-positive tumors of our series of MPM also indicates that in these lesions an important deregulation of both epigenetic control of chromatin assembly and proliferation-linked DNA repair has been established.

Although biological therapies are still in the early phases of development, it may ultimately be possible to positively interfere with the natural history of HPV-linked deregulation of the epigenetic control of cell proliferation. Our preliminary data remain to be confirmed by larger and statistically significant series in order to determine the usefulness of careful screening the primary tumors of MPM patients for the presence of high-risk HPV. Identification of this sub-group of patients who are homogeneous for viral infection and epigenetic changes will allow the biological aggressiveness of these tumors and of the preneoplastic lesions to be determined, and the most appropriate treatment options to be addressed. It will also shed light on the natural history of these lesions, the risk of other viral-linked primary malignancies, the prevention of transmission, and methods for their prevention and detection.

We think that "the viral pathway to cancerogenesis" represents a promising alternative perspective for improving our understanding of the biological behavior of at least a subgroup MPM. The study of the epigenetic changes in these tumors may lead to the identification of "epigenetic markers" to be used in the early diagnosis, prognostic evaluation and therapy of HPV-linked MPM.

References

1. Yamamoto S, Yoshimura K, Ri S et al (2006) The risk of multiple primary malignancies with colorectal carcinoma. Dis Colon Rectum 49:S30-36
2. Colangelo LA, Gapstur SM, Gann PH et al (2004) Cigarette smoking and colorectal carcinoma mortality in a cohort with long-term follow-up. Cancer 100:288–293
3. Otani T, Iwasaki M, Yamamoto S et al (2003) Alcohol consumption, smoking, and subsequent risk of colorectal cancer in middle-aged and elderly Japanese men and female: Japan Public Health Center-based prospective study. Cancer Epidemiol Biomarkers Prev 12:1492–1500
4. Syrjänen S (2007) Human papillomaviruses in head and neck carcinomas. N Engl J Med 356: 1993–1995
5. Mork J, Lie AK, Glattre E et al (2001) Human papillomavirus infection as a risk factor for squamous-cell carcinoma of the head and neck. N Engl J Med 344:1125–1131
6. Bosch FX, Lorincz A, Munoz N (2002) The causal relation between human papillomavirus and cervical cancer. J Clin Pathol 55:244–265
7. Wright TC, Schiffman M, Solomon D et al (2004) Interim guidance for the use of human papillomavirus DNA testing as an adjunct to cervical cytology for screening. Obstet Gynecol 103:304–308
8. Schiffman M, Kjaer SK (2003) Natural history of anogenital human papillomavirus infection and neoplasia. J Natl Cancer Inst Monogr 31:14–19
9. Castellsague X, Munoz N (2003) Cofactors in human papillomavirus carcinogenesis –role of parity, oral contraceptives, and tobacco smoking. J Natl Cancer Inst Monogr 31:20–28
10. Palefsky JM, Holly EA (2003) Immunosuppression and co-infection with HIV. J Natl Cancer Inst Monogr 31:41–46
11. Kreimer AR, Clifford GM, Boyle P et al (2005) Human papillomavirus types in head and neck squamous cell carcinomas worldwide: a systematic review. Cancer Epidemiol Biomarkers Prev 14:467–475
12. Polo SE, Yheocharis SE, Klijaieko J et al (2004) CAF-1, a marker of clinical value to distinguish quiescent from proliferative cells. Cancer Res 64:2371–2381
13. Staibano S, Mignogna C, Lo Muzio L et al (2007) Chromatin assembly factor-1(CAF-1) mediated regulation of cells proliferation and DNA repair: a link with the biological behavior of squamous cell carcinoma of the tongue. Histopathology 50:911–919
14. Staibano S, Mascolo M, Mancini FP et al (2008) Chromatin Assembly Factor-1 (CAF-1) "a prostate cancer progression marker?" (In press)
15. Staibano S, Mascolo M, Scalvenzi M (2008) Detection of biological profile of cutaneous malignant melanoma by CAF-1 proteins expression. (In press)
16. Staibano S, Mascolo M, Nugnes L et al (2008) CAF-1 and chromatin states in the cervical cancer: is there a correlation?" (In press)
17. Lo Muzio L, Staibano S, Pannone G et al (2001) Expression of the apoptosis inhibitor survivin in aggressive squamous cell carcinoma. Exp Mol Pathol 70:249–254
18. Li HP, Leu YW, Chang YS (2005) Epigenetic changes in virus-associated human cancers. Cell Research 15:262–271
19. Matsukura T, Sugase M (2001) Relationship between 80 Human papillomavirus genotypes and different grades of cervical intraepithelial neoplasia: Association and causality. Virology 283:139–147
20. Woodman CB, Collins SI, Young LS (2007) The natural history of cervical HPV infection: unresolved issues Nat Rev Cancer 7:11–22
21. Sedjo RL, Inserra P, Abrahamsen M et al (2002) Human papillomavirus persistence and nutrients involved in the methylation pathway among a cohort of young women. Cancer Epidemiol Biomarkers Prev 11:353–359
22. Kim K, Garner-Hamrick PA, Fisher C et al (2003) Methylation patterns of papillomavirus DNA, its influence on E2 function, and implications in viral infection. J Virol 77:12450–12459

23. Badal S, Badal V, Calleya-Macias IE et al (2004) The human papillomavirus-18 genome is efficiently targeted by cellular DNA methylation. Virology 324:483–492
24. Turan T, Kalantoni M, Calleya-Macias IE et al (2006) Methylation of the human papillomavirus-18 L1 gene: a biomarker of neoplastic progression? Virology 349:175–183
25. Badal V, Chuang LS, Tan EH et al (2004) CpG methylation of human papillomavirus type 16 DNA in cervical cancer cell lines and in clinical specimens: genomic hypomethylation correlates with carcinogenic progression. J Virol 77:6227–6234
26. Kang GH, Lee S, Kim WH et al (2002) Epstein-Barr virus-positive gastric carcinoma demonstrates frequent aberrant methylation of multiple genes and constitutes CpG island methylator phenotype-positive gastric carcinoma. Am J Pathol 160:787–794
27. Vo QN, Geradts J, Gulley ML et al (2002) Epstein-Barr virus in gastric adenocarcinomas: association with ethnicity and CDKN2A promoter methylation. J Clin Pathol 55:669–675
28. Yang B, Guo M, Herman JG et al (2003) Aberrant promoter methylation profiles of tumor suppressor genes in hepatocellular carcinoma. Am J Pathol 163:1101–1107
29. Li X, Hui AM, Sun L et al (2004) p16INK4A hypermethylation is associated with hepatitis virus infection, age, and gender in hepatocellular carcinoma. Clin Cancer Res 10:7484–7489
30. Kim NR, Lin Z, Kim KR et al (2005) Epstein-Barr virus and p16INK4A methylation in squamous cell carcinoma and precancerous lesions of the cervix uteri. J Korean Med Sci 20:636–642
31. Suzuki M, Toyooka S, Shivapurkar N et al (2005) Aberrant methylation profile of human malignant mesotheliomas and its relationship to SV40 infection. Oncogene 10:1302–1308
32. Gasco M, Crook T (2003) The p53 network in head and neck cancer. Oral Oncol 39:222–231
33. Dong SM, Sun DI, Benoit NE et al (2003) Epigenetic inactivation of RASSF1A in head and neck cancer. Clin Cancer Res 9:3635–3640
34. Torland EC, Myers SL, Persing DH et al (2000) Human papillomavirus type 16 integrations in cervical tumors frequently occur in common fragile sites. Cancer Res 60:5916–5921
35. Thorland EC, Myers SL, Gostout BS et al (2003) Common fragile sites are preferential targets for HPV16 integrations in cervical tumors. Oncogene 22:1225–1237
36. Marsit CJ, McClean MD, Furniss CS et al (2006) Epigenetic inactivation of the SFRP genes is associated with drinking, smoking and HPV in head and neck squamous cell carcinoma. Int J Cancer 119:1761–1766
37. Chan AO, Peng JZ, Lam SK et al (2006) Eradication of Helicobacter pylori infection reverses E-cadherin promoter hypermethylation Gut 55:463–468
38. Esteller M (2006) Epigenetics provides a new generation of oncogenes and tumour-suppressor genes. Br J Cancer 94:179–183
39. Monk BJ, Wiley DJ (2004) Human papillomavirus infections: truth or consequences. Cancer 100:225–227
40. Woodman CB Collins S Winter H et al (2001) Natural history of cervical human Papillomavirus infection in young women: a longitudinal cohort study. Lancet 357:1831–1836
41. Syrjänen S (2004) HPV infections and tonsillar carcinoma. J Clin Pathol 57:449–455

Chapter 8
The Hereditary Syndromes

Nicola Carlomagno, Luigi Pelosio, Akbar Jamshidi, Marius Yabi,
Francesca Duraturo, Paola Izzo, Andrea Renda

Introduction

Within the ambit of multiple tumors, an important issue is that of already identified hereditary syndromes, a group of anatomical-clinical entities that have been well distinguished and studied for years. Such diseases have a common etiopathogenetic mechanism, mostly represented by a genetic mutation. It is easy to understand how a patient, who has in his or her genetic history a genomic alteration, could develop multiple tumors.

A close examination of such pathologies is, in our opinion, indispensable to the study of multiple primary malignancies (MPM). In these syndromes, the main manifestations are: colonic adenomas for familial adenomatous polyposis (FAP), colorectal cancer for hereditary nonpolyposis colorectal cancer (HNPCC), and medullar thyroid cancer (MTC) for multi-endocrine neoplasia type 2 (MEN2). They can be compared to an "index tumor," alongside which other synchronies and/or metachronous tumors can develop.

Biomolecular studies have confirmed that hereditary syndromes have a common etiopathogenetic process, represented in a specific genetic mutation. This knowledge together with an awareness of the clinical presentations of these diseases forms the basis of a correct diagnostic-therapeutic approach. It is likely that similar mechanisms can be ascribed to "sporadic" MPM, such that closer examination of the accumulated experience in treating patients with hereditary syndromes will alter the clinical approach to MPM. For these reasons, we have carried out a detailed study of the clinical and genetic aspects of the most frequent hereditary syndromes: MEN 1, 2a, and 2b, colorectal cancer (FAP and HNPCC), and hereditary breast and ovarian cancers (HBOC).

Clinical Manifestations

Familial Adenomatous Polyposis

Identification of the adenomatous polyposis coli (APC) gene, responsible for the transmission FAP, came a century after the original clinical description, although the first report of FAP was precisely due to Menzel in 1721. Virchow (1863) coined the term "polypoid colitis" in describing a 15-year-old boy with signs of multiple colonic adenomas, and Cripps (1881) described the familial characteristics of the disease. Cockayne (1927) defined the mode of transmission as autosomal dominant, while Dukes was the first to devise a registry by interviewing family members, as also reported by Lockhart-Mummary in 1930. Diverse clinical presentations in association with specific extracolonic manifestations (ECM), with the definition of distinct syndromes, were later described [1, 2].

FAP has an estimated incidence in Italy of 1:7,000–23,000 [3]. The average patient age is 25 years and the classic clinical presentation is the occurrence of 100–1,000 adenomas along the entire colon. The tumors are small (<1 cm), sessile or peduncular, tubular, villous, or tubulovillous (Fig. 8.1) and become symptomatic in patients in their early 30s (hematic and mucous diarrhea, abdominal cramps).

The progression of these tumors to cancer in untreated patients occurs within 10 years of symptom onset [4], with a topographical distribution of the tumors analogous to those of sporadic cancer. The disease is identified in 90% of affected individuals before they reach age 50, but in 20–46% of cases the proband is unknown because there is no family history ("de novo" mutation) [5]. The natural course of FAP is not the same in all families, as the number, localization, and age of onset of colonic adenomas and CRC, as well as the presence of some ECM greatly vary. Patients with the variant attenuated familial polyposis coli (AFAP), or hereditary flat adenoma syndrome, have relatively few adenoma (<50) (Fig. 8.2) and the disease is of later onset (10–15 years) than the classic form, with the cancer mostly localized to the proximal tract of the colon [6].

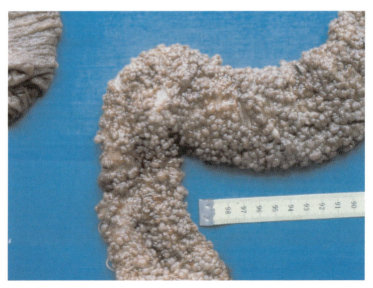

Fig. 8.1 Familial adenomatous polyposis (FAP): severe polyposis with hundreds of adenomas

8 The Hereditary Syndromes

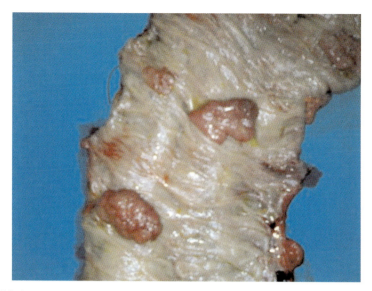

Fig. 8.2 Attenuated FAP with only a few colonic adenomas

Alongside the colonic adenomas, several ECM (often oncological) are observed, such as desmoids, gastric polyps, and duodenal adenomas, as well as other benign or malignant neoplasms (periampallary carcinoma, pancreatic cancer, cancer of the stomach, adrenals, thyroid, hepatoblastomas, carcinoid, osteogenic sarcoma, CNS tumors) dental abnormalities, dermoid cysts, osteomas, and congenital hypertrophy of epithelium pigmentation of the retina (CHRPE). ECM occurring before the colonic adenomas serve as a clinical marker, and some have an important prognostic role (Fig. 8.3).

Peutz-Jeghers Syndrome

This is an extremely rare (1/200,000) autosomal dominant syndrome characterized by the presence of numerous intestinal hamartomas and cutaneous-mucus pigmentations. The clinical outset is generally in the second decade of life, with abdominal pain, bowel obstruction (intussusceptions), and digestive-tract hemorrhages. The diagnosis is suspected in patients who present with more than two hamartomas or with a single hamartoma against a background of a family history of PJS or with the characteristic cutaneous pigmentation. The prognostic importance of PJS is related to the occurrence of adenocarcinoma not only of the digestive tract (colon [20%], stomach [5%], small bowel and pancreas) but also of other sites (lungs, breast, ovaries, uterus, testicles), with a risk of 80–90% during the patient's lifetime [8].

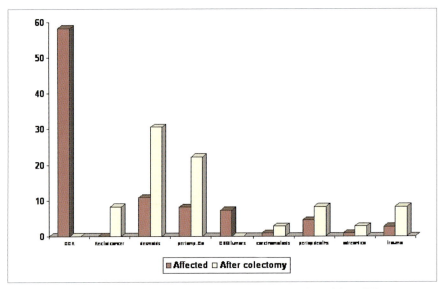

Fig. 8.3 FAP-related deaths before and after total colectomy (adapted from [7])

Hereditary Nonpolyposis Colorectal Cancer

Although a connection between inherited polyposis coli and cancer was established at the end of the 19th century, hereditary CRC without polyposis was only recognized at the end of the 20th century. Henry T. Lynch, of the Preventive Medicine Dept. of the University of Nebraska (USA), was credited for drawing attention to this association; in recognition of his work, the two forms of HNPCC are also known as Lynch's syndromes I and II. In 1971, Lynch [9] resumed earlier research of Warthin's (1913) [10, 11] in focusing his work on HNPCC. A seamstress who worked for Whartin had told him that she expected to die at a young age from colonic or endometrial cancer, as this had been the case in many members of her family [12]. Lynch recognized two forms of HNPCC. In site-specific HNPCC, or Lynch syndrome I, there is autosomal dominant transmission of nonpolyposis colorectal cancer, with an early age of occurrence (25% at 50 years and 70–80% within 70 years), predilection for the proximal colon (60–80%), and high rates of metachronous colorectal cancer (30% at 10 years and 50% at 15 years from the first tumor). Cancer family syndrome, or Lynch syndrome II, has the same characteristics but also extracolonic tumors involving the uterus (25–60%), ovaries (8–14%), stomach (13%), and urinary tract (4%) [12].

HNPCC accounts for 5–15% of all colorectal cancers, although the true incidence is unknown, confounded by incomplete penetrance (<80%), the rapid progression of adenoma to progression (<5 years), the development of extracolonic neoplasms, and the inter- and, occasionally, intra-familiar heterogeneity of the lesions [13].

In HNPCC, the adenomas have the same frequency as in sporadic cases, but a more rapid progression to carcinoma. Due to the deficiency in DNA-repair genes, adenomas accumulate mutations about three times faster than in sporadic disease.

Multiple Endocrine Neoplasia

These complex disorders arise from the hyper-function of two or more endocrine glands. The three main syndromes were described by Wermer (1954), Sipple (1961), and Williams and Pollock (1966), who, respectively, characterized the association of parathyroid adenomas, pituitary and endocrine tumors of the pancreas and gastrointestinal tract (MEN 1), and of MTC and pheochromocytomas (PHEO) with hyperparathyroidism (MEN 2a) and multiple mucosal neuromas and marfanoid habitus (MEN 2b).

The clinical expression of MEN1 generally occurs in the third to fourth decade of life; the appearance of signs and symptoms is rare in patients less than 10 years of age. Men and women are equally affected, consistent with autosomal dominant transmission. However, MEN1 also has been described in numerous geographical areas and in diverse ethnic groups but with no racial predilection. Penetrance of the disease is close to 100% but with a variable expressiveness, such that patients may express some but not necessarily all the components of the syndrome. The majority of patients, if observed for an extended period of time, eventually show involvement of all three endocrine tissues, as was the case in a study in which all three endocrine tissues were shown to be affected in 90% of MEN1 patients studied at autopsy [14–18].

The clinical manifestations of patients with MEN1 depend on the endocrine tissue and on the overproduction of a specific hormone, e.g., due to the presence of neuroendocrine duodenopancreatic or pituitary tumors. The most common anomaly is not represented a tumor but rather parathyroid hyperplasia. In 90–97% of MEN1 patients there are biochemical signs of hyperparathyroidism. Importantly, MEN1 causes MPM: neuroendocrine duodenopancreatic tumors (30–80%), [14–20] furthermore gastrinomas (50–70%), and insulinomas (20–40%), glucagonomas, VIPomas, and somatostatinomas [15]. Pancreatic tumors are even more frequent as autoptic targets (>80%), representing the definitive and most relevant prognostic factor [21, 23]. Wilkinson's retrospective analysis [24] conducted on the Tasmanian population over a period spanning 130 years and a Mayo Clinic series [25] covering the period of 1951–1997 have highlighted that many cases of pancreatic tumors are diagnosed at post-mortem examination. Other studies have shown a prognostic role for these tumors, as they, rather than the adverse effects of peptic disease, are the main cause of death [26, 27] (Fig. 8.4). Pituitary adenoma is relatively less frequent (15–50%) [14]: prolactinomas (20%), GH-, ACTH-, and TSH-secreting tumors (5, 2, and <2%, respectively).

Other neoplasm without endocrine functions are rarely present: bronchial

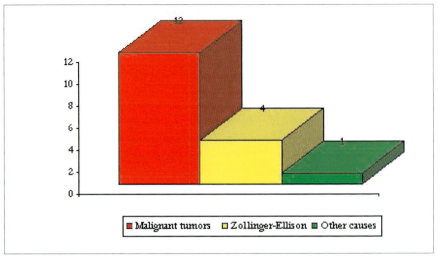

Fig. 8.4 Main causes of death in multiple endocrine neoplasia type 1 (MEN1) (adapted from [27])

carcinoid (2%), thymic tumors,(2%), benign thyroid tumors (<1%), benign or malignant medullary adrenal tumors (<25%), lipomas (30%), facial angiofibromas (85%), collagenomas (70%), and CNS ependymomas (1%) [15, 21].

MEN2A is a rare dominant autosomal hereditary syndrome, affecting <1,000 families worldwide, with a prevalence of 1:30,000 [28]. Almost all such patients contract MTC, while only 30–50% develop a bilateral and/or multifocal PHEO, or adrenal medullary hyperplasia and hyperparathyroidism as a consequence of hyperplasia or parathyroid adenoma (15–30%) [14, 28, 29].

MEN2b is much less common (<5% of all MEN2 cases) [14, 28], but is much more aggressive than MEN2A. In MEN2b, the MTC is precocious, generally appearing 10 years earlier than MEN2A with rapid metastases and alongside PHEO. Hyperparathyroidism is not present, but patients may have multiple neurinomas of the mucus membranes, ganglioneuromatosis of the gastro-enteric mucosa (responsible for abdominal distension, megacolon, constipation, or diarrhea), skeletal deformations (increased lordosis, scoliosis), flexural elasticity, myelinated corneal nerves, and a characteristic marfanoid habitus [28].

Nearly all MEN2A and MEN2B patients have MTC (6% of all thyroid carcinomas, of which about 20–30% are the inherited form), which is usually the first expression of the syndrome [14, 28]. In MEN2A, biochemical signs of MTC appear in patient 5–25 yeas of age [30]. In some rare variants, paraneoplastic syndromes occur before MTC (i.e., lichen amyloidosis cutaneous in the upper part of the back or excessive production of corticotrophins) [31]. In the familial MTC subtype, no tumors are associated with MTC. The severity of MTC decreases from MEN2B to MEN2A to familial MTC [32]. It originates as multifocal hyperplasia of the thyroid C cells, with the progression to cancer extremely variable (up to years) [33]. It has a natural tendency to metastasize locally (central and lateral, cervical, and mediastinal nodes) and at a distance (liver, bone, lung) [34]. Clinically, there is swelling or pain in the neck at 15–20 years and, in cases of elevated plasmatic levels of calcitonin or in the presence of metastatic forms, diarrhea.

The other main expression of MEN2 is PHEO, with its specific symptomatology of hypertension, episodic headache, palpitations, nervousness, and cutaneous paleness all of which are due to excessive synthesis of epinephrine, norepinephrine, and dopamine by adrenal chromaffin cells [28].

The chronological relation between these MTC and PHEO is shown in Fig. 8.5.

Hereditary Breast and Ovarian Cancer

Since HBOC is discussed in-depth elsewhere in this monograph, the discussion here is limited to the main concepts. In 1994, breast cancer gene 1 (BRCA1) was identified and associated with HBOC. In 1995, a second gene, BRCA2, was discovered. Based on these findings, a new field emerged in the treatment of breast and ovarian cancer. Detection of these genes has prompted new challenges and concerns, such as identifying patients who are candidates for genetic testing, informing them about the advantages and disadvantages of testing, and determining the appropriate treatment for those with positive results.

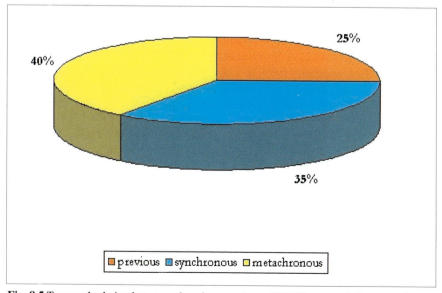

Fig. 8.5 Temporal relation between pheochromocytoma (PHEO) and medullary thyroid carcinoma (MTC) in multiple endocrine neoplasia type 2 (MEN2) (adapted from [28, 35–37])

In western countries, one out of nine women is at risk of developing breast cancer during her lifetime. Of all such cases, ~5–10% are the result of a hereditary predisposition. Transmission of BRCA1 and BRCA2 is autosomal dominant. Women with germline BRCA1 or BRCA2 mutations are at higher risk of breast and ovarian cancer than the general population. Carriers of BRCA1 mutation have a 40–85% lifetime risk of mammary cancer and a 20–50% risk of ovarian cancer. For carriers of a BRCA2 mutation, the likelihood of a breast tumor is the same, but is 15–20% for ovarian cancer [38–42].

Evidence is mounting that hereditary carcinomas have specific morphological patterns, suggesting that their natural histories differ from those of sporadic cases. In particular, BRCA1-associated breast cancers are highly proliferating and poorly differentiated tumors. Surprisingly, despite these elements suggestive of a poor prognosis, the overall survival rates among patients with hereditary breast cancer and inherited ovarian carcinomas are almost the same or even better than in sporadic forms [43]. Another characteristic of hereditary breast cancer is its propensity to younger women, with a 49 and 28% risk by age 50 for carriers of BRCA1 and BRCA2 mutation, respectively. A similar, but less dramatic, predilection for early-onset (by age 50) is present also for ovarian cancer: 23–29% (BRCA1) and 0.4–3.3% (BRCA2) [44].

Genetics

During the 1990s, an explosion of discoveries regarding hereditary cancer syndromes included the identification and cloning of several of the relevant genes [45] (Table 8.1).

Mutation of the oncosuppressor APC gene, on chromosome 5, (5q21), results in FAP. The cDNA is 8535 bp long and consists of 16 exons encoding a single, very complex protein (2843 amino acids) with no homologies to already known proteins. In the homodimer form, it is able to bind cytoskeletal microtubules and other proteins, including beta-catenin, glycogen synthetase kinase (GSK3b), the DLG protein (human homologue of the oncosuppressor protein of Drosophila discs large tumor suppressor), and the microtubule-associated protein EB1.

The main role of APC is to regulate the beta-catenin concentration, but it also is involved in cell-cell adhesion, microtubule stability, cell cycle regulation, and probably in apoptosis as well.

Since APC gene expression affects growth control in colonic cells, the first phenotypic manifestation of a mutation is represented by the onset of multiple small benign tumors. Each adenoma can slowly accumulate successive mutations of other genes (RAS, p53, etc); due to the large number of such adenomas, it is probably that one or more will progress to carcinoma.

It has been suggested that APC also mediates the apoptotic control of cellular migration within the colonic mucosa, regulating the balance between cell formation at the base and cell death at the summit of the crypts. Mutations in the APC gene are very heterogeneous, dispersed along all 16 exons, and the major-

8 The Hereditary Syndromes

Table 8.1 Inherited neoplastic syndromes

Syndrome	Gene (year of identification)	Multiple primary malignancy (MPM)
Retinoblastoma	RB (1985)	Retinoblastoma, osteosarcoma
Neurofibromatosis-1	NF1 (1987)	Neurofibromas multiple, glioma ottica, neurofibrosarcoma
Li Fraumeni syndrome	TP53 (1990)	Leukemia, sarcomas, breast, adrenal and CNS tumors
FAP	APC (1991)	Colorectal and extracolonic tumors
Gorlin's syndrome	NBCCS (1992)	Basaloma
		Schwannoma, meningioma, acustic neurinoma
Neurofibromatosis-2	NF2 (1993)	
MEN2a	RET (1993, 1994)	Medullar thyroid, pheocromocytoma
HNPCC	hMSH2, hMLH1, hPMS1, hPMS2, MET(1993–1997)	Colorectal and extracolonic tumors
Von Hippel Lindau	VHL (1993)	Kidney, pheochromocytoma, hemangioblastoma
Familial melanoma	CDKNp16 (1994)	Melanoma, glioblastoma, lung
HBOC	BRCA1, BRCA2 (1994, 1996)	Breast, ovary, prostate
Ataxia-telangiectasia	ATM (1995)	Breast
Cowden's syndrome	PTEN (1997	Breast, thyroid, kidney, hamartomatosis
MEN1	MEN1 (1997)	Parathyroid, pancreas, pituitary
MEN2	RET (1993)	Medullary thyroid carcinoma, pheochromocytoma
"Familial gastric cancer"	ECAD (1998)	Stomach
Peutz-Jeghers's syndrome	STK11 (1998)	Colon, ileal and extracolonic tumors

ity of them are confined to single pedigrees. In 95% of cases, the mutations consist of small deletions or insertions (65% in the germline), altering the context and determining the formation of premature stop codons and thus of truncated proteins. There are nonsense point mutations (28% in the germline) and 2% of germinal alterations are missense and/or splicing site mutations. Rearrangements of the APC locus are rare. Two mutational hot spots are present at codons 1061 and 1309.

A significant number of families with classic FAP (>100 colonic adenomas) and AFAP (15–100 adenomas) do not carry APC mutations. In fact, genetic tests do not show alterations in the gene in over 20% of classic FAP and in an even higher percentage of AFAP cases [46]. In this variation diverse mutations have been identified extremely 5' and 3' of the APC gene [4]. Recent studies emphasized that a subgroup of these APC-negative families, above all with those with AFAP, have alterations in the MYH-repair gene [47, 48]. MYH-related FAP is transmitted as a recessive autosomal condition and is characterized by multiple colorectal adenomas with a high risk of cancerization [49]. The data collected in some studies indicate a single recessive polyposis MYH-associated syndrome. [50–55]. Biallelic mutations of MYH can affect other genes involved in colorectal cancer, such as APC [51] and Ki-ras [56]. Sieber's multicenter study [54] highlighted that one-third of AFAP patients and 7.5% of classic FAP patients have biallelic MYH mutations [57].

In HNPCC, the altered genes control DNA repair and are responsible for correct DNA synthesis during replication; they include the yeast mutS homologues hMSH2, GTBP (hMSH6) and hMSH3, which form a functional complex with hMLH1 and hPMS2 [1]. Errors in the repair genes cause nucleotide mismatches.

Germline mutations in the hMLH1 and hPMS2 genes have been frequently implicated in HNPCC and are associated, in 90% of cases, with microsatellite instability in tumor tissues. Microsatellites are small insertions or deletions that are present in repetitive coding or noncoding genomic regions.

The mutations described thus far are heterogeneously dispersed in codifying sequences although there is no evidence for a mutational hot spot. They result in missense and nonsense mutations as well as small and/or large deletions or insertions that alter the length of the protein or its splice sites.

MEN1 and MEN2 are caused by alterations of the MEN1 and RET genes, respectively. MEN1 has almost a 100% penetrance [26]. The mutation responsible for MEN1 was identified in 1988 and is located in the q13 region of chromosome 11 [58, 59]; the gene was cloned in 1997. It is an oncosuppressor gene formed by 10 exons that span >9 kb of genomic DNA; the encoded protein, menin, is made up of 610 amino acids [58, 59] and is expressed in lymphocytes, thymus gland, pancreas, thyroid, gonads, and other tissues. In a manner analogous to that of other oncosuppressor proteins menin is located in the nucleus [14], where it interacts with proteins that regulate cell proliferation, including cme JunD [60, 61], Smad 3 [62], and the activator of the S-phase kinase [60, 63]. The latter is a crucial regulator of cdc7 kinase, required for the start of DNA replication [64, 65].

The genetic defect leading to MEN2, a mutation in the proto-oncogene cRET, was identified in 1993 [66, 67]. The gene is located in the pericentromeric region of chromosome 10 (10q12.2) and encodes the 21 exons of the RET protein, a subunit of a multimolecular complex. Germline mutations of c-RET [32] have been detected in 98% of patients and occur in exons 10, 11, 13, 14, 15, and 16. Mutations of exon 8 have been recently described in familial MTC [28, 68].

When triggered by its ligand, wild-type RET receptors are induced to dimerize and this dimerization activates RET kinase activity followed by signal transduction [69]. This sequence of events is altered in cells with cRET mutations, the oncogenicity of which depends on the site of the amino acid change. Cysteine substitution by several other residues in the cysteine-rich domain is believed to prevent the formation of intramolecular disulfide bonds, enabling ligand-independent receptor dimerization and thus constitutive kinase activation. Thus, cysteine point mutations in MEN2A and FMTC have a "gain of function" effect on RET. In MEN2A and familial MTC, mutated RET receptors into which an extracellular cysteine residue has been inserted are constitutively dimerized, i.e., they function independent of ligand binding.

Mutations at cysteine 634 result in a stronger transforming ability than those at other extracellular cysteines. In contrast, in most MEN2B cases one of two intracellular tyrosine kinase domains is altered. Regardless, little is known about how mutations in the tyrosine kinase domains activate RET. RET-phosphorylated tyrosines interact with the docking protein FSR2, causing downstream activation of the mitogen-activated protein kinase (MAPK) signaling cascade. Thus, mutations at this level may alter regulation of MAPK pathways [70, 71]. Microarray expression analysis of PHEO and MTC tissues from patients with MEN2A and MEN2B demonstrated differences in their gene expression profiles, possibly explaining the more aggressive nature of MEN2B [28,72].

Genetic factors account for only a few cases (5%) of breast cancers, but in 25% of patients <30 years of age. In 1988, a group of studies by Marie-Claire King provided evidence of genetic transmission in families at high risk for cancer, and in 1990 a region of the long arm of chromosome 17 (17q21) with genes susceptible to mutations was identified.

The BRCA1 gene was characterized in 1994. The BRCA1 protein acts as a tumor suppressor, probably by negatively regulating cell growth or by being involved in the search and repair of genome damage or spontaneous mutations. The latter result in the inactivation of a single BRCA1 allele and precede a somatic event in breast epithelia cells, which eliminates the remaining BRCA1 allele. BRCA is a large gene with 24 exons, making mutational analyses particularly complex.

In the same period in which BRCA1 was identified, a second susceptible locus was found on chromosome 13. This gene, called BRCA2, is responsible for more than 30% of familiar breast tumors. Like BRCA1, it is a large and complex gene and its functions are not yet entirely known. Together, BRCA1 and 2 account for 50–75% of familiar breast cancers. The penetrance of BRCA1 and BRCA2 refers to the possibility that the mutations generate a breast tumor. Initial estimation of the penetrance of these mutations was very high (80–90%) but is currently thought to be about 56% (40–73%).

Important mutations of the two genes are very rare in normal populations, but with interesting geographic variations (1/1,000 in the American population, 1/100 of Ashkenazi Jewish/Eastern European women).

Other high-risk genes known to predispose women to breast cancer tend to be rare and associated with specific clinical, diagnostic features: Li–Fraumeni syndrome (also associated with soft-tissue sarcoma, adrenocortical carcinoma, glioblastoma and lung cancer, gene TP53), Peutz-Jeghers syndrome (diagnosed from the association of gastrointestinal tract hamartomas and skin and mucosal pigmentation, LKB1/STK11 gene), and Cowden disease (usually associated with macrocephaly, trichilemmomas and other features, PTEN gene) [73].

Genotype-Phenotype Correlations

The tremendous genetic heterogeneity, with hundreds of mutations in each gene having been identified, has made it difficult to correlate genetic information with phenotypic expression, or to associate a genotype with a specific syndrome or the particularly aggressive behavior of a disease. Nonetheless, knowledge of the patient's genotype can influence the clinical, diagnostic, and therapeutic approach.

In FAP >300 mutations [5] in the APC gene have been described and all are associated with specific ECM [74–94]. Table 8.2 lists the main associations.

The mutations responsible for HNPCC (>100, mostly in hMSH2 and hMLH1) have not yet been characterized in detail, but the prognosis and the disease phenotype have been preliminarily associated with specific mutations of MMR genes.

Literature reports [95] have tracked geographic differences in the occurrence of certain mutations. In the USA, hMSH2 and hMLH1 mutations are equally distributed, while in other countries (Spain, Korea, China, Sweden, and Finland)

Table 8.2 FAP: genotype-phenotype correlations in the literature [73–94]

Phenotype	Mutation (site)
CHRPE+	10–15 proximal, 463–1387, 457–1444 codons
CHRPE-	Exons 1–8, 15 distal
Diffuse polyposis	1250–1464 codons
Severe polyposis	1309, 1336 codons
Early-onset polyposis	835. 1309 codons
Late onset polyposis	1061 codon
High rates of colorectal cancer	1250–1450 codons
Multiple extracolonic manifestations	1309, 1402–1578, 1465, 1546, 2621 codons
Attenuated FAP	Exons 1–4
Desmoids	1445–1578 codons
Osteomas	1403, 1444 codons
Duodenal adenomas	479, 976–1067, 1700 codons

8 The Hereditary Syndromes

most mutations involve hMLH1. There are also differences regarding sex, as men present more frequently than women with MSH2 mutations (96% vs. 39%).

The probability of developing extracolonic cancers and/or MPM, the topography of these tumors, and the nodal involvement of colorectal cancer seem related to specific MMR gene mutations, but the data are too limited to draw definitive conclusions. Compared to hMLH1, mutations in hMSH2 are associated with a higher percentage of both extracolonic cancer (63% hMSH2 vs. 35% hMLH1, $p = 0.003$) and MPM (42% MSH2 vs. 18% hMLH1, $p = 0.004$).

Over 600 germline mutations of the MEN1 gene are currently known, but they have not been matched with specific clinical manifestations [15]. For MEN2, there is a strong genotype-phenotype correlation (Table 8.3). The three main pathological expressions (MTC, PHEO, and hyperparathyroidism) can be associated with specific mutations of the RET gene, which simplifies the management of these patients in that prophylactic total thyroidectomy is now the standard approach. In addition, surveillance programs can be differentiated on the basis of the genetic risk linked to the specific clinical expression of a disease.

Table 8.3 MEN2: genotype-phenotype correlations in the literature [11, 14, 18, 28, 32]

Mutations	Phenotype
Six cysteines in the extracellular cysteine-rich domain of RET: 609, 611, 618, 620, 630 at exon 10); 790, and 791 at exon 13	MEN2A (93–98%) and FMTC (80–96%); infrequent hyperparathyroidism
Codon 634 at exon 11	MEN2A 85% and FMTC 30%, pheochromocytoma strictly associated and high risk of hyperparathyroidism
Intracellular domain of RET:768, 790 and 791 at exon 13, 804 and 844 at exon 14, 891 at exon 15	Rare MEN2A and FMTC
631 at exon 10	FMTC
Intracellular tyrosine kinase receptor domains of RET: M918T mutation at exon 16,	MEN2B >95%
Harbor the A883F substitution at exon 15 Missense mutations: 804 and 806 at exon 14, 904 at exon 15, 922 at exon 16	MEN2B 5% MEN2B
All RET proto-oncogene mutations except those in codons 609, 768, val804met, and 891	Pheochromocytoma
Codon 768, val804met, and 891	Hyperparathyroidism rare
883, 918, or 922	MEN2B, no hyperparathyroidism

In HBOC, the breast cancers are usually infiltrating ductal carcinomas, with some authors reporting an increased frequency of medullary and atypical medullary types. The tumors are often poorly differentiated, although there may be subtle differences between BRCA1- and BRCA2-associated disease in this regard. BRCA-associated cancers are often aneuploid, with high proliferative rates, as shown by flow cytometry or Ki-67 staining. BRCA1-associated cancers are usually, but not always, hormone-receptor-negative, in contrast to BRCA2-associated tumors. HER-2/neu overexpression appears to be uncommon, particularly in BRCA1, but p53 mutations are common and may be directly relevant to the pathogenesis of BRCA-associated cancer [44].

Carriers of BRCA1 and BRCA2 mutations have the same lifetime risk of breast cancer (23–85%), but ovarian (20–50% vs. 15–20%) and prostate (25% vs. 5–7.5%) cancer are more frequent for BRCA1 [39–42, 44] and male breast cancer for BRCA2 [96]. Other associations (colon for BRCA1 and stomach and head and neck tumors for BRCA2) have been suggested but not proven [44].

Our Experience

Analysis of Mutations in Patients with FAP and HNPCC

At our institution, beginning in 2000 and currently ongoing, 65 families with a history of FAP and 84 with a history of HNPCC, all from southern Italy, have been analyzed for mutations in the APC and MYH genes (FAP) and for mutations in MMR-genes for HNPCC. Genetic mutations were analyzed by PCR, followed by single strand conformation polymorphism (SSCP), protein truncation test (PTT), denaturing high-performance liquid chromatography (DHPLC), and DNA sequencing. Of the 65 families with FAP, 32 different APC mutations were identified in 40 of them (62%) (Table 8.4). Of the 84 families with HNPCC, 17 different mutations in MLH1 and MSH2 were identified in 28 of them (33%) (Table 8.5). For those families with a clinical diagnosis of FAP or HNPCC diagnosis in whom molecular analysis failed to reveal mutations in APC or MLH1-MSH2 respectively, mutational analyses of other genes also involved in these syndromes were carried out.

In the probands of the remaining 25 families with a clinical diagnosis of FAP but without APC mutation, the MYH gene was analyzed: 11 mutations were identified in seven FAP patients, four of whom were found to be heterozygotes (Table 8.6). In the probands of the 56 HNPCC families negative for MLH1 and MSH2, other MMR genes (MLH3, MSH6, and MSH3) were searched for mutations. Accordingly, seven mutations of the MSH6 gene, one in the MLH3 gene, and two in the MSH3 gene were found in 13 families (Table 8.7). For some patients, the presence of one or more MMR mutations could result in an additive effect for the development of cancer. Importantly, we were able to identify a large number of carriers (35/61 FAP and 52/96 HNPCC), apparently in good health, but belonging to a family at risk.

8 The Hereditary Syndromes

Table 8.4 Germline point mutations found in the APC gene in FAP families from southern Italy (phenotype: attenuated = 10–100 polyps, classical = 100–1,000 polyps; aggressive >5,000 polyps)

Exon	Mutation	Protein change	Phenotype
5	591-592delAG	Stop at codon 250-251	Classic
5	595insG	Stop at codon 250-251	Aggressive, desmoids, CHRPE-
8	893-894delAC	Stop at codon 325-326	Classic, CHRPE+
14	1797C>A	C599X	Classic, CHRPE+
14	1879-1882delAACA	Stop at codon 629-630	Classic, CHRPE+
15	2119insT	Stop at codon 732-733	Classic
15	2520-2523insCTTA	Stop at codon 860-861	Aggressive, CHRPE+
15	2626C>T	R876X	Aggressive
15	2638delA	Stop at codon 915-916	Classic, CHRPE+
15	2800-2803delACTT	Stop at codon 954-955	Classic
15	2804insA	Stop at codon 938-939	Classic, CHRPE+
15	3183-3187delACAAA	Stop at codon 1063-1064	Classic
15	3186-3187delAA	Stop at codon 1063-1064	Attenuated, CHRPE+
15	3202-3205delTCAA	Stop at codon 1125-1126	Classic
15	(3225T>A; 3226C>A)	(Y1075X; P1076T)	Classic, CHRPE+
15	3577-3578delCA	Stop at codon 1206-1207	Classic, CHRPE+
15	3927-3931delAAAGA	Stop at codon 1313-1314	Aggressive, desmoids, CHRPE+
15	3982C>T	Q1328X	Classic
15	(4145-46delTC; 4148-50delTGT)	Stop at codon 1384-1385	Classic, CHRPE+
15	4526-4527insT	Stop at codon 1512-1513	Attenuated, gastric polyps, desmoids, osteomas
15	4621C>T	Q1541X	Classic, gastric polyps, desmoids, osteomas
*	del locus APC	-	Classic FAP
*	del locus APC	-	Classic, FAP
6	c.697delC	Q233fs59X	AFAP, thyroid nodules
15	c.4006G>T	R1336X	Classic FAP
	RNA alteration	-	AFAP
15	c.3927-31delAAAGA	G1309-I1311fs3X	

continue →

continue **Table 8.4**

Classic FAP			
15	c.4909G>A	D1637N	AFAP
15	c.3865delT	Cys1289fs16X	Classic FAP
15	c.3161-62delAC	H1054fs1X	Classic FAP
6	c.694C>T	R232X	Classic FAP
15	c.2522T>A	L841X	Classic FAP

CHRPE, Congenital hypertrophy of the retinal pigment epithelium

Table 8.5 Germline point mutations found in the MLH1 and MSH2 genes in hereditary non-polyposis colorectal cancer (HNPCC) families from southern Italy

Exon and gene	Mutation	Protein change	Phenotype (family number)
11- MLH1	954delC	Stop at codon 366	Lynch II (1) Lynch I (7) Lynch I (13) Lynch I (46) Lynch II (77)
7- MLH1	c.579T>C	Ser193Pro	Lynch I (2) Lynch II (66)
3- MLH1	c.231T>C	Cys77Arg	Lynch I (3) Lynch II (49) Lynch II (59)
16- MLH1	c.1854_55AA>GC	Lys618Ala	Lynch II (37)
12- MLH1	c.1323G>A	Ala441Thr	Lynch II (28)
19- MLH1	c.2248T>C	Leu 749Pro	Lynch II (32)
1- MSH2	InsC191/92	Stop codon 81/82	Lynch II (34) Lynch I (52) Lynch II (64)
9- MSH2	c.1467G >T	Stop codon 489	Lynch I (8)
1- MLH1	63delG	Stop codon 380	Lynch II (27)
10- MSH2	1576delA	Stop codon 542	Lynch II (48) Lynch II (73)
16- MLH1	1854_56del AAG	del618Lys	atypical Lynch, (only the proband is affected) (16)
5- MSH2	a>t 942+3	del in frame exon 5	Lynch II (68) Lynch II (81)
5- MSH2	t>a 942+2	del in frame exon 5	Lynch I (83)
5- MSH2	delAAAAAAAAAAAAA 942+3-16	RNA alteration	Lynch I (57)
13- MSH2	c.2135_36insT	Stop codon 716	Lynch II (44)
3- MLH1	c.304G>A	Splice defect	atypical Lynch, (proband's parents healthy) (55)
10- MLH1	c.2379C>T	Arg793Cys	Lynch II (67)

8 The Hereditary Syndromes

Table 8.6 Germline point mutations in the MYH gene of FAP families from southern Italy

Phenotype inheritance	Type of manifestation	Extracolonic colon polyps	Number of mutation	APC mutation	MYH
Classic FAP	R	NO	100–1000	N.F.	c.494A→G (p.Y165C); c.692G→A (p.R231H)
Classic FAP	R	NO	100–1000	N.F.	c.502C→T (p.R168C); c.1395-97 delGGA (p.466delE)
AFAP	N.I.	NO	7	N.F.	c.1145G→A (p.G382D); c.270C→A (p.Y90X)
AFAP	N.I.	NO	25	N.F.	c.972G→C (p.Q324H)
AFAP	N.I.	Lymphoma (proband's father: 53 years old)	24	N.F.	c.310C→T (p.R231H); c.494A→G (p.Y165C)
AFAP	N.I.	NO	5–100	N.F.	c.1145G→A (p.G382D)
AFAP	N.I.	NO	50–100	N.F.	c.1145G→A (p.G382D)

Classic FAP: >100 polyps; AFAP 2–4/99 polyps; *R*, recessive inheritance; *D*, dominant inheritance; *N.I.*, no inheritance; *N.F.*, mutation not found; the blood test indicates a novel mutation

Table 8.7 Germ line point mutations found in the MSH6, MLH3 and MSH3 genes in HNPCC families from southern Italy

Patient	Mutations in MSH6	Mutations	Mutations in MSH3	Phenotype in MLH3
05/1	Ex2 431g>t (Ser→Ile)	NO	NO	No family history, early onset
95/25	Ex4 2633t>g (Val→Ala)	IVS7–9 T>C	NO	Amsterdam I
04/10	Ex4 2633t>g (Val→Ala)	Ex21 3110G>A . (Arg→Gly); IVS6 -63C>T	NO	Amsterdam I

continue →

continue **Table 8.7**

04/14	NO	Ex21 3110G>A (Arg→Gly)	NO	Amsterdam I
02/10	Ex4 2941a>c (Ile→Val)	Ex21 3110G>A (Arg→Gly)	NO	Amsterdam I
02/11	Ex4 2941a>c (Ile →Val)	NO	Ex1 3010t>c (Ser→Pro)	Amsterdam I; early onset
04/16	NO	NO	Ex1 3010t>c (Ser→Pro)	Amsterdam I
04/19	NO	NO	Ex1 3010t>c (Ser→Pro)	Amsterdam I
01/3	Ex5 3261_62Insc (Phe→stop)	NO	no	Amsterdam I; late onset
01/5	Ex5 3295_97deltt (Ile→stop)	NO	IVS3+37 del TCTT; IVS8 +66 g >a; IVS10 +13 c >g.	Amsterdam I; early onset
00/13	Ex7 3639t>a (Asp→Glu)	NO	NO	Amsterdam I
04/9	IVS2 +33 insgtgt RNA alteration	NO	NO	Amsterdam I
95/2	NO	Ex12 1947G>C (Tyr→Asn)	NO	Amsterdam I; late onset

References

1. Renda A, Izzo P, D'Armeinto F et al (2004) Chirurgia oncologica "Dna-guidata". Archivio e Atti SIC, Pozzi, Rome, 1:141–172
2. Rolandelli RH, Roslin JJ (2003) Colon. In: Sabiston DC (ed) Trattato di chirurgia. Le basi biologiche della moderna pratica chirurgica, prima edizione italiana sulla sedicesima americana. Delfino Editore, Rome, pp 662–696
3. Bertario L, Russo A, Sala P et al (2003) Multiple approach to the exploration of genotype-phenotype correlations in familial adenomatous polyposis. J Clin Oncol 21(9):1698–1707
4. Soravia C, Berk T, Madlensky L et al (1998) Genotype-phenotype correlations in attenuated adenomatous polyposis coli. Am J Hum Genet 62(6):1290–1301
5. Lal G, Gallinger S (2000) Familial adenomatous polyposis. Semin Surg Oncol 18(4):314–323
6. Lynch HT, Smyrk TC, McGinn T et al (1995) Attenuated familial adenomatous polyposis (AFAP): a phenotypically and genotypically distinctive variant of FAP. Cancer 76:2427–2433
7. Arvanitis ML, Jagelman DG, Fazio VW et al (1990) Mortality in patients with familial adenomatous polyposis. Dis Col & Rectum 33(8):639–642
8. Giardiello FM, Brensinger JD, Tersmette AC et al (2000) Very high risk of cancer in familial Peutz-Jeghers syndrome. Gastroenterology 119:1447–1453
9. Lynch HT, Krush AJ (1971) Cancer family G revisited: 1895–1970. Cancer 27:1505–1511
10. Warthin AS (1913) Heredity with reference to carcinoma. Arch Intern Med 12:546–555
11. Warthin AS (1925) The further study of a cancer family. J Cancer Res 9:279–286
12. Rijcken FE, Mourits MJ, Kleibeuker JH et al (2003) Gynecologic screening in hereditary nonpolyposis colorectal cancer. Gynecol Oncol 91(1):74–80

8 The Hereditary Syndromes

13. Moslein G (2003) Clinical implications of molecular diagnosis in hereditary nonpolyposis colorectal cancer. Recent Results Cancer Res 162:73–78
14. Moley JF, Wells SA Jr (2003) Ipofisi e surreni. In: Sabiston DC (ed) Trattato di chirurgia. Le basi biologiche della moderna pratica chirurgica, prima edizione italiana sulla sedicesima americana. Delfino Editore, Rome, pp 662–696
15. Lévy-Bohbot N, Merle C, Goudet P et al (2004) Prevalence, characteristics and prognosisof MEN 1-associated glucagonomas, VIPomas,and somatostatinomas Study from the GTE (Groupe des Tumeurs Endocrines) registry. Gastroenterol Clin Biol 28:1075–1081
16. Calender A, Cadiot G, Mignon M (2001) Néoplasie endocrinienne multiple de type 1: aspects génétiques et cliniques. Gastroenterol Clin Biol 25:B38-B48
17. Chanson P, Cadiot G, Murat A (1997) Management of patients and subjects at risk for multiple endocrine neoplasia type 1: MEN 1. GENEM 1. Groupe d'Etude des Neoplasies Endocriniennes Multiples de type 1. Horm Res 47:211–220
18. Marx S, Spiegel AM, Skarulis MC et al (1998) Multiple endocrine neoplasia type 1: clinical and genetic topics. Ann Intern Med 129:484–494
19. Cadiot G, Mignon M, Gresze (2003) Diagnostique des tumeurs endocrines de la région duodéno-pancréatique. Gastroenterol Clin Biol 27:S6-S14
20. Skogseid B, Oberg K, Benson L et al (1987) A standardized meal stimulation test of the endocrine pancreas for early detection of pancreatic endocrine tumors in multiple endocrine neoplasia type 1 syndrome: five years experience. J Clin Endocrinol Metab 64:1233–1240
21. Triponez F, Dosseh D, Goudet P et al (2006) Epidemiology data on 108 MEN 1 patients from the GTE with isolated nonfunctioning tumors of the pancreas. Ann Surg 243:265–272
22. Brandi ML, Gagel RF, Angeli A et al (2001) Guidelines for diagnosis and therapy of MEN type 1 and type 2. J Clin Endocrinol Metab 86:5658–5671
23. Doherty GM, Thompson NW (2003) Multiple endocrine neoplasia type 1: duodenopancreatic tumours. J Intern Med 253:590 –598
24. Wilkinson S, Teh BT, Davey KR et al (1993) Cause of death in multiple endocrine neoplasia type 1. Arch Surg 128:683–690
25. Dean PG, van Heerden JA, Farley DR et al (2000) Are patients with multiple endocrine neoplasia type I prone to premature death? World J Surg 24:1437–1441
26. Ebeling T, Vierimaa O, Kyto S et al (2004) Effect of multiple endocrine neoplasia type 1 (MEN1) gene mutations on premature mortality in familial MEN1 syndrome with founder mutations. J Clin Endocrinol Metab 89(7):3392–3396
27. Geerdink EAM, Van der Luijtl RB, Lips CJ (2003) Do patients with multiple endocrine neoplasia benefit from periodical screening? Eur J Endocrinol 149:577–582
28. Marini F, Falchetti A, Del Monte F et al (2006) Multiple endocrine neoplasia type 2. Orphanet J Rare Dis 1:45
29. Farnebo F, Kytola S, Teh BT et al (1999) Alternative genetic pathways in parathyroid tumorigenesis. J Clin Endocrinol Metab 84:3775–3780
30. Lips CJ, Landsvater RM, Hoppener JW et al (1994) Clinical screening as compared with DNA analysis in families with multiple endocrine neoplasia type 2A. N Engl J Med 331:828–835
31. Robinson MF, Furst EJ, Nunziata V et al (1992) Characterization of the clinical features of five families with hereditary primary cutaneous lichen amyloidosis and multiple endocrine neoplasia type 2. Henry Ford Hosp Med J 40:249–252
32. Brandi ML, Gagel RF, Angeli A et al (2001) Guidelines for diagnosis and therapy of MEN type 1 and type 2. J Clin Endocrinol Metab 86:5658–5671
33. Papotti M, Botto Micca F et al (1993) Poorly differentiated thyroid carcinomas with primordial cell component. A group of aggressive lesions sharing insular, trabecular, and solid patterns. Am J Surg Pathol 17:291–301
34. Carling T (2005) Multiple endocrine neoplasia syndrome: genetic basis for clinical management. Curr Opin Oncol 17:7–12
35. Eng C (1996) The RET proto-oncogene in multiple endocrine neoplasia type 2 and Hirschsprung's disease. N Engl J Med 335:943–951

36. Dralle H, Gimm O, Simon D et al (1998) Prophylactic thyroidectomy in 75 children and adolescents with hereditary medullary thyroid carcinoma: German and Austrian experience. World J Surg 22:744–750
37. Neumann HP, Bausch B, McWhinney SR et al (2002) Freiburg-Warsaw-Columbus Pheochromocytoma Study Group. "Germ-line mutations in nonsyndromic pheochromocytoma. N Engl J Med 346:1459–1466
38. Yarden RI, Papa MZ (2006) BRCA1 at the crossroad of multiple cellular pathways: approaches for therapeutic interventions. Mol Cancer Ther 5(6):1396–1404
39. Schmeler KM, Sun CC, Bodurka DC et al (2006) Prophylactic bilateral salpingo-oophorectomy compared with surveillance in women with BRCA mutations. Obstet Gynecol 108:515–520
40. Ford D, Easton DF, Stratton M et al (1998) Genetic heterogeneity and penetrance analysis of the BRCA1 and BRCA2 genes in breast cancer families. The Breast Cancer Linkage Consortium. Am J Hum Genet 62:676–689
41. Struewing JP, Hartge P, Wacholder S et al (1997) The risk of cancer associated with specific mutations of BRCA1 and BRCA2 among Ashkenazi Jews. N Engl J Med 336:1401–1408
42. Antoniou A, Pharoah PD, Narod S et al (2003) Average risks of breast and ovarian cancer associated with BRCA1 or BRCA2 mutations detected in case series unselected for family history: a combined analysis of 22 studies. Am J Hum Genet 72:1117–1130
43. Eisinger F (1998) Recommendations for medical management of hereditary breast and ovarian cancer: The French National Ad Hoc Committee. Ann Oncol 9:939–950
44. Robson ME (2002) Clinical considerations in the management of individuals at risk for hereditary breast and ovarian cancer. Cancer Control 6:457–465
45. Peterson G (1999) Genetic testing for cancer: the surgeon's critical role. Clinical cancer genetics: 1998 (what's available to you in your practice). J Am Coll Surg 188(1):89–93
46. Hernegger GS, Moore HG, Guillem JG (2002) Attenuated familial adenomatous polyposis: an evolving and poorly understood entity. Dis Colon Rectum 45:127–136
47. Lindahl T (1993) Instability and decay of the primary structure of DNA. Nature 348:709–715
48. Ames BN, Gold LS (1991) Endogenous mutagens and the causes of aging and cancer. Mutat Res 250:3–16
49. Al-Tassan N, Chmiel NH, Maynard J et al (2002) Inherited variants of MYH associated with somatic G:C fi T:A mutations in colorectal tumors. Nat Genet 30:227–232
50. Enholm S, Hienonen T, Suomalainen A et al (2003) Proportion and phenotype of MYH-associated colorectal neoplasia in a population-based series of Finish colorectal cancer patients. Am J Pathol 163:827–832
51. Halford SE, Rowan AJ, Lipton L et al (2003) Germline mutations but not somatic changes at the MYH locus contribute to the pathogenesis of unselected colorectal cancers. Am J Pathol 162:1545–1548
52. Jones S, Emmerson P, Maynard J et al (2002) Biallelic germline mutations in MYH predispose to multiple colorectal adenoma and somatic G:C fi T:A mutations. Hum Mol Genet 11:2961–2967
53. Sampson JR, Dolwani S, Jones S et al (2003) Autosomal recessive colorectal adenomatous polyposis due to inherited mutations of MYH. Lancet 362:39–41
54. Sieber OM, Lipton L, Crabtree M et al (2003) Multiple colorectal adenomas, classic adenomatous polyposis, and germ-line mutations in MYH. N Engl J Med 348:791–799
55. Venesio T, Molatore S, Cattaneo F et al (2004) High frequency of MYH gene mutations in a subset of patients with familial adenomatous polyposis. Gastroenterology 126:1681–1685
56. Jones S, Lambert S, Williams GT et al (2004) Increased frequency of the k-ras G12C mutation in MYH polyposis colorectal adenomas. Br J Cancer 90:1591–1593
57. Leite JS, Isidro G, Martins M et al (2005) Is prophylactic colectomy indicated in patients with MYH-associated polyposis? Colorectal Dis 7:327–331
58. Chandrasekharappa SC, Guru SC, Manickam P et al (1997) Positional cloning of the gene for multiple endocrine neoplasia-type 1. Science 276:404–407

59. Lemmens I, Van de Ven WJ, Kas K et al (1997) Identification of the multiple endocrine neoplasia type 1 (MEN1) gene. The European Consortium on MEN 1. Hum Mol Genet 6:1177–1183
60. Schnepp RW, Chen YX, Wang H et al (2006) Mutation of tumor suppressor gene Men1 acutely enhances proliferation of pancreatic islet cells. Cancer Res 66(11):5707–5715
61. Agarwal SK, Novotny EA, Crabtree JS et al (2003) Transcription factor JunD, deprived of menin, switches from growth suppressor to growth promoter. Proc Natl Acad Sci USA 100:10770–10775
62. Kaji H, Canaff L, Lebrun JJ et al (2001) Inactivation of menin, a Smad3-interacting protein, blocks transforming growth factor type h signalling. Proc Natl Acad Sci U S A 98:3837–3842
63. Schnepp RW, Hou Z, Wang H et al (2004) Functional interaction between tumor suppressor menin and activator of S-phase kinase. Cancer Res 64:6791–6796
64. Kumagai H, Sato N, Yamada M et al (1999) A novel growth- and cell cycle-regulatedprotein, ASK, activates human Cdc7-related kinase and is essential for G1/S transition in mammalian cells. Mol Cell Biol 19:5083–5095
65. Masai H, Matsui E, You Z et al (2000) Human Cdc7-related kinase complex. In vitro phosphorylation of MCM by concerted actions of Cdks and Cdc7 and that of a critical threonine residue of Cdc7 bY Cdks. J Biol Chem 275:42–52
66. Howe JR, Moley JF, Goodfellow P, Wells SA Jr (1993) Mutations in the RET proto-oncogene are associated with MEN 2A and FMTC. Hum Mol Genet 2:851–856
67. Mulligan LM, Kwok JB, Healey CS et al (1993) Germ-line mutations of the RET proto-oncogene in multiple endocrine neoplasia type 2A. Nature 363:458–460
68. Da Silva AM, Maciel RM, Da Silva MR et al (2003) A novel germ-line point mutation in RET exon 8 (Gly(533)Cys) in a large kindred with familial medullary thyroid carcinoma. J Clin Endocrinol Metab 88:5438–5443
69. Jing S, Wen D, Yu Y et al (1996) GDNF-induced activation of the ret protein tyrosine kinase is mediated by GDNFR-alpha, a novel receptor for GDNF. Cell 85:1113–1124
70. Santoro M, Melillo RM, Carlomagno F et al (2004) RET: normal and abnormal functions. Endocrinology 145:5448–5451
71. Santoro M, Carlomagno F, Melillo RM, Fusco A (2004) Dysfunction of the RET receptor in human cancer. Cell Mol Life Sci 61:2954–2964
72. Jain S, Watson MA, DeBenedetti MK et al (2004) Expression profiles provide insights into early malignant potential and skeletal abnormalities in multiple endocrine neoplasia type 2B syndrome tumors. Cancer Res 64:3907–3913
73. Thull DL, Vogel VG (2004) Recognition and management of hereditary breast cancer syndromes. Oncologist 9:13–24
74. Carlomagno N, Scarano MI, Gargiulo S et al (2001) Familial colonic polyposis: effect of molecular analysis on the diagnostic-therapeutic approach. Ann Ital Chir 72(2):207–214
75. Traboulsi EI, Apostolides J, Giardiello FM et al (1996) Pigmented ocular fundus lesions and APC mutations in familial adenomatous polyposis. Ophthalmic Genet 17(4):167–174
76. Olschwang S, Laurent-Puig P, Thuille B et al (1992) Frequent polymorphism in the 13th exon of the adenomatous polyposis coli gene. Hum Genet 90:161–163
77. Nagase H, Miyoshi Y, Horii A et al (1992) Correlation between the location of germ-line mutations in the APC gene and the number of colorectal polyps in familial adenomatous polyposis patients. Cancer Res 52:4055–4057
78. Wu JS, Mc Gannon EA, Church JM (1998) APC genotype, polyp number and surgical options in familial adenomatous polyposis. Ann Surg 227:57–62
79. Nordling M, Engwall Y, Wahistrom J et al (1997) Novel mutations in APC gene and clinical features in Swedish patients with polyposis coli. Am Cancer Res 17:4275–4280
80. Caspari R, Friedi W, Mandl M et al (1994) Familial adenomatous polyposis: mutation at codon 1309 and early onset of colon cancer. Lancet 343:629–632
81. Presciuttini S, Varesco L, Sala P et al (1994) Age of onset in familial adenomatous polyposis: heterogeneity within families and among APC mutations. Ann Hum Genet 58:331–342

82. Giardiello FM, Krush AJ, Petersen GM et al (1994) Phenotypic variability of familial adenomatous polyposis in 11 unrelated families with identical APC gene mutation. Gastroenterology 106(6):1542–1547
83. Giardiello FM, Brensinger JD, Luce MC et al (1997) Phenotypic expression of disease in families that have mutations in the 5' region of the adenomatous polyposis coli gene. Ann Intern Med 126(7):514–519
84. Cunningham C, Dunlop MG (1996) Molecular genetic basis of colo-rectal cancer susceptibility. Br J Surg 83:321–329
85. Leggett BA, Young IP, Biden K et al (1997) Severe upper gastrointestinal polyposis associated with sparse colonie polyposis in a familial adenomatous polyposis family with an APC mutation at codon 1250. Gut 41:518–521
86. Nugent KP, Phillips RK, Hodgson SV et al (1994) Phenotypic expression in familial adenomatous polyposis: partial prediction by mutation analysis. Gut 35:1622–1623
87. Spirio L, Otterud B, Stauffer D et al (1992) Linkage of a variant or attenuated form of adenomatous polyposis coli to the adenomatous polyposis coli (APC) locus. Am J Hum Genet 51(1):92–100
88. Olschwang S, Tiret A, Laurent-Puig P et al (1993) Restriction of ocular fundus lesions to a specific subgroup of APC mutations in adenomatous polyposis coli patients. Cell 75(5):959–968
89. Caspari R, Olschwang S, Friedl W et al (1995) Familial adenomatous polyposis: desmoid tumours and lack of ophthalmic lesions (CHRPE) associated with APC mutations beyond codon 1444. Hum Mol Genet 4(3):337–340
90. Davies DR, Armstrong JG, Thakker N et al (1995) Severe Gardner syndrome in families with mutations restricted to a specific region of the APC gene. Am J Hum Genet 57(5):1151–1158
91. Moisio A-L, Jarvinen H, Peltomaki P (2002) Genetic and clinical characterisation of familial adenomatous polyposis: a population-based study. Gut 50:845–850
92. Gebert JF, Dupon C, Kadmon M et al (1999) Combined molecular and clinical approaches for the identification of families with familial adenomatous polyposis coli. Ann Surg 229:350–361
93. Friedl W, Caspari R, Sengteller M et al (2001) Can APC mutation analysis contribute to therapeutic decisions in familial adenomatous polyposis? Experience from 680 FAP families. Gut 48:515–521
94. Matsumoto T, Lida M, Kobori Y et al (2002) Genetic predisposition to clinical manifestations in familial adenomatous polyposis with special reference to duodenal lesions. Am J Gastroenterol 97:180–185
95. Umar A, Boland CR, Terdiman JP et al (2004) Revised Bethesda Guidelines for hereditary nonpolyposis colorectal cancer (Lynch syndrome) and microsatellite instability. J Natl Cancer Inst 96(4):261–268
96. Eccles DM (2004) Hereditary cancer: guidelines in clinical practice. Breast and ovarian cancer genetics Ann Oncol 15(Suppl 4): iv133-iv138

Chapter 9
Multifocal and Multicentric Tumors

Carlo de Werra, Ivana Donzelli, Mario Perone, Rosa Di Micco, Gianclaudio Orabona

Multifocality

Multifocal tumors are not multiple tumors; they originate from a unique cellular clone and grow multifocally in a single organ (liver, kidney, thyroid, etc.). These tumors are not included as multiple primary malignancies (MPM), but they can represent a single event of this syndrome. Multicentric tumors are also different because they develop simultaneously in more than one organ (e.g, breast, mono- or bilaterally in the kidney), but without a clonal relationship with respect to their carcinogenesis. The differential diagnosis is often very difficult. Examples of multifocality are mammary carcinoma, renal cell carcinoma, hepatocellular carcinoma, and esophageal adenocarcinoma.

The mechanism by which such multifocal cancers are generated and their relation to the stage and metastatic potential of the cancer are not fully understood; yet, this knowledge is important for decisions regarding treatment and surgery. Multifocal cancers can be generated through the dynamic interplay between tumor-promoting and tumor-inhibiting factors. Mathematical modeling indicates that somatic evolution away from tumor inhibition and towards tumor promotion results in the transition from a small contained tumor to multi-focal tumors, and finally to a large tumor mass within a tissue. Several studies have identified tumor-promoting and tumor-inhibiting factors, produced either by the tumor cells themselves or by the cells of the surrounding tissue. An obvious example is angiogenesis inhibition and promotion, in which simple mutations can change the balance away from inhibition and to favor promotion. Other inhibiting factors that are not related to angiogenesis have also been described, although their exact identity and function remain unknown. In this context, observations of the pattern of cancer growth have shown that at early stages of cancer progression the balance between inhibitors and promoters favors inhibition, until an initiating population of transformed cells produces more promoters or reduces the production of inhibitors; in the same way, other mutants are produced at a relatively high frequency.

At this point in the process there are three possibilities by which multifocal cancer can progress:

1. Tumor inhibition is strong or slightly shifted in favor of promotion, with growth initially producing a unifocal and self-contained lesion
2. The first mutation strongly shifts the balance towards promotion, which is sufficient to result in the generation of multiple focal lesions
3. Tumor inhibition is weaker upon initiation, such that cancer growth occurs as a single lesion rather than as several lesions, until the entire tissue is invaded

According to this model, multifocal cancer represents an intermediate stage in cancer progression, as the tumor evolves away from inhibition and towards promotion. Several lesions do not occur; instead, the tumor first grows as a single and self-limited lesion. Then, if the degree of promotion is large enough relative to the degree of inhibition, this lesion bifurcates to give rise to two or more lesions. In both cases 1 and 2, many lesions can appear, but in the first case in addition to the mutation, which slightly shifts the balance towards tumor formation, further mutations in an oncogene or a tumor suppressor gene are required so that the mutant can grow to sufficiently high numbers. In the second case, no further mutations are required because multiple foci arise from the splitting and migration of a single lesion. The higher the number of foci, the further advanced the stage of cancer progression; so that the concept of multifocality becomes linked to the process of metastasis.

Several studies that investigated the metastatic potential of multifocal compared to unifocal cancers, were able to show that multifocality correlates with an increased chance that metastatic cells will grow rather than remain dormant. This is also due to the reduced inhibition, which allows tumors to grow; this is why the therapeutic use of inhibitors should be further explored [1].

Molecular and Immunological Basis of Cancer

Genetic mutations are the molecular basis of cancer and they are largely responsible for the generation of malignant cells. Both in multiple and single lesions, these mutations alter the quantity or function of protein products that regulate cell growth and division and DNA repair. In other words, the molecular basis of multifocality is the same as that of cancerogenesis in general (see Chapter 2); nevertheless, that balance between promoters and inhibitors is important at molecular level too, so that mutations that favor a more invasive phenotype increase the probability of multifocality.

In multifocal advanced cancer, the invasive phenotype is associated with dynamic changes in several marker of the cellular and local tumoral microenvironment. Studies of ErbB receptors have proved that overexpression of ErbB heterodimers is associated with the most aggressively growing tumors. ErbB receptors (ErbB-1/epidermal growth factor receptor, ErbB-2, ErbB-3, and ErbB-4) were stably overexpressed in a polyclonal cell population either alone or as paired combinations in murine and human breast cell models. The broad diversity of ErbB-regulated cancer-associated genes and the several novel targets they revealed may have therapeutic applications for targeting tumor progression involving aberrations of ErbB receptors [2].

Another finding of potential therapeutic interest is the hypermethylation of the tumor-related genes in gastric carcinoma [3].

The immune system is linked to the development of cancer because its dysfunction, as a result of genetic mutation, acquired disease, aging, or immunosuppressants, interferes with normal immune surveillance of early tumors. Known cancer-associated immune disorders include ataxia-telangiectasia (acute lymphocytic leukemia, brain tumors, gastric cancer); Wiskott-Aldrich syndrome (lymphoma, acute lymphocytic leukemia); X-linked agammaglobulinemia (lymphoma and acute lymphocytic leukemia); immune deficiency secondary to immunosuppressants or HIV infection (large-cell lymphoma, Kaposi's sarcoma); rheumatologic conditions, such as systemic lupus erythematosus, rheumatoid arthritis, and Sjögren's syndrome (B-type lymphoma); and general immune disorders (lymphoreticular neoplasia). According to the theory of immune surveillance, the immune system continually recognizes and eliminates tumor cells; when a tumor escapes immune surveillance and grows too large for the immune system to kill, cancer is the result. Multifocality is commonly linked to the lack of tumor rejection by an intact immune systems; it is not always due to the absence of recognizable antigens or to the absence of T cells able to recognize those antigens. In fact, tumor-specific lymphocytes can be found in the blood, draining lymph nodes, and the tumor itself of patients with actively growing tumors. These lymphocytes can kill tumor cells in vitro but fail to do so in vivo. Progress in our knowledge about tumor-specific antigens (TSA, also called tumor-specific transplantation antigens, TSTA, or tumor rejection antigens, TRA), tumor-associated antigens (TAA), immunotherapies, and vaccines represents will provide novel strategies in the treatment of single and multiple tumors [4].

Liver

Hepatocarcinoma (HCC) is a highly malignant tumor that is generally associated with a poor prognosis. This disease is highly prevalent in Asia but relatively rare in developed countries, although the incidence is increasing in both the United States and Japan. Recent studies in molecular biology have shown that some HCCs are multicentric. Clinically, it is important to determine whether multiple tumors in the liver are multicentric or represent metastases from a main tumor since the results of treatment for single (unicentric), multicentric, and intrahepatic metastatic HCCs differ (Fig. 9.1).

In one variant of multicentric hepatocellular carcinoma, at least one tumor is a well-differentiated HCC, whereas in a separate region the tumor(s) are moderately or poorly differentiated HCC. In another variant, there is a well-differentiated HCC with less differentiated tumors at other hepatic sites. Studies on the outcome of patients with these tumor variants showed that the cumulative survival rate was significantly higher in patients with multicentric HCC than in

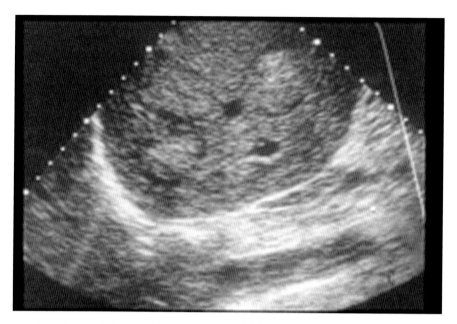

Fig. 9.1 Multifocal hepatocellular carcinoma (HCC) of the right lobe of the liver. Two hyperechoic lesions with hypoechoic halos are seen

those with multifocal HCC (associated with intrahepatic metastases). Thus, according to Cox's proportional hazard model, multicentricity is not a relevant factor influencing outcome. The risk of multicentric occurrence increases with the progression of chronic liver disease. Univariate analysis showed that there are several risk factors for multicentricity: age, male sex, alcohol abuse, history of blood transfusion, liver cirrhosis, and hepatitis. The odds ratios for the factors hepatitis virus infection, male sex, history of blood transfusion, and liver cirrhosis were all more than 2.0. Also, hepatic AST and ALT activities were significantly higher in patients with multicentric HCC than in patients with a single HCC, and the risk of multicentric carcinogenesis increased as ICGR15 (indocyanine green retention rate at 15 min), AST, ALT, and total bilirubin increased and the platelet count and albumin level decreased (Table 9.1). These results indicate that the potential of multicentric carcinogenesis increases with the progression of chronic liver disease and that chronic hepatitis is responsible for this form of carcinogenesis. The prevalence of hepatitis C virus (HCV) was significantly higher in patients with multicentric HCCs than in patients with single HCC or in patients with intrahepatic metastasis; thus, HCV seems to be a stronger risk factor than HBV in multicentric HCCs. This may explain the higher incidence of HCC development in patients with HCV (about 7% per year in Japan) than in patients with HBV, despite suggestions of an interaction between HCV and HBV in multicentric carcinogenesis. Some investigators have found that co-infection with HCV and HBV has a synergistic effect on HCC development (Table 9.1).

9 Multifocal and Multicentric Tumors

Table 9.1 Correlation between viral infection and incidence of multicentric liver tumors

HCV	HBsAg	HBcAg	N	Patients with multicentric tumors (%)
+	-	-	65	7 (11)
+	-	+	108	28 (26)
+	+	+	10	0 (0)
-	-	-	15	1 (7)
-	-	+	15	0 (0)
-	+	+	38	1 (3)

N, Number of patients; *HCV*, hepatitis C virus; *HbsAg*, hepatitis B surface antigen; *HbcAg*, hepatitis B core antigen

Recent analysis of HBV DNA sequences showed that the HBx gene is sometimes detected in HCC and in noncancerous tissues of patients without HBsAg. HBV DNA is integrated into the cellular genome. This leads to rearrangements of the cellular DNA, insertional mutagenesis, production of truncated HBV proteins such as preS2/S and X proteins, activation of cellular proto-oncogenes, and inhibition of p53, which together may lead to carcinogenesis. In one possible mechanism, genetic changes or carcinogenesis caused by the integration of HBV could become more deleterious in the presence of continuous hepatitis caused by HCV. The likelihood of multicentric carcinogenesis is low in patients with HBsAg because HCC often develops before cirrhosis. In this light, the clinicopathological criteria for multicentric HCC are of practical value in the selection of treatment in that the viral state of the patient must be taken into consideration. The different risk factors have relevance regarding the development of multicentric HCCs, even after resection of HCC [5].

Although other therapeutic approaches to HCC have been introduced, surgery remains the treatment of choice. The progression and outcome of truly relapsed HCC compared with a second primary tumor are distinct, and clonal analysis of the initial and recurrent HCC therefore of clinical significance. Recently, one group reported frequent mtDNA mutations in HCC and in the noncancerous tissue of these patients. The high frequency of mutations within the control region of mtDNA allowed determination of the clonal origin of multiple HCCs in individual patients. Accordingly, if the first tumor but not the second tumor has a mutation, they should be considered independent lesions.

Although there are some discrepancies between mtDNA mutation status and clinical diagnosis, these mutations can help establish the clonal relationship of the tumors and thus the selection of an appropriate treatment strategy for new primary tumors or recurrent cancers. This molecular approach requires minimal DNA from each tumor and can be used to analyze routine needle biopsies. Finally, the high frequency of control region mtDNA mutations in HCC provides significant information in determining the clonality of multiple HCCs. Indeed, these mutations may serve as sensitive markers to distinguish metastatic disease from the occurrence of multiple independent primary tumors [6].

Despite enormous research efforts, relatively little is known about the entire mechanism of human hepatocarcinogenesis. During the multistep carcinogenesis of human cancers, numerous genetic abnormalities accumulate, including the activation of oncogenes and genes related to cell growth and the inactivation of tumor suppressor genes. In HCC cells, the CD24 gene is often overexpressed. This glycoprotein antigen is composed of a short peptide core of only 31–35 amino acids and a very high carbohydrate content. The antigen is present on the cell membrane of immature B cells and modulates the cellular response to signal activation. CD24 mRNA was found to be overexpressed in 66% of unicentric HCCs and in 68% of tumor nodules from patients with multicentric HCC. Analysis of the expression of CD24 mRNA in combination with AFP mRNA expression, p53 gene mutation, and hepatitis B virus DNA integration pattern may allow determination of the clonal origin of multicentric HCC [7].

Intraoperative ultrasound (IOUS) is of diagnostic benefit in multifocal tumors because apart from highlighting the tumor itself, it can reveal the presence of new nodules. It also allows evaluation of the exact anatomy of the liver and the relationships of the lesion with vasculobiliary structures, detects neoplastic portal thrombi, and identifies the limits of the injury, ensuring proper resection (Fig. 9.2).

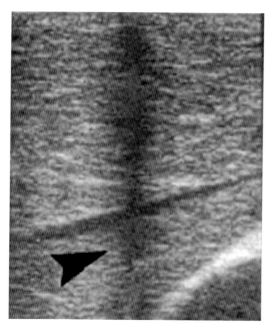

Fig. 9.2 Intraoperative ultrasound of small multifocal HCC detected in the VII hepatic segment, behind the right hepatic vein

Breast

Multicentricity refers to the presence of separate independent foci of carcinoma within the breast separate from the lesion which is clinically or mammographically evident. The separate foci reflect the de novo development of malignant epithelium and must be distinguished from multifocal carcinomas, which can result from intraductal spread from a single, primary carcinoma. Surgically defined, lesions are considered multicentric if they are situated in different quadrants of the breast or more than 5 cm apart or in the other breast, and multifocal if situated in the same quadrant as the primary lesion or less than 5 cm apart. One hypothesis to explain this pattern of tumor growth and extension is that both multicentric and multifocal breast cancers result from intraductal spread, in which case the lesions should be genetically similar. An alternative explanation is the developmental hypothesis: genetic hits to epithelial stem cells during breast development are transmitted to daughter cells during growth, such that further genetic hits will predispose some areas of the breast to malignant transformation [8]. According to the a literature review, the prevalence of multicentricity and multifocality in the breast varies from 9 to 75%; this variability is due to several important factors, including the difficulty of correctly defining these tumors following anatomic and pathologic evaluation of biopsy samples; differences in patient selection, especially patient age, among the various studies; and the definition of clinical vs. subclinical lesions.

The factors associated with an increased risk of multicentricity are a lesion located in the nipple or aureole and the presence of ductal or lobular carcinoma in situ. The relationship between tumor dimension and multicentricity is controversial, but dimension does not represent a risk factor, neither does patient age. Instead, the tumor istotype is the most important variant in multicentricity, in that in situ lesions are more frequently multicentric. Ductal carcinoma in situ (DCIS) tends to evolve towards multicentricity and can affect large areas of the breast. Similarly, invasive carcinomas have large numbers of DCIS lesions. Lobular carcinoma in situ (LCIS) is also characterized by multicentricity; its distribution is nonrandom and mostly involves radial mammary sectors, often skipping contiguous radii; this suggests that LCIS is distributed along ductal systems. According to Rosen [9], the risk of multicentricity of DCIS varies from 35 to 48%, whereas Silverstein [10] recently concluded that DCIS is predominately monocentric rather than multicentric. It is therefore clear that multicentricity and multifocality should be evaluated whenever the decision is made to conservatively treat operable breast tumors. In this context it is fundamental to follow the indications obtained by imaging modes such as echography, mammography, and magnetic resonance imaging (MRI) (Fig. 9.3).

The true importance of identifying mammographically occult multicentric or multifocal tumor preoperatively is not well established in terms of either survival or a decreased rate of local recurrence. The best way to diagnose a multicentric breast cancer seems to be MRI (Figs. 9.4, 9.5) [11].

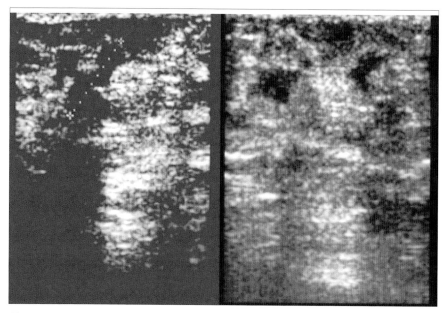

Fig. 9.3 Echography of multicentric breast cancer

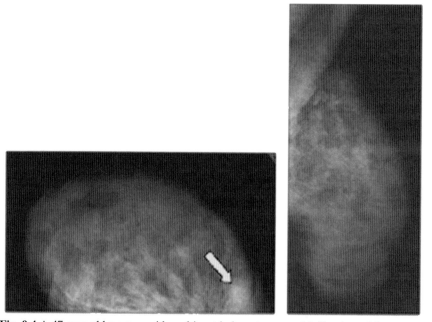

Fig. 9.4 A 47-year-old woman with multicentric breast cancer. (**a**) Craniocaudal mammogram shows round hyperdense opacity (arrow) at external quadrants; (**b**) mediolateral oblique mammogram does not clearly detect the tumor

9 Multifocal and Multicentric Tumors

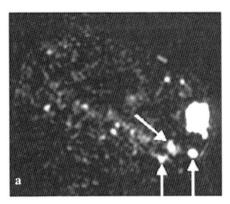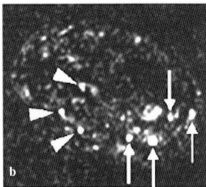

Fig. 9.5 A 47-year-old woman with multicentric breast cancer. **a** Contrast-enhanced subtracted coronal magnetic resonance (MR) image (first dynamic phase) shows the major tumor as a large round area of contrast uptake with irregular borders at external quadrants as well as three small satellites (*arrows*) indicative of multifocal cancer. **b** Subtracted coronal image (first dynamic phase), obtained in a plane anterior to that shown in (**a**) confirms multifocality at external quadrants (arrows); however, three other small foci (arrowheads) of contrast uptake are detected at internal quadrants, and thus evidence of multicentric cancer

The results of several studies have shown an increased risk of local recurrence of 25–40% when the initial disease is multifocal or multicentric, compared with an 11% recurrence rate when the initial tumor is unifocal [12]. According to many studies, patients with multifocal tumors have a higher rate of positive axillary nodes than those with unifocal tumors, so that multifocality represents a significant predictor of node positivity when the largest tumor focus is classified (Table 9.2) [13].

Thyroid

Papillary thyroid carcinoma is the most common cancer of the thyroid gland, with approximately 20,000 cases annually in the United States. Its pathogenesis involves mutations in the RET, NTRK1, RAS, and BRAF genes. The first sign of a papillary cancer is often the occurrence of a thyroid nodule that does not take up radioactive iodine or an enlarged lymph node containing a metastasis. In patients undergoing surgical treatment for papillary thyroid cancer, pathological analysis commonly identifies multiple noncontiguous tumor foci in individual

Table 9.2 clinical and histological characteristics of patients with multifocal breast cancer

Characteristics	Multifocal tumors N	%	Unifocal tumors N	%
All women	94	11.1	754	88.9
Age				
<50	33	35.1	231	30.6
≥50	61	64.9	523	69.4
Histology				
Ductal	70	74.5	614	81.4
Lobular	15	16	73	9.7
Mixed ductal/lobular	4	4.3	15	2
Tubular	4	4.3	17	2.3
Other	1	1.1	35	4.6
Tumor grade				
I	18	19.1	155	20.6
II	36	38.3	284	37.7
III	27	28.7	242	32.1
Hormone receptor				
ER+	24	63.2	159	76.1
Node positivity	49	52.1	283	37.5

N, Number of patients

glands. Estimates of the frequency of such tumors vary between 18 and 87%, depending on the techniques used. The pathologic picture of this kind of cancer is typically a primary tumor >1 cm in diameter; with most of the additional foci measuring <1 cm in diameter (microcarcinomas). Multifocal tumors have been associated with increased risks of lymph-node and distant metastases, persistent local disease after initial treatment, and regional recurrence. All these features suggest that patients with multifocal papillary thyroid cancer should receive aggressive treatment. The phenomenon of X-chromosome inactivation, in which either the maternal or paternal X chromosome in women is inactivated, makes it possible to determine whether a tumor arose from one or multiple progenitor cells because the inactivated X chromosome is stably transmitted from parent cell to progeny cell. For this reason, all the cells in a clonal population have the same inactivated X chromosome, maternal or paternal. Studies of X-chromosome inactivation patterns have advantages over methods that compare specific changes in DNA or gene expression in papillary carcinoma, because such changes could arise as late events in separate subclones of the original tumor and lead to the mistaken interpretation that clonally related tumor foci are unrelated

(Fig. 9.6). The discovery of small foci that are histologically identical to a larger cancer nodule in the same gland suggests that the smaller tumors are metastases of the larger tumor. This interpretation is also favored by the anatomy of the thyroid, since this gland has a unique lymphatic drainage system, with the two lobes and the isthmus enclosed in a capsule containing an abundant network of intralobular lymphatic vessels.

The finding that multifocal tumors in papillary thyroid cancer are of independent origins has implications for pathogenesis. Since neoplastic transformation is usually a rare event, it is unlikely that many cells within the same gland would undergo transformation independently without some predisposing influence, such as an environmental insult, a mutation, or polymorphisms. Exposure to radiation is one well-known predisposing factor, but the frequent presence of multifocal papillary thyroid cancer in patients who have not been exposed to radiation suggests other influences. Recent studies have shown that any thyroid tissue remaining after surgical removal of a papillary thyroid cancer in patients with multifocal disease may contain – or is likely to develop – additional foci of cancer that could become recurrences. Thus, establishing that foci of papillary cancer have independent origins provides theoretical support for the appropriateness of total thyroidectomy and radioablation of remaining tissue [14]. Multicentric tumors can also involve the thyroid gland in the context of familial

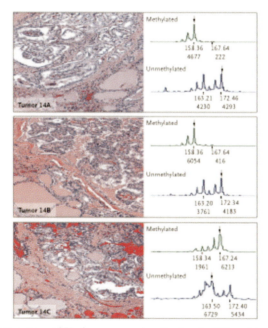

Fig. 9.6 Discordant pattern of X-chromosome inactivation in different tumor foci. The tissue was obtainde from a patient with multifocal papillary thyroid tumor, as revealed by methylation-specific PCR

papillary carcinoma, in which the probability of multiple lesions is higher. The characteristics of familial thyroid carcinoma are: (a) predominantly papillary type, (b) early age of cancer onset (mean age about 35 years), and (c) smaller tumor size and higher frequency of multicentricity. This disease is often characterized by mutations in the proto-oncogenes encoding RET, its tyrosine kinase receptors (TKRs and NTRK1), thus establishing that the familial occurrence has a genetic basis. Of interest is the fact that in these cases the alterations are germline mutations, predisposing a higher number of cells to develop tumors and explaining why multiple tumors are more commonly found [15]. RET seems to play a very important role in carcinogenesis in the thyroid and its expression correlates strongly with the likelihood of developing multiple lesions. Furthermore, albeit less commonly, multifocality may occur in medullary thyroid carcinoma (MTC). For example, MTC in the context of MEN2A is associated with multifocal RET mutations and C-cell hyperplasia [16].

Bladder

A strong association between the nuclear accumulation of p53 protein (due to mutations in the p53 gene) and tumor progression in transitional-cell carcinoma of the bladder has been recognized since the early 1990s. This accumulation predicts a significantly increased risk of recurrence and death, independent of tumor grade, stage, and lymph node status [17]. Bladder cancer is often characterized by a multifocal growth pattern; about one-third of all bladder cancers occur as several simultaneous tumors appearing at different sites of the bladder wall. This phenomenon gave rise to the "field cancerization" hypothesis, according to which individual cells of the bladder urothelium are primed to undergo transformation because of environmental mutagens, thereby leading to the development of independent multiclonal tumors. This theory is mainly based on morphological and immunohistochemical mapping studies that demonstrated areas of modified cells adjacent to the sites of the tumors. In contrast, genetic studies have suggested a monoclonal origin of the tumors because: (a) all tumors of a single patient with multifocal disease revealed the same X chromosome inactivation pattern; (b) mostly the same patterns of loss of heterozygosity as well as identical tp53 mutations were detected. Most investigators have therefore concluded that intraluminal seeding or the intraepithelial migration of cells originating from a single primary tumor is responsible for multifocal tumor occurrence. Bladder cancer is characterized by highly complex chromosomal changes in cells surrounding the tumors as well as at distant sites. In comparative genomic hybridization studies of multifocal bladder cancer, the average number of aberrations per tumor (20.4) was remarkably higher than that reported for pT2–4 (7.9 aberrations) or grade 3 carcinomas (7.8 aberrations), suggesting an exceptionally high degree of genomic instability in multifocal bladder cancer. One or more currently unknown genes located on chromosome 17p may exert an influence on multifocality by inhibiting cell migration capabilities in healthy urothelium. A similar effect may be induced by gains involving chromosome 20p. This latter finding was surprising as this alteration is described only rarely (9%) in monofocal bladder cancer. Interestingly, cytogenetically closely related tumors revealed a close spatial relationship, thus raising questions regarding the mechanism of tumor cell spread leading to multifocal bladder cancer. Immunohistochemistry studies aimed at the detection of cells accumulating the tp53 protein in tumors and normal urothelium located between the tumors have been carried out to address this issue. Based on the cytogenetic and immunohistochemical data, it can be speculated that the ability of a neoplastic cell population to become multifocal depends on the order in which particular genetic defects are acquired. In monofocal cancer, there may be a growth advantage such that tumor formation is the initial step, followed by genetic instability, invasion capability by lysis of the lamina propria, migration into the muscularis mucosae and blood vessels attributable to loss of cell adhesion, and, finally, metastatic settlement. In contrast, genetic instability and loss of cell adhesion may be the initial events in multifocal tumors, leading to the migration of neoplastic cells through wide areas of the urothelium. This process may be driven by specific genetic changes, including the loss of 17p which in turn might inactivate genes that would otherwise prevent the lateral spread of cells throughout the urothelium or maintain genetic stability. The close spatial relationship of tumors revealing identical genetic features, tp53 mutations, and patterns of chromosomal aberrations, as well as the detection of tumor cells within continuous areas of the urothelium, reflect the migration of tumor cells of clonal origin throughout the bladder epithelium [18].

Kidney

Multifocality is a common feature of papillary renal-cell carcinomas that are not sporadic but occur in familial syndromes. In contrast to sporadic renal-cell carcinoma, fewer steps are required for the development of inherited forms of the disease, because all of the patient's cells have a predisposing mutation. As a result, carcinomas associated with the familial syndromes occur earlier and are often multifocal. These familial renal-cancer syndromes are autosomal dominant and the tumors often have defined histologic features. Most commonly, they are papillary lesions covered by small cells with pale cytoplasm and small oval nuclei with indistinct nucleoli. The mutation causing hereditary papillary renal carcinoma occurs in a gene located on chromosome 7 and encoding MET, a receptor tyrosine kinase that is normally activated by hepatocyte growth factor. Patients with hereditary renal-cell carcinoma should be closely monitored. Computed tomography (CT) before and after the administration of contrast material is the best method to detect and assess renal masses, with gadolinium-enhanced MRI as an alternative. The studies can be performed at intervals ranging from every 3–6 months to every 2–3 years, depending on the size of the lesions and the type of syndrome, with larger masses requiring more frequent evaluation. Because small masses are usually of low grade, they can be observed until they reach 3 cm, at which point they should be removed. These lesions are ideal candidates for minimally invasive percutaneous ablative therapy, especially in patients with multifocal tumors [19].

References

1. Wodarz D, Iwasa Y, Komarova NL (2004) On the emergency of multifocal cancers. J Carcinogen 3:13
2. Alaoui-Jamali MA, Song DJ, Benlimame N (2003) Regulation of multiple tumor microenvironment markers by overexpression of single or paired combinations of ErbB receptors. Cancer Res 63:3764–3774
3. Leung WK, yu J, Ng EKW et al (2001) Concurrent hypermetilation of multiple tumor – related genes in gastric carcinoma and adjacent normal tissue. Am Cancer Soc 91:2294–2301
4. Janeway CA (2003) Immunobiology. Piccin, Padua
5. Kubo S, Nishiguchi S, Hirohashi K et al (1998) Clinicopathological criteria for multicentricity of hepatocellular carcinoma and risk factors for such carcinogenesis. Jpn J Cancer Res 89:419–426
6. Nomoto S, Yamashita K, Koshikawa K et al (2002) Mithocondrial D-loop mutations as clonal markers in multicentric hepatocellular carcinoma and plasma. Clin Cancer Res 8:481–487
7. Huang L, Hsu H (1995) Cloning and expression of CD24 gene in human hepatocellular carcinoma: a potential early tumor marker gene correlates with p53 mutation and tumor differentiation. Cancer Res 55:4717–4721
8. Sharpe CR (1998) A developmental hypothesis to explain the multicentricity of breast cancer. Can Med Ass J 158:55–59
9. Rosen P.P, Senie R, Schottenfeld D (1979) Non invasive breast carcinoma: frequency of unsuspected invasion and implication for treatement. Ann Surg 189:377
10. Silverstein MJ (ed) (2000) Ductal carcinoma in situ of the breast. Lippincott Williams & Wilkins, Philadelphia, pp 287–300
11. Berg WA, Gilbreath PL (2000) Multicentric and multifocal cancer: whole-breast US in preoperative evaluation. Radiology 214:59–66
12. Sardanelli F, Giuseppetti GM, Panizza P et al (2004) Sensitivity of MRI versus mammography for detecting foci of multifocal, multicentric breast cancer in fatty and dense breasts using the whole-breast pathologic examination as a gold standard. AJR Am J Roentgenol 183:1149–1157
13. Coombs NJ, Boyages J (2005) Multifocal and multicentric breast cancer: does each focus matter? J Clin Oncol 23:7497–7502
14. Shattuck TM, Westra WH, Ladenson PW (2005) Independent clonal origins of distinct tumor foci in multifocal papillary thyroid carcinoma. N Engl J Med 352:2406–2412
15. Mihajlović-Boćić V, Tatiać S, Paunović I (2001) Familial papillary thyroid carcinoma. Arch Oncol 8(3):135–136
16. Diaz-Cano S.J, de Miguel M, Blanes A et al (2001) Germline RET 634 mutation positive MEN 2A-related C-cell hyperplasias have genetic features consistent with intraepithelial neoplasia. J Clin Endocrinol Metab 86:3948–3957
17. Esrig D, Elmajian D, Groshen S et al (1994) Accumulation of nuclear p53 and tumor progression in bladder cancer. N Engl J Med 331:1259–1264
18. Simon R, Eltze E, Schäfer KL et al (2001) Cytogenetic analysis of multifocal bladder cancer supports a monoclonal origin and intraepithelial spread of tumor cells. Cancer Res 61:355–362
19. Cohen HT, McGovern FJ (2005) Renal-cell carcinoma. N Engl J Med 353:2477–2490

Chapter 10
The Cancer Spectrum Related to Hereditary and Familial Breast and Ovarian Cancers

Matilde Pensabene, Rosaria Gesuita, Ida Capuano, Caterina Condello,
Ilaria Spagnoletti, Eleonora De Maio, Flavia Carle, Stefano Pepe,
Alma Contegiacomo

Hereditary Breast Cancer

Multiple factors are associated with an increased risk of developing breast cancer, including age, family history, exposure to reproductive hormones, dietary factors, benign breast diseases, and environmental factors. Recently, increasing interest has been devoted to the interaction between environmental and genetic factors. Family history has been recognized as an important risk factor for developing breast cancer. Individuals with a first-degree family member affected with breast cancer have a relative risk of 2.1 (95% CI = 2.0–2.2). Moreover, risk varies with the age at which the affected relative was diagnosed, the number of affected and unaffected family members and, finally, the closeness of the relationship [1].

In the mid-1990s, developments in the molecular genetics of cancer led to the identification of predisposing hereditary breast and/or ovarian cancer genes. Studies of linkage analysis showed that there is an autosomal dominant predisposition to breast cancer and led to the identification of several highly penetrant genes; these included BRCA1 and BRCA2, which cause inherited cancer in many breast-cancer-prone families.

Overall, 5–10% of primary breast cancers are inherited and 15–20% are familial [1, 2]. Hereditary and familial forms are identified by the individual and the family history. In familial forms, members of some families are prone to developing breast cancer in the absence of identifiable carcinogenic exposure. Affected individuals in these families may represent clustering of sporadic occurrences, multifactorial inheritance, the presence of low-penetrance genes, or common habits and similar life style. Close relatives are at moderately increased risk of developing that type of malignancy. However, the average age of onset is usual similar to that observed in the general population.

The family features that suggest a hereditary predisposition to breast cancer include: (a) multiple cases of breast and ovarian cancer in different generations of a family, suggesting an autosomal dominant transmission (vertical transmission) according to the Lynch criteria; (b) an early age of onset; (c) multiple primary cancers in the same individual (i.e., bilateral breast cancer or breast and ovarian cancer); (d) male breast cancer. The presence of both breast and ovarian cancer in a family increases the likelihood of a cancer-predisposing mutation.

About 84% of hereditary breast cancers derive from BRCA1 and BRCA2 mutations that are characteristic of the hereditary breast/ovarian cancer (HBOC) syndrome, in which there is an autosomal dominant pattern of transmission, incomplete penetrance, and variable expressivity [2]. To date, for each of the BRCA genes approximately 3,400 sequence variants have been identified. Some specific mutations have been observed in defined ethnic groups, suggesting a founder effect. The most common in the United States are the three mutations commonly found in the BRCA1 (185delAG and 5382insC) and BRCA2 (6174delT) genes in Ashkenazi Jews. Founder mutations in other populations, including those from Iceland, Poland, and in Dutch kindreds also have been identified. Founder mutations have been described as well in geographically restricted areas of Italy [3–5].

Other known susceptibility genes, such as ATM, PTEN, p53, and STK11, are involved in hereditary breast cancer syndromes with a well-defined cancer spectrum. Unknown low-penetrance genes also seem to be involved in other, less frequent hereditary breast cancers [2]. Mutations in each of these genes produce different clinical phenotypes of specific cancers and, in some instance, other non-malignant abnormalities associated with different hereditary syndromes known to involve the breast as a tumor site within the cancer spectrum. These syndromes include Li-Fraumeni syndrome, Cowden's syndrome, ataxia-telangiectasia, and Peutz-Jeghers syndrome [6, 7].

BRCA1- and BRCA2-Associated Breast and Ovarian Cancers

Recently, Chen and Parmigiani reported a meta-analysis of BRCA1 and BRCA2 penetrance. The mean cumulative risk at age 70 years was 57% (95% CI, 47–66%) for breast cancer and 40% (95% CI, 35–46%) for ovarian cancer in BRCA1 mutation carriers. In carriers of BRCA2 mutations, the mean cumulative risk at age 70 years was 49% (95% CI, 40–57%) for breast cancer and 18% (95% CI, 13–23%) for ovarian cancer [8].

Mutations in BRCA1 and BRCA2 particularly increase the risk of early-onset breast carcinoma. Whereas a woman's likelihood of developing breast cancer before age 50 is normally only 2%, the risk is 33–50% for a woman with a mutation in one of the two genes. In women with breast cancer, mutations in BRCA1 have been associated with a 64% cumulative risk of contralateral breast cancer by age 70.

The variation in cancer risk among the studies involving families assessed for breast cancer clustering suggests allelic heterogeneity. Moreover, the variation in risk within families and over time suggests a role for genetic and epigenetic modifying factors. Nongenetic factors, such as menstrual and reproductive histories, contraceptive and hormone use, exercise and body weight, and environmental and occupational exposure, might explain some portion of the variation in breast cancer incidence, as these factors significantly influence the penetrance even of high-penetrance mutations [9].

BRCA1-associated breast cancers are usually high-grade, poorly differentiated, and infiltrating ductal carcinomas. Atypical medullary carcinomas, a phenotype characterized by abundant lymphocytic infiltrate and a smooth margin, also occur more frequently in patients with BRCA1 mutations. These tumors frequently show a basal-cell-like phenotype, characterized by estrogen receptor (ER), progesterone receptor (PgR), and HER2/neu negativity and the expression of basal-cell cytokeratins 5, 6, and 14 [10, 11]. BRCA2-associated breast cancers do not have a phenotype or behavior distinct from that of sporadic breast cancers [7, 10].

BRCA1 ovarian cancers usually are serous and papillary; less frequently, they are endometrioid or of the clear cell variety. Borderline tumors of the ovary also have been associated with hereditary breast and/or ovarian cancer syndrome.

Several studies found that there were no significant differences among BRCA1- and BRCA2-associated and sporadic breast cancer with respect to outcome [12, 13].

Cancer Related to BRCA1 and BRCA2 Mutations Other Than Breast and Ovarian Cancer

Data concerning the risk of cancer at sites other than breast and ovary in carriers of mutations in BRCA1 and BRCA2 genes are contradictory. The Cancer Genetics Studies Consortium reported an increased life-time cumulative risk for ovarian cancer (44%), colorectal cancer (6%), and prostate cancer (8%) in BRCA1 mutation carriers [14]. In a second study, conducted in families ascertained for BRCA1 mutations, the Breast Cancer Linkage Consortium reported an increased relative risk for several cancers, including pancreatic cancer (RR = 2.26; 95% CI = 1.26–4.06), cancer of the uterine body (RR=2.65, 95% IC 1.69–4.16) and cervix (RR=3.72, 95% IC 2.26–6.10), and prostate cancer in men under 65 years of age (RR=1.82; 95% IC 1.01–3.29) [15].

The Breast Cancer Linkage Consortium also observed increased risks for several other cancers in carriers of BRCA2 mutations. In particular, statistically significant increases in risks were reported for prostate cancer (RR= 4.65; 95% CI= 3.48–6.22), pancreatic cancer (RR= 3.51; 95% CI= 1.87–6.58), gallbladder and bile-duct cancer (RR= 4.97; 95% CI= 1.50–16.52), stomach cancer (RR =2.59; 95% CI=1.46–4.61), and melanoma (RR= 2.58; 95% CI =1.28–5.17). The relative risk for prostate cancer for men below the age of 65 years was 7.33 (95% CI = 4.66–11.52) (Table 10.1) [16].

Bermejo and Hemminki confirmed the association of BRCA1 and BRCA2 mutations with ovarian, pancreatic, prostate, and stomach cancers at a population level. In families with a history of bilateral breast cancer or two cases of breast cancer in family members age 50 years, there is concern about early-onset

Table 10.1 Risk for cancer at sites other than the breast in carriers of BRCA1 and BRCA2 mutations

	Cumulative risk (%) BRCA 1	Relative risk BRCA1	BRCA2
Colorectal	6	–	–
Pancreas	–	–	–
Ductal biliary tract	–	2.26	–
Stomach	–	–	4.97
Uterine body	–	–	2.59
Cervix	–	2.65	–
Ovary	44	3.72	–
Prostate	8	–	4.65
Melanoma	–	1.82	2.58

pancreatic cancers. Prostate cancers are also in excess in these families but the risk is only moderate. Most cases of ovarian cancer in families with male breast cancer, and in families with at least two cases of breast cancer diagnosed before age 50 years are probably attributable to BRCA1/2 mutations [17].

The relationship between BRCA1 mutations and the development of colon cancer remains puzzling. Recently, Garber reported that the risk of colon cancer in BRCA1 mutation carriers is, on the basis of studies published, not a matter of concern. An increased risk of colorectal cancer in BRCA1 carriers may yet be demonstrated, but it seem increasingly likely that it will be a small increase, if that, or limited to a particular subset of carriers. Intensified targeted colorectal cancer screening and prevention should be directed only to the subset of BRCA1 mutation carriers who have remarkable medical histories either personally or with respect to familial colorectal cancer or other risk factors. Moreover, effects of modifying factors, such as diet and exposure to other environmental factors, should be considered. Epigenetic modifications of DNA were recently reported to be responsible for reversible and clonally heritable alterations in transcription state, producing a phenotype equivalent to that resulting from an inactivating germline mutation [18, 19].

The various studies published in this field did not report childhood cancers in families with hereditary breast cancer. In the most of those studies, the onset is earlier for hereditary breast, prostate and pancreatic cancer than for sporadic cancers.

Cancer Genetic Counseling

Scientific developments in the field of the genetics of cancer have led to new scenarios in the setting of prevention, diagnosis, and management of hereditary and familial cancers. Given the necessity to identify and adequately manage the genetic and familial risk in oncology, ad hoc clinical services have been implemented in many countries. Their aim is to offer cancer genetic counseling to support individuals in any decision-making process concerning their own risk.

As the public's awareness of cancer susceptibility genes has grown markedly in recent years, the demand for genetic services to assess familial cancer risk and for genetic testing have increased accordingly. Almost all centers provide genetic testing services not only to cancer patients and their families but also to individuals concerned with risk. Most genetic counseling services in Europe and the USA also include medical evaluation, cancer risk assessment, genetic counseling and pedigree analysis [20].

In 1975 genetic counseling was defined by the American Society of Human Genetics as "a communication process which deals with human problems associated with the occurrence or risk of occurrence of a genetic disorder in a family." Genetic counseling in the oncological setting (cancer genetic counseling) should also provide sufficient information to enable the user to make a fully informed choice of action, particularly regarding prevention, in case of a familial cancer risk or the identification of a mutation in a family. The goal is risk assessment, the promotion of awareness, genetic testing for susceptibility genes, and the management of high-risk subjects and family members by offering adequate preventive measures.

As the leading organization representing cancer specialists involved in patient care and clinical research, the American Society of Clinical Oncology (ASCO) is committed to integrating cancer risk assessment and management, including molecular analysis of cancer predisposing genes, into the practice of oncology and preventive medicine. In particular, the ASCO has made recommendations regarding indications of genetic testing, the testing of children for cancer susceptibility, medical-management counseling after testing, regulation of genetic testing, protection against discrimination by insurers or employers, coverage of services, confidentiality and communication of familial risk, educational opportunities in genetics, and special issues relating to genetic research on human tissue. Another important aspect concerns oncologists involved in the management of at-risk subject with respect to oncogenetic counseling, including the discussion of possible risks and benefits of prevention modalities [21]. Within the setting of prevention, knowledge of the typical cancer spectrum related to hereditary breast cancer syndromes is relevant in individualizing subject management, based on the cancer risk profile.

Familial cancer clinics are continuing to develop across Europe, with considerable similarity in the organization of their activities, including breast-cancer risk assessment, mutation testing, and management within counseling. In the most European centers, genetic counseling is led by medical specialists with expertise in cancer genetics. Formal training in the field of hereditary cancers and cancer genetics is established in the UK and Netherlands but is not available in France, Germany, and Italy. Similarities among centers include the provision of a multidisciplinary team including the psychologist with a specific expertise in hereditary and familiar cancer issue, albeit with varying degrees of integration. Surveillance and management protocols are generally based on recommendations that largely have relied on expert opinion rather than on international guidelines [22].

A Model of Oncogenetic Counseling in Italy

In Italy, between 1999 and 2005, the Ministry of Research supported a national project entitled the "Development of a National Network for the Study of Hereditary Breast Cancer." This multistep model of oncogenetic counseling was designed and promoted at the Screening and Follow-up for Hereditary and Familial Cancer Unit at "Federico II" University in Naples, and was validated by five clinically oriented centers of the Italian Network [22]. The different steps of the model are aimed at promoting awareness in individuals identified as being at hereditary or familial risk (Fig. 10.1) and to apply a global approach to patients

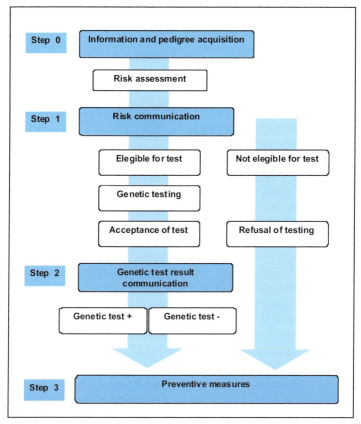

Fig. 10.1 The multistep oncogenetic counseling model designed at the Screening and Follow-Up for Hereditary and Familial Cancer Unit, University, Federico II, Naples, Italy. (Modified from [24])

affected by cancer and to disease-free at-risk subjects through multidisciplinary team involvement. Oncogenetic counseling is led by the oncologists of the team, who are trained to assess risk, propose diagnostic/therapeutic strategies, and explain these to the user considering his or her health or disease status. The model foresees structured sessions with the psycho-oncologist in order to discuss benefits, risks, and limitations of oncogenetic counseling, inquire about the consultant's motivations and expectations for pursuing genetic testing, assess psychological functioning, and facilitate emotional expression. Moreover, the psychological intervention allows the identification of psychological determinant of adjustment problems after test disclosure and full awareness of the medical risks and the various management options [23]. This counseling model entails risk identification, risk definition, and risk management of subjects with suspected hereditary breast cancer and their family members. It favors the management of at-risk subjects through prevention measures based on the risk profile and cancer spectrum [24].

At the proband intake, the family history of at least three generations is acquired by pedigree construction, including maternal and paternal lines; the individual clinical history is registered and consanguinity is reported.

For each subject, a risk profile (hereditary, familial and personal) is defined by widely used predictive models [25]. Hereditary and familial risks are clinically defined according to the Modena criteria, including familial clustering for breast and/or ovarian cancers, first- and second-degree affected family members, age of onset of breast cancer less than 40 years, and bilateral breast cancers. Breast cancer before the age of 35 years, male breast cancer, and synchronous breast and ovarian cancers are all definitions of a hereditary risk without familial clustering [26].

The a priori genetic risk of BRCA1/2 mutations is assessed according to the Frank criteria and BRCApro model, the latter specifically implemented for penetrance estimates in the Italian population [27–29]. Applying the BRCApro model to the Italian population, carrier probabilities of BRCA1 and BRCA2 gene mutations, including information on the proband's first- and second-degree relatives, were calculated using the CancerGene software.

Genetic testing for BRCA1 and BRCA2 mutations was recommended in the following conditions: a priori hereditary risk ≥10% according to the Frank criteria; a priori hereditary risk ≥10% according to the BRCApro model; hereditary risk with or without clustering according to the Modena model. Testing was carried out according to the ASCO policy statement [21] and the Italian guidelines for genetic testing and performed at the laboratories of the Italian Network. The testing procedure consisted of direct automatic DNA sequencing, with single-strand conformation polymorphism (SSCP) and protein truncation test (PTT) analyses in some cases.

When a disease-free subject requested counseling, it was necessary that the affected family member, generally the youngest, also underwent genetic testing to maximize the likelihood of obtaining a useful and informative test result, if a hereditary risk was suspected. If someone with a cancer diagnosis and a family history of cancer is tested and found to have a BRCA1/2 mutation, other family members can undergo counseling and be tested for the specific mutation identified in the family.

Spectrum of Related Tumors in Hereditary and Familial Breast Cancer: Experience in Naples

Here we describe the evaluation of a spectrum of related tumors in hereditary/familial breast cancer in a series of families selected from subjects who were referred for cancer genetic counseling to the Screening and Follow-up for Hereditary and Familial Cancer Unit at "Federico II" University in Naples, Italy, between 2000 and 2007. This study group consisted of: (1) subjects with a personal history suggesting a genetic risk (e.g., early-onset breast cancer, male breast cancer, breast and ovarian cancer in the same subject, and multiple cancers beside breast and ovarian cancers in the same subject), (2) cancer patients with a family history of breast and/or ovarian cancer; and 3) disease-free subjects in families clustering breast and/or ovarian cancers. All subjects derived from Italy and of Caucasian ethnicity.

For each pedigree, data regarding the family composition were recorded. In particular, for affected subjects, data concerning cancer, including site, date of diagnosis, residence at diagnosis, and histological confirmation, were reported. Probands gave their informed consent at each step of counseling and for research use of the data.

The cancer spectrum and the age-standardized incidence rates of tumors were evaluated in a series of 104 families referred for counseling. Moreover, mutational analysis for BRCA1 and BRCA2 genes was carried out in 68 families of the sample.

We considered three cohorts of individuals belonging to the following risk categories according to Modena model: hereditary with clustering, hereditary without clustering, and familial. Moreover, of the individuals who were offered genetic testing, the subset of families with a mutated BRCA1/2 genotype was included.

The pedigrees comprised a total of 4,100 individuals (2,117 females, 1,983 males), including probands and their I–IV degree family members and excluding non-consanguineous members such as spouses. Of the 104 families, 41 were grouped as hereditary with clustering (39.4%), 27 as hereditary without clustering (26%), and 36 as familial (34.6%). Of the 587 independent events of cancer, 294 were detected in the hereditary with clustering group, 103 events in the hereditary without clustering group, and 190 in the familial group.

Primary breast cancers were recorded in 312 cases (177 cases in hereditary with clustering group, 54 cases in hereditary without clustering group, and 81 in familial group). The percentage distribution of breast cancer was considered for the three risk categories as a function of both mean age at diagnosis and sex. The age at diagnosis of breast cancer was 39 years in the hereditary without clustering group, which was earlier than the age at diagnosis of breast cancer in either the hereditary with clustering or the familial group (48 years and 57 years, respectively). Male breast cancer seemed to cluster to a greater extent, albeit not statistically significant, in the hereditary groups than in the familial group (3% vs. 2.4%).

Tumors other than breast cancer were registered in 275 cases, of which 117 were in the hereditary with clustering group, 49 in the hereditary without clustering group, and 109 in the familial group. Figure 10.2 shows the percentage distribution of tumors for sites in each of the three risk categories. The percentage distribution of ovarian (15%), prostate (9%), and stomach (10%) cancers was higher in the hereditary with clustering group than in the other two groups (8, 6, and 0% in the hereditary without clustering group and 8, 5, and 3% in the familial group). The percentage distribution of kidney cancer in the hereditary without clustering group was double that of the other two groups (10% vs. 5%, respectively). Colorectal cancer and lung cancer did not show a typical distribution pattern in the spectrum of cancers related to hereditary and familial breast cancer. The high percentage distributions of colorectal and lung cancers in each of the three groups (11, 16, and 16% for colorectal cancer, and 13, 18, and 15% for lung cancer in the hereditary with clustering, hereditary without clustering, and familial groups, respectively) may be representative of the high frequency of these tumors in the general population. Uterine cancer is associated with the two groups specifically characterized by the clustering of breast cancer, i.e., the hereditary with clustering and familial groups (11 and 12% respectively). Finally, various tumors were detected in each of the three groups, including cancer site unknown, hemangioblastoma, bone cancer, and cancer of the adrenal gland in the hereditary with clustering group; cancer site unknown, ganglioneuroblastoma, myeloma, mesothelioma, bone cancer, and central nervous system (CNS) cancer in the hereditary without clustering group; and cancer site unknown, anal cancer, esophageal cancer, neuroblastoma, bone cancer, retinoblastoma, and CNS cancer in the familial group.

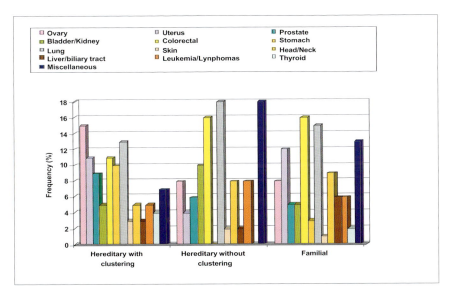

Fig. 10.2 Cancer spectrum in hereditary with/without clustering families and in those with familial breast cancers

The age-standardized incidence for cancer at a site other than breast cancer, during the period 1930–2007 did not differ statistically regarding risk categories and sex (Fig. 10.3). In our series, statistical analysis did not show a cancer spectrum that was typical for hereditary and familial breast cancers. At the evaluation of standardized incidence rates for other cancer, the age of onset of the different-site cancers was the same as for these cancers in sporadic cases (data not shown). A few cases of childhood cancers, such as a case of leukemia, hemangioblastoma, ganglioneuroblastoma, and retinoblastoma have been reported.

Among the 68 subjects at hereditary risk, 44, belonging to different families, were screened for germline BRCA1 and/or BRCA2 mutations. In the 43 subjects tested for BRCA1, 10 distinct mutations (23.2%) were identified; in the 30 subjects tested for BRCA2, there were six distinct mutations (0.2%).

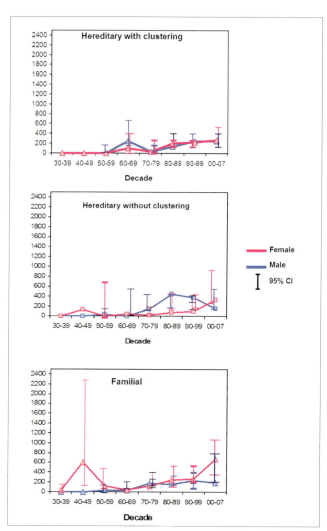

Fig. 10.3 Standardized incidence rates (× 100,000 individuals) of cancer at sites other than the breast according to risk category (hereditary with clustering, hereditary without clustering, and familial), sex, and decade (1930–2007)

10 The Cancer Spectrum Related to Hereditary and Familial Breast and Ovarian Cancers

Figure 10.4 shows the percentage distribution of tumors other than breast cancer in families with BRCA1 and BRCA2 genotypes. Fifty tumors were detected, of which 36 involved the BRCA1 genotype and 14 the BRCA2 genotype. Kidney/bladder cancer and stomach cancer were only detected in BRCA1 families, both with a percentage distribution of 11%, while prostate cancer was only detected in BRCA2 families, with a percentage distribution of 14%. Ovarian, uterine, and colorectal cancers clustered in both BRCA1 and BRCA2 families but with a different percentage distribution. The percentage distribution of ovarian cancer was higher in BRCA1 families (33%) than in BRCA2 families (22%), whereas for uterine and colorectal cancers the percentage distribution was higher in BRCA2 (22 and 14%) than in BRCA1 (8 and 5%) families. A high frequency of lung cancer was registered in each of the two genotype families. In BRCA1 families, miscellaneous tumors included skin cancer, cancer of the head and neck, liver and ductal biliary tract tumors, bone cancer, leukemia and lymphomas, neuroblastoma and cancer site unknown, each with a 3% distribution. In BRCA2 families, the miscellaneous tumors were represented by skin cancer, leukemia and lymphomas, and cancer site unknown, each with a 7% distribution.

Our experience suggests that maximum care must be taken in specific clinical surveillance carried out on the basis of risk categories and mutation status, until data derived from population-based studies become available.

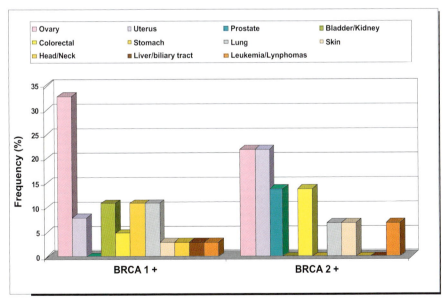

Fig. 10.4 Cancer spectrum in families with BRCA1 and BRCA2 genotypes

References

1. Pharoah PD, Antoniou A, Bobrow M et al (2002) Polygenic susceptibility to breast cancer and implications for prevention. Nat Genet 31:33–36
2. Antoniou A, Pharaoh PD, Narod S et al (2003) Average risk of breast and ovarian cancer associated with BRCA1 or BRCA2 mutations detected in case series unselected for family history: a combined analysis of 22 studies. Am J Hum Genet 72:1117–1130
3. Cipollini G, Tommasi S, Paradiso A et al (2004) Genetic alterations in hereditary breast cancer. Ann Oncol 15(Suppl 1):I7-I13
4. Ottini L, Marsala G, D'Amico C et al (2003) BRCA1 and BRCA2 mutation status and tumor characteristics in male breast cancer: a population-based study in Italy. Cancer Res 63(2):342–347
5. Marroni F, Cipollini G, Peissel B et al (2008) Reconstructing the genealogy of BRCA1 founder mutation by phylogenetic analysis. Ann Hum Genet 72(3):310–318
6. Robson M, Offit K (2007) Clinical practice. Management of an inherited predisposition to breast cancer. N Engl J Med 357(2):154–162
7. Garber JE, Offit K (2005) Hereditary cancer predisposition syndromes. JCO 23(2):276–292
8. Chen S, Parmigiani G (2007) Meta-analysis of BRCA1 and BRCA2 penetrance. J Clin Oncol 25(11):1329–1333
9. King MC, Marks JH, Mandell JB for the New York Breast Cancer Study Group (2003) Breast and ovarian cancer risks due to inherited mutations in BRCA1 and BRCA2. Science 302(24):643–646
10. Lakhani SR, Jacquemier J, Sloane JP et al (1998) Multifactorial analysis of differences between sporadic breast cancer involving BRCA1 and BRCA2 mutations. J Natl Cancer Inst 90:1138–1145
11. Narod SA, Foulkes WE (2004) BRCA1 and BRCA2: 1994 and beyond. Nat Rev Cancer 4:665–676
12. Brekelmans CT, Seynaeve C, Menke-Pluymers M et al (2006) Survival and prognostic factors in BRCA1-associated breast cancer. Ann Oncol 17(3):391–400
13. Rennert G, Bisland-Naggan S, Barnett-Griness O et al (2007) Clinical outcomes of breast cancer in carriers of BRCA1 and BRCA2 mutations. N Eng J Med 357:115–123
14. Burke W, Daly M, Garber J et al (1997) Recommendations for follow-up care of individuals with an inherited predisposition to cancer. II. BRCA1 and BRCA2. Cancer Genetics Studies Consortium. JAMA 277(12):997–1003
15. Thompson D, Easton DF and the Breast Cancer Linkage Consortium (2002) Cancer incidence in BRCA1 mutation carriers. J Natl Cancer Inst 94(18):1358–1365
16. Breast Cancer Linkage Consortium (1999) Cancer risks in BRCA2 mutation carriers. J Natl Cancer Inst 91(15):1310–1315
17. Bermejo JL, Hemminki K (2004) Risk of cancer at sites other than the breast in Swedish families eligible for BRCA1 or BRCA2 mutation testing. Ann Oncol 15:1834–1841
18. Garber JE, Syngal S (2004) One less thing to worry about: the shrinking spectrum of tumors in BRCA founder mutation carriers. J Natl Cancer Inst 96(1):2–3
19. Niell BL, Rennert G, Bonner JD et al (2004) BRCA1 and BRCA2 founder mutations and the risk of colorectal cancer. J Natl Cancer Inst 96(1):15–21
20. Epplein K, Koon KP, Ramsey D, Potter JD (2005) Genetic services for familial cancer patients: a follow-up survey of National Cancer Institute Cancer Centers. J Clin Oncol 23(21):4713–4718
21. American Society of Clinical Oncology (2003) American Society of Clinical Oncology policy statement update: genetic testing for cancer susceptibility. J Clin Oncol 21 (15):2397–2406
22. Hopwood P, van Asperen CJ, Borreani G et al (2003) Cancer genetics service provision: a comparison of seven European centres. Community Genet 6:192–205
23. Condello C, Gesuita R, Pensabene M et al (2007) Distress and family functioning in onco-genetic couselling for hereditary and familial breast and/or ovarian cancers. J Genet Couns 16(5): 625–634

24. Contegiacomo A, Pensabene M, Capuano I et al on behalf of the Italian Network on Hereditary Breast Cancer (2004) An oncologist-based model of cancer genetic counseling for hereditary breast and ovarian cancer. Ann Oncol 15(5):726–732
25. Domchek SM, Eisen A, Calzone K et al (2003) Application of breast cancer risk prediction model in clinical practice. J Clin Oncol 21(4):593–601
26. Cortesi L, Turchetti D, Marchi I et al (2006) Breast cancer screening in women at increased risk according to different family histories: an update of the Modena Study Group experience. BMC Cancer 6:210
27. Frank TS, Deffenbaugh AM, Reid JE et al (2002) Clinical characteristics of individuals with germline mutations in BRCA1 and BRCA2: analysis of 10,000 individuals. J Clin Oncol 20(15):1480–1490
28. Berry DA, Iversen ES, Guadbjartsson DF et al (2002) BRCApro validation, sensitivity of genetic testing of BRCA1/BRCA2 and prevalence of other breast cancer susceptibility genes. J Clin Oncol 20(11):2701–2712
29. Marroni F, Aretini P, D'Andrea E et al (2004) Evaluation of widely used models for predicting BRCA1 and BRCA2 mutations. J Med Genet 41:278–285

Chapter 11
The Role of Genetic Predisposition and Environmental Factors in the Occurrence of Multiple Different Solid Tumors. The Experience of the University Hospital of Sienna

Francesco Cetta, Armand Dhamo, Annamaria Azzarà, Laura Moltoni

This work is supported by the University of Sienna, PAR Project, and by the Comune di Milano, PROLIFE Flagship Project.

Introduction

An inherited predisposition and environmental factors are the main determinants of human malignancies. Although uniquely, they represent the two outer boundaries of cancerogenesis, in most cases they act in combination, in particular when multiple tumors concomitantly affect the same individual or the same kindred. Inherited multi-tumoral syndromes are caused by germline mutations of tumor suppressor genes, which can result in either malignant or benign tumors as well as various nontumoral alterations. However, multiple tumors, i.e. solid tumors that are not causally related to each other, are increasingly observed in the same individual in the absence of genetically determined syndromes. This may simply be due to the increased life expectancy and/or to improvements in the early diagnosis and treatment of tumors, and thus an improved long-term survival after removal of the first tumor. However, at least three modern-day conditions may act as independent factors for the increased occurrence of multiple solid tumors in the same individual:

1. Radiotherapy and/or chemotherapy, or a combination of both, are increasingly used at the highest doses. Powerful antimetabolic, antiblastic, antibiotic drugs, together with immunosuppression and immunomodulation facilitate the occurrence of second tumors, sometimes within the first decade after treatment.
2. Environmental pollution or inappropriate waste treatment has increased our exposure to carcinogens and other toxic agents. This has lead to increased frequencies of some cancers, particularly in subjects genetically more sensitive to these agents. Polycyclic aromatic hydrocarbons, nitrosamines, aromatic amines are known carcinogens found in cigarette smoke and in air pollution. Transitional metals (Fe, Cr, Cu, Pb, Cd, V), fibers such as asbestos,

pollutants from metropolitan areas, as well as long-term and long-distance side-effects of nuclear accidents (such as Chernobyl or similar nuclear disasters) are certainly responsible for an increased number of tumors, i.e., in addition to those usually occurring in the natural history of each individual.
3. Patients undergoing organ transplantation, such as liver transplantation, in the treatment of malignant disease require immunosuppression. In these patients, in addition to recurrence of the primary tumor, new tumors, related to chronic immunosuppression, may develop.

This chapter focuses on four different topics, all deriving from the authors' recent personal experience at a surgical referral center (University of Sienna) for inherited multi-tumoral syndromes. Firs, we present an analysis of a personal series (collected during a multi-centric study) of extracolonic manifestations of familial adenomatous polyposis (FAP), including papillary thyroid carcinoma, primary liver tumors, and brain tumors. All these tumors were observed in siblings belonging to a FAP kindred. Next, we analyze the occurrence of second (and third) tumors after retinoblastoma. These patients were tracked by the National Registry of Retinoblastoma, created in Siena many years ago. These tumors are peculiar in that they develop in predisposed subjects with germline mutations of the RB1 gene. However, there is a superimposed effect of chemotherapy and radiotherapy administered during treatment of the primary, pediatric tumor. Third, a small personal series of patients with multiple solid tumors (i.e., excluding lymphomas or leukemia), in the absence of transplantation and/or related immunosuppression, is presented. This series, while small, is of particular interest because the data were collected in a tertiary referral center for inherited multi-tumoral syndromes. Therefore, even if some of these patients may be index cases for a new, yet unknown multi-tumoral syndrome, they carefully checked for the "proxy" inherited syndromes (FAP, HNPCC, MEN 1 and 2, Cowden disease, Li-Fraumeni syndrome, Carney complex, Peutz-Jeghers syndrome), which were subsequently excluded in every case. Finally, the lessons to be learned from the health impact of environmental factors in metropolitan areas are discussed, including the preliminary experience with the side-effects of air pollution in the metropolitan area of Milan.

Inherited multi-tumoral syndromes are rare diseases in which various tumoral and non-tumoral manifestations are found in the same individual because of a germline mutation in a tumor suppressor gene. The treatment of these patients requires a combined approach by surgeons, oncologists, and molecular biologists. Early diagnosis permits surgical treatment in the pre-invasive stage, before full development of the malignant phenotype, with obvious advantages in terms of both the avoidance of radical treatment and better prognosis [1–3].

In particular, in some inherited multi-tumoral syndromes, such as FAP, hereditary non-polyposis colon cancer (HNPCC) and Peutz–Jeghers Syndrome (PJS), colorectal carcinoma is a manifestation integral to the syndrome. In such cases, the timing of the various therapeutic options, tumor selection (i.e., which must be treated earlier), the ideal timing for surgery, and the extent of surgery, are often unresolved questions that may be best-answered by genotype-phenotype correlations [1–3].

Germline mutations of mismatch repair genes (MSH, MLH) are thought to be the cause of HNPCC (Lynch syndrome), which includes colorectal carcinoma, breast cancer, endometrial carcinoma, and ovarian carcinoma. By contrast, PJS is an autosomal dominant syndrome characterized by melanotic mucocutaneous pigmentation and associated with multiple polyps of the gastrointestinal tract. It is determined by germline mutations of the gene STK11/LKB1, which encodes a serine-threonine kinase. Mutations of this gene are detected in 30–80% of cases at chromosome 19p13.3. The overall risk that an affected patient will develop cancer at an age of 70 is 85%. The most frequent neoplasms include those of the esophagus, stomach, small bowel, colon rectum, and pancreas. Less frequent neoplasms are those of the breast, ovary, endometrium, cervix, and lung. Patients with evident clinical PJS, but in whom a germline mutation of STK11 at chromosome 19p13.3 has not been detected, show a very high incidence of cholangiocarcinomas (40%).

Analysis of a Personal Series, Collected during a Multi-centric Study, of Patients with Extracolonic Manifestations of FAP

The autosomal dominant hereditary syndrome FAP is characterized by the presence of hundreds to thousands of colorectal adenomatous polyps, which, if not surgically treated, develop into colorectal cancer (CRC) in 100% of cases. The prevalence of FAP is 1:5,000–10,000, affecting both genders equally and with a uniform worldwide distribution. In FAP, colorectal adenomatous polyps begin to appear in affected individuals at a mean age of 16 years (range 7–36), invariably evolving into carcinomas in those between 30 and 50 years of age.

FAP is determined by germline mutations of the adenomatous polyposis coli (APC) gene, mapped at chromosome 5q21 [4]. APC consists of 15 transcribed exons, and the APC gene product of 2843 amino acids, yielding a protein with a molecular mass of 311.8 kDa. Because mutations tend to accumulate within the 5' end of exon 15, between codons 1250 and 1513, this region has been termed the "mutation cluster region" (MCR), and it is the site of approximately 60% of reported somatic mutations.

The APC protein is essential for the Wnt pathway. It is part of a protein complex, modulated by the Wnt signaling pathway, that regulates the phosphorylation and degradation of beta-catenin. Wnts are a family of secreted glycoproteins that bind to the 7-transmembrane receptor "frizzled" and its co-receptors. Activation of the Wnt signaling pathway leads to inhibition of GSK-3b, by dissociating the enzyme from a multi-protein complex that involves axin, APC, and beta-catenin.

Germline mutations of tumor suppressor genes, in this case the APC gene, are responsible for a wide range of phenotypic alterations occurring at various ages of life, depending either on biallelic inactivation of the gene, i.e., loss of function of the residual allele, or on interactions with modifier genes, environmental factors, sex-related factors (hormones, etc.), all of which variously effect the function of the APC protein.

In particular, studies of genotype–phenotype correlation have shown that several types of colonic polyposis are prominently related to the site of APC germline mutation [1–3]. Severe (classical) FAP, with thousand of colorectal polyps, occurring early, sometimes within the first or second decade of life, and usually determining an onset of carcinoma before age 35, is usually associated with germline mutations in the MCR, i.e., between codons 1250 and 1464, whereas intermediate FAP is associated with APC mutations between codons 157–311 and 412–1597 (except 1250–1464). Finally, attenuated FAP (AFAP), with less than 100 polyps, late onset of polyps (4th to 5th decade) and carcinoma (delayed), is associated with mutations 5' to codon 157 or 3' to codon 1596.

On the basis of these correlations, it has been suggested that, in the planning of surgical treatment, colectomy should be the intervention of choice, with primary ileorectal anastomosis (IRA) for patients with APC germline mutations before codon 1250, whereas primary proctocolectomy with ileopouch anastomosis (IPAA) is recommended for patients with APC germline mutations between codons 1250 and 1464 [1, 3]. This strategy is based on the results of Wu et al. [2] in a study of 34 patients with IRAs who were followed up for decades. Of the eight patients, who required re-operation, seven had APC mutations beyond codon 1250 [2].

Disruption of the Wnt pathway due to a germline APC mutation, i.e., one that is present since birth in all cells, not only determines the occurrence of colonic polyps and subsequent malignant transformation, but the inherited genetic abnormality also is responsible for numerous extracolonic manifestations. They include the occurrence of benign and malignant tumors in other sites, such as gastric and duodenal polyps and cancers [5], liver tumors [6–11], pancreatobiliary tumors [12], thyroid carcinoma [13–21], tumors of the central nervous system (CNS) [22–25], desmoid tumors [26], ovarian and adrenocortical gland tumors, as well as non-malignant manifestations, such as congenital hypertrophy of the retinal pigment epithelium (CHRPE) [27], epidermoid cysts, lipomas, and dental and bone abnormalities. This association between benign and malignant abnormalities of various anatomic sites is typical of all inherited multi-tumoral syndromes. Therefore, early diagnosis followed by proper and timely treatment requires that clinicians are well aware of the sites of the various extracolonic manifestations, the typical age of onset, and the genotype-phenotype correlations. Here, three peculiar, even if unusual, extracolonic manifestations of FAP are extensively analyzed: (1) hepatoblastoma (HB) and primary liver tumors [6–11]; (2) thyroid carcinoma [13–21]; and (3) brain tumors [22–25].

Genotype-phenotype correlations in patients with FAP-associated HB are shown in Table 11.1. HB is a rare embryonic tumor that occurs in children, with an average age of onset of 2–3 years. An increased relative risk of HB has been found in FAP patients and their first-degree relatives (relative risk RR = 847.95: confidence limits 230 and 2,168) [6]. Despite this increased risk, FAP-associat-

Table 11.1 Genotype-phenotype correlations in patients with familial adenomatous polyposis (FAP)-associated hepatoblastoma

Patient number	Sex	Age (years)	CHRPE	APC germline mutation Exon	Codon	Wild-type seequence	Mutant sequence
1	M	3.8	–	3	141	GTCATTGC	GTCTGC
2	2F	2.3	–	4	Intron 3	G	T
3	M	4.0	–	5	213	CGA	TGA
4	F	0.1	–	5	215	CAG	TAG
5	M	3.2	–	8	279	GGTTAA	GGTAA
6	M	0.7	–	8	302	CGA	TGA
7	M	4.6	–	13	541	CAG	TAG
8	M	3.1	+	13	554	CGA	TGA
9[a]	F	3.5	+	15	1061	AAACAAAGT	AAGT
10[a, b]	F	2	+	15	1061	AAACAAAGT	AAGT
11[a]	M	3.3	+	15	1061	AAACAAAGT	AAGT
12	M	3.4	+	15	1061	AAACAAAGT	AAGT
13	M	2.4	+	15	1105	CGGGGA	CGGGA
14	M	9.9	+	15	1189	GATATTCCT	–
15[c]	M	2.5	+	15	1230	CAG	TAG
16[c]	F	1.4	+	15	1230	CAG	TAG

CHRPE, Congenital hypertrophy of the retinal pigment epithelium
[a] Thyroid carcinoma associated in one member of the kindred
[b] Thyroid carcinoma associated in 3 members of the kindred
[c] Siblings belonging to the same kindred

ed HB is very rare; for example, only 33 cases (24 men, 9 women) were reported by Giardiello et al. [6]. Table 11.1 lists genotype-phenotype correlations in 15 patients with APC germline mutations: seven of these patients were recruited during our international cooperative study [7, 10]. It is noteworthy that all of these germline mutations were located 5' to codon 1230, most at codon 1061. Other mutations were located at codons 141, 213, 215, 275, and 302, i.e., in the very 5' portion of the gene.

Interestingly, one patient who had right-liver resection at age 2 after neoadjuvant treatment for HB underwent subsequent resection for hepatocellular carcinoma (HCC) at age 14. Therefore, in the same liver, HB occurred at age 2, and HCC, i.e., a completely different tumor, at age 14 [7, 8, 10].

Table 11.2 lists the patients in our personal series who had FAP-associated papillary thyroid carcinoma (PTC) ($n = 18$) [13–21]. Literature reports describe 150 such patients [11]. There is a striking female prevalence (F:M ratio >17:1 vs. 2.5:1 in sporadic tumors). The mean age at diagnosis was 24.8 years in our

Table 11.2 A personal series of cases comprising patients with FAP-associated papillary thyroid carcinoma (PTC)[a]

Patient number	Sex	Age	Histologic variant	Codon number	Exon number	CHRPE	LOH APC gene activation	Ret/PTC	BTP
1	F	30	papillary	140	3	–	np	np	–
2	F	19	Encapsulated follicular	593	14	+	np	np	–
3	F	22	Solid	778	15	+	–	+	+
4	F	31	Cribriform	937	15	+	–	+	–
5	F	18	Papillary	976	15	+	np	np	–
6	F	27	Cribriform	993	15	+	np	np	–
7	F	39	papillary	1105	15	+	np	np	–
8	F	34	Mixed	1105	15	+	np	np	–
9	F	25	Cribriform	1068	15	+	–	+	–
10	F	26	Cribriform	1061	15	+	–	+	–
11[b]	F	22	Papillary with cribriform areas	1061	15	+	–	+	–
12[b]	F2	20	Cribriform with solid areas	1061	15	+	–	+	+
13[b]	F	36	papillary	1061	15	+	–	–	–
14	F	24	Mixed	1061	15	+	–	–	–
15	F	20	Encapsulated follicular variant	1309	15	+	–	+	–
16	F	27	Papillary	1309	15	na	np	np	–
17	F	22	Cribriform follicular	na	15	na	np	np	–
18	F	20	Solid	na	na	na	np	np	–

LOH, Loss of heterozygosity; *np*, not performed; *na*, not available
[a] In two patients, also with brain tumors
[b] Hepatoblastoma and hepatocellular carcinoma in a member of this kindred

series and 28 years in patients described in the literature [13]. In about one-third of the patients, FAP and PTC were diagnosed concomitantly, in another third FAP was diagnosed first, and in the remaining third the first diagnosis was PTC. The histologic type of PTC was almost always (at least two third of patients) "conventional" papillary; however, an unusual pattern, the so-called cribriform morular pattern, which is very infrequent in sporadic tumors (<0.16%), was found in one-third of these patients [16–20]. Interestingly, in a comparison of patients with and without PTC, most, i.e. 22 out of 24, had APC germline mutations located before codon 1220 ($p = 0.005$) [13].

Noteworthy, there was no loss of heterozygosity for APC in the thyroid tumoral tissue [15], suggesting a dominant negative mechanism or a role for concomitant environmental factors (e.g., ionizing radiation) [21]. Most patients had RET/PTC activation [16].

Table 11.3 lists the incidence of FAP-associated brain tumors and PTC in the same patient or kindred. Brain tumors (BTs) were recognized by Turcot [22] as a component of the inherited polyposis colorectal syndrome. However, Turcot's syndrome included BT polyposis associated with FAP (mostly medulloblastoma) and with HNPCC (mostly glioblastoma) [23, 24]. Attard et al. [25] showed that most of these FAP-associated BTs co-segregated with HB. In our series, we found that FAP-associated BTs not only co-segregate in the same genomic area as HB, but also that there are individual patients, or patients belonging to the same kindred, who concomitantly have colonic polyps, PTC, and BT. Most of these patients also have CHRPE. Interestingly, in addition to

Table 11.3 Brain tumors associated with PTC in the same patients or FAP kindred

Author (year)	Sex	Age[a]	APC mutation	Brain tumor Histotype	PTC Patient age	CHRPE
Crail (1994)	M	24	1061	Medulloblastoma	24	+[b]	nr
Lynch (2001)	F	29	1061	Medulloblastoma	30	+[c]	nr
Fenton (2001)	F	29	1061	Medulloblastoma	6	+[b]	+
Plawski (2004)	nr	35	608	Cerebral falx tumor	na	+[c]	nr
	nr	10	608	Brain fibromatoses	10	+[c]	nr
Gadish (2006)	F	21	1061	Pinealoblastoma	18	+[c]	nr
Our series	F	22	778	Craniopharyngioma	16	+[b]	+
	F	36	1061	Medulloblastoma	32	+[c]	+
	F	20	1061	–	–	+[c]	+
	F	22	1061	–	–	+[c]	+

nr, Not reported
[a] Age (years) of first diagnosis of colonic polyps
[b] In the same patient
[c] In another member of the same kindred

medulloblastomas, other malignant tumors, such as pinealoblastomas or astrocytomas, and even benign tumors, such as brain fibromatoses, pinealoma, pineal cysts, and cystic tumors of the CNS, are observed. Therefore, even if FAP-associated BTs usually do not include glioblastomas or other aggressive histotypes, the prognosis of FAP patients with BT is often dismal, because in these patients, as well as in those with HB or primary liver tumors, the occurrence of the tumors precedes that of colonic polyps, and tumor recurrence is frequent.

While PTC in FAP may also recur, recurrence is infrequent (<10% of cases) and usually many years later. One of the main findings of the present study is that BTs co-segregate with PTC in patients with FAP. In particular, intensive screening for HB before age 2, for BT after age 2, and for thyroid nodules after age 15 is recommended, when a single patient or an entire kindred has CHRPE or mutations in exon 15. Like any other extracolonic manifestation, HB, PTC, and BT may precede clinical diagnosis of FAP. Whether patients with HB, PTC, and BT usually have APC mutations in the same genomic area needs further confirmation. However, this observation could facilitate early diagnosis, better treatment, and a deeper insight into genotype-phenotype correlations in patients with FAP. For example, in addition to more informed selection of the proper surgical procedure, other choices can be made according to the germline mutations, including age at which endoscopic surveillance should begin, intensity of rectal surveillance, or whether surveillance is required only after colectomy and ileorectal anastomosis [28, 29].

In FAP patients, the severity of the disease cannot be defined simply on the basis of the number or early onset of colonic polyps. In fact, FAP is not merely a pre-neoplastic disease of the colon, but a genetically determined multi-tumoral syndrome. The diversity and the relative importance of the various tumors differ, even in terms of patient survival.

In a relevant subset of APC patients, 7–23% who were negative for APC mutation and had a phenotype overlapping that of attenuated FAP (AFAP) there were associated biallelic germline variants of the MYH gene. MYH is a DNA glycosylase involved in the repair of oxidative guanine damage, (MIM #604933). Recognition of this autosomal recessive form of adenomatous polyposis suggests the genetic heterogeneity of adenomatous polyposis. Screening for both APC and MYH mutations should be considered in patients who do not have a family history of thyroid tumors. Extracolonic manifestations such as osteomas and desmoid tumors are less frequently associated with MYC mutations [30].

There is legitimate hope that, in patients with inherited multi-tumoral syndromes, genetic analysis will eventually guide not only intensive screening, but also surgical practice. Particularly in FAP patients, surgical treatment, in terms of extent of colon resection and the choice of the reconstructive procedure, as well as the overall therapeutic strategy for patients who may have five or more extracolonic manifestations, cannot be planned without an accurate preoperative genetic analysis. However, when specific oncogenetic alterations have already involved a given tissue (such as ret-PTC activation in patients with FAP-associated thyroid carcinoma), caution is required in speculating on the risk of occurrence of one type of tumor instead of another, or in attempting to establish the severity of the multi-tumoral syndrome simply on the basis of the germline mutation. There is wide phenotypic variability, both within different kindreds carrying the same APC mutation and within the same kindred. Modifier genes and environmental factors, especially for peculiar tumors such as thyroid carcinoma, play a major role in the occurrence of the malignant phenotype. In these cases, the germline APC mutation may only serve to give an overall greater propensity to tumor development [13, 21].

Despite the use of tyrosine-kinase inhibitors, such as imanitib mesylate in the treatment of chronic myeloid leukemia and gastrointestinal stromal tumors, as genetically targeted drugs, genetic treatment of cancerous diseases is not around the corner. In fact, clinically evident tumors usually manifest a multi-step carcinogenetic mechanism that develops over a period of years and consists of alterations in multiple genes as well as the disruption of different pathways. Therefore, genetic replacement of multiple abnormalities does not seem feasible, at least in the near future. While intensive genetic screening is suggested in cases involving specific tumors that have an increased incidence in patients with a given germline mutation, we advise caution before extrapolating surgical guidelines from mutational analysis and the avoidance of surgical treatment planning simply on the basis of germline mutations.

Analysis of Second (and Third) Tumors after Retinoblastoma: A Study Based on Patients Enrolled in the Siennese National Registry of Retinoblastoma

Data from the Italian Retinoblastoma Registry ($n = 1,111$; 703 sporadic and 408 hereditary retinoblastomas) were recently reported [31, 32]. Patients were recruited between 1923 and 2003. About a quarter of them were recruited at our institution (University Hospital of Sienna). In 35 unrelated patients, we identified retinoblastoma (RB1) mutations (RB1 gene mapped at chromosome 13p14) in six out of nine familial cases (66%) and in seven out of 26 patients without a family history of RB (27%). Screening the entire coding region of the RB1 gene by single strand conformation polymorphism (SSCP) analysis revealed 11 novel mutations, including three nonsense, five frameshift, and four splice-site mutations. Only two of these mutations had been previously reported [31].

The second malignant neoplasm was located inside the radiation field in 21 patients and outside the radiation field in 17 patients. Soft-tissue sarcomas were observed in 12 patients; specifically, nine osteosarcomas and three rhabdomyosarcomas) (Table 11.4). Whereas the rhabdomyosarcomas were all within the radiation field, of the three leiomyomas, two were outside of the radiation field, suggesting an inherited predisposition through the germline RB mutation.

Table 11.4 Second tumors in patients with previous retinoblastoma (University of Sienna series)

Second tumor histotype	Number of affected patients
Osteosarcoma	9 (5 lower limbs, 2 upper limbs, 2 skull and face)
Soft-tissue sarcoma	6
Rhabdomyosarcoma	3
Leiomyosarcoma	2
Brain, CNS tumors	4
Meningioma	2
Myeloid leukemia	3
Samll intestine	2
Melanoma	2
Seminoma	1
Breast	1
Ovarian sarcoma	1
Prostate carcinoma	1
Kidney carcinoma	1

Similar data were reported by Kleinerman et al. [33–36], who estimated the risk based on the histologic type of soft-tissue sarcomas in a large cohort (n = 963) of long-term survivors, coming from two institutions after diagnosis of hereditary RB. Between 1930 and 1959, 306 patients were diagnosed; between 1960 and 1969, 312 patients; and between 1970 and 1984, 345 patients. Of the 69 soft tissue sarcomas observed in 68 patients, ten were soft-tissue sarcomas (14.5%), eight rhabdomyosarcomas (11.6%), 13 fibrosarcomas (12 histiocytomas (17.1%), three liposarcomas (4.3%), and 23 leiomyosarcomas, i.e., malignant tumors of smooth muscle (33.3%). Fourteen of these 23 were located outside the radiation field. Furthermore, the site of occurrence was influenced by sex. In males, seven of 11 tumors (64%) were located mainly in the head and face, whereas in females seven of 12 (58%) were in the pelvic area (5 in the corpus uteri, 1 in the pelvis, and 1 in the retroperitoneum). Interestingly, one patient, after RB, had cutaneous melanoma 20 years before developing leiomyosarcomas, suggesting an underlying genetic susceptibility to both tumors. Other patients developed lung cancer late in life [34]. In general, the age at which the sarcoma occurred was approximately equivalent to the expected age of distribution for individual subtypes of sarcomas in the general population, with rhabdomyosarcoma and fibrosarcoma occurring mainly within 10 years after RB diagnosis, i.e., before age 20, and leiomyosarcomas arising later. Eighteen of the 23 leiomyosarcomas (78%) were diagnosed 30 or more years after RB.

Soft-tissue sarcomas represented, together with bone sarcomas, 76% of all cancers diagnosed before age 25, and 48% of all cancers diagnosed at older ages. Brain cancer and nasal-cavity tumors were also found as second tumors in RB patients. Brain, nasal-cavity, bone, and soft-tissue sarcomas in the head and neck may have been, at least partly, related to radiation, which was associated with surgery in 88% of cases; however, the occurrence of leiomyosarcoma in the pelvis, i.e., outside of the radiation field, suggested that the RB1 gene confers susceptibility to uterine leiomyosarcoma without radiation or at very low doses [37–40].

The data suggest that alterations of the RB gene are mainly responsible for the development of RB in the retinal epithelium, but they also confer a specific susceptibility to soft-tissue sarcomas, namely, leiomyosarcomas, which can occur at distant sites and long after the initial diagnosis. Therefore, it is important that survivors continue to undergo regular surveillance for sarcomas, particularly those of the uterus, even 30 years after RB diagnosis. Cumulative data concerning RB, including our own, suggest that, in addition to second-cancer susceptibility driven by germline RB mutations, second tumors after RB are also determined by treatment-related factors, such as concomitant radio- and chemotherapy. Therefore, early diagnosis, the key factor determining the need for radical surgery without adjuvant therapy, and new therapeutic approaches, such as local administration of drugs to minimize systemic side-effects, should be additional major goals in the overall RB treatment strategy [31–40].

Analysis of a Small Personal Series of Patients with Multiple Solid Tumors

Data concerning patients with multiple tumors, including colorectal cancer, occurring in the absence of inherited multitumoral syndromes are reported in Table 11.5. During the last 3 years (beginning in 2005), five patients (4 with colon cancer, 1 with rectal carcinoma) with second or third tumors have been admitted to our institution.

Such data are of particular interest to surgeons as they must be aware that, in a patient with a previous cancer, a new solid tumor may occur either as a part of or in the absence of an inherited multitumoral syndrome. The treatment of patients with multi-tumoral syndromes or second tumors involves coordination of the timing and the various procedures with other specialists. Familiarity with the occurrence of second tumors and the ability to suspect them will ensure early and effective diagnosis. In addition, a word of caution is required concerning "extended" surgical resection or extended radio- or chemotherapy in these patients, since, even in the absence of a known inherited multi-tumoral syndrome, they are highly susceptible to second tumors. Therefore, an additional medically induced decrease of their immune defenses could be inappropriate.

Early diagnosis, either in patients with inherited syndromes or those with second tumors, is facilitated by thorough knowledge of the most frequent sites

Table 11.5 Multiple tumors, including colorectal cancer, in the absence of known inherited multi-tumoral syndromes

Patients n.	Age (years)	Sex	Follow-up	Colon cancer	Year of onset	Other tumors no. (year of onset)
1	71	M	Alive and disease-free after multiple surgical procedures and multiple cycles of chemotherapy (5FU, GEM)	Left colonic flexure	2007	Ductal infiltrating pancreatic cancer (1999) Liver metastases (2002) Prostatic carcinoma (2004)
2	69	F	Dead due to metastases from colon cancer 7 years after left-side hepatectomy	Sigmoid	2006	Breast cancer (1997) Thyroid tumor (1980) Cholangiocarcinoma/ Klatskin tumor (1999)
3	67	F	Alive and disease-free after multiple chemotherapy (GEM) cycles	Right side colon	2005	Endometrial carcinoma (1985) Cholangiocarcinoma (2000)
4	69	M	Alive without clinically evident disease	Left side colon	2005	Ampulloma (2000)
5	62	M	Dead due to diffuse abdominal carcinomatosis 30 months after colostomy. He also had left-side pleural mesothelioma recurrence (previous pleurectomy + chemo- and radiotherapy)	Colorectal	2005	Right-side pleural mesothelioma (2004)

of related tumors, such as in RB patients. Noteworthy is the complete absence of clinical symptoms in patients with second or third tumors who comprised our small series, at least as observed during the last 3 years. All four patients developed colorectal cancer, in some case "locally advanced" (T3 with local lymph node involvement in 2 patients) (Table 11.5). Even in the patients who underwent regular follow-up with clinical examination every 3–6 months, ultrasound every 6 months, and computed tomography (CT) every year, the earliest altered marker was an increase of CEA, which increased from <10 units to ≥20 units. However, in the presence of elevated CEA levels, the first suspected diagnosis was recurrence of a previous abdominal cancer (ductal carcinoma of the pancreas, ampulloma, cholangiocarcinoma). Imaging examination was negative (ultrasound, CT). The patients underwent upper GI endoscopy and colonoscopy as completion procedures, in the absence of symptoms suggesting enteric involvement. Interestingly, CEA values returned to within physiologic levels immediately after surgery and remained "normal" excluding the patient who died due to a recurrence of sigmoid cancer. In this patient, colonic cancer was the fourth solid tumor.

Lessons from the Health Impact of Environmental Factors in Metropolitan Areas

Advancements in science and technology, more health-conscious life styles, and living in metropolitan areas in which there are diagnostic and therapeutic referral centers have facilitated early diagnosis and treatment of many diseases, including cancer, and thereby have increased our life expectancy. However, at the same time it is clear that living in densely populated metropolitan area likely increases the incidence of second tumors. This is especially true in predisposed children with a history of RB or other pediatric malignancies and in the frail elderly. Despite much research and speculation, at present, there is no clear-cut evidence that living in close vicinity to waste-treatment plants or highly polluted sites increases significantly the risk of malignancies in the absence of genetic predisposition, particularly when compared with exposure to other known carcinogens, such as tobacco smoke and asbestos exposure. Nonetheless, recent studies concerning the roles of environmental exposures and gene regulation in disease etiology have shown that physical (radiation, asbestos) or chemical pollutants influence a diverse array of molecular mechanisms and consequently alter disease risk.

New perspectives, including those addressing the "plasticity" of the genome and its regulation, have provided support for genomic reaction and adaptation in response to environmental stimuli. In particular, chemicals deposited in the environment by human activities can and do promote disease by altering gene expression. Epigenetic studies have improved our knowledge concerning the fetal origin of adult disease, while offering novel possibilities for the investigation of acquired and potentially heritable genetic variation and disease susceptibility. For example, recent studies have examined why a given chemical can have multiple modes of action and why sensitivity to chemical exposure varies among individuals. Most important, these studies have led to new ways of thinking about disease etiology, showing that disease risk is best predicted by considering genetic and environmental factors in tandem. According to this view, phenotypic expression of some manifestations of inherited multi-tumoral syndromes can be determined by epigenetic factors. Examples of this are the striking female prevalence of papillary thyroid carcinoma in FAP patients (F:M=17:1), which is certainly related to hormonal differences, and the increased incidence of thyroid tumors 8–12 years after the Chernobyl accident [21], suggesting a long-term and long-distance effect of nuclear disasters, at least in the subgroup of frail and genetically predisposed subjects, with FAP or other inherited tumoral syndromes, who are highly susceptible to radiation [21]. Similar comments can be made concerning the role of external radiation in the occurrence of primary or second tumors in some individuals instead of others, even if they have had the same professional exposure or live in the same area or building, or even belong to the same kindred.

Molecular biology may soon be able to explain the mechanisms behind long-term survivals (even for usually rapidly evolving tumors, such as pancreatic carcinoma) and therapeutic procedures, and how they interact with the biological behavior of a tumor in association with individual host predisposition. Evidence is accumulating that exposure to some xenobiotics determines genotoxic changes that not only facilitate the occurrence of tumors in exposed individuals, but may also be transmitted to offspring.

Chemical and Dietary Factors

The persistent and widespread environmental contaminant 2-3-7-8 tetrachloro benzo-p-dioxin (TCDD) is a potent carcinogen with multiple modes of action. Among these, TCDD promotes carcinogenesis by stabilizing the mRNA of urokinase plasminogen activator (uPA), a serine protease that contributes to matrix turnover and the growth of tumor cells. High uPA mRNA concentrations are found in tumors such as hepatocellular carcinoma but not in healthy tissues; similarly, survival time is inversely related to uPA mRNA levels. In rat liver cells, the TCDD-induced stabilization of uPA mRNA is mediated by a 50-kDa cytoplasmic protein (p50) that binds specifically to sites in the 3' untranslated region of uPA mRNA. Based on the finding that p50 is activated rapidly (in 15 min) by dioxin-mediated phosphorylation. it has been suggested that the protein stabilizes uPA mRNA by protecting nuclease cleavage sites from attack. In another study, dioxin exposure reduced the half-life of luteinizing hormone receptor (LH-R) mRNA in rat granulosa cells, which may influence steroidogenesis, luteinization, and ovulation by reducing granulosa cell sensitivity to circulating LH. Therefore dioxin could affect the production or activity of regulatory proteins that destabilize LH-R mRNA [41]. Exposure to TCDD is also correlated with an increased number of circulating F(14;18)-positive lymphocytes, facilitating the occurrence of childhood leukemia and follicular non-Hodgkin's lymphoma (NHL). In fact, in follicular NHL, the anti-apoptotic B-cell-leukemia/lymphoma 2 (*bcl2*) gene, normally found on chromosome 18, translocates to the immunoglobulin heavy chain locus on chromosome 14. This F(14;18) translocation places *bcl2* under the control of the heavy chain enhancer, resulting in the gene's overexpression and, consequently, increased cell survival and lymphomagenesis. It is well-established that exposure to TCDD, as well to many other pesticides, including dieldrin, atrazine, and fungicides, can increase the frequency of the F(14;18) translocation, both in terms of number of people affected and the number of affected lymphocytes. Interestingly, the translocation frequency depends on the frequency of pesticide exposure occurs, such that the risk of NHL increases with the resulting, cumulative genetic instability. Therefore, variability in environmental exposure, coupled with genetic events like translocation, alters disease risk [41, 42].

Perhaps even more interesting are animal studies showing that parental diet and other exposures can influence fetal DNA methylation patterns, with permanent effects on outcome in later life. Moreover, there is evidence that environmentally induced changes in DNA methylation patterns are heritable through generations [43–46]. DNA methylation occurs in two modes: dynamic methylation and theoretically permanent methylation, such as X chromosome inactivation and genomic imprinting. DNA methylation/demethylation reactions switch genes on or off throughout the life of an organism. The more permanent, although not necessarily irreversible, methylation patterns are determined during early embryogenesis and continue to adjust through the neonatal period. For instance, genes that predispose a person to obesity (and, in turn, related to many forms of cancer) can be affected by maternal diet. In rats, dietary intake of genistein (the major phytoestrogen in soy) during gestation in mice increased methylation of a retrotransposon (non-codifying portion of genome) located upstream of a gene, thus reducing its expression (number of copies of the gene). Altered transcription of this gene determines obesity and tumorigenesis. Since the degree of DNA methylation is similar in endodermal, mesodermal, and ectodermal tissues, genistein likely acts during early embryonic development. These observations suggest an active role for retrotransponsons in cancerogenesis, e.g., by misregulation of their original developmental role later in life.

Behavioral influences after birth also play a role in somatic cell methylation patterns as part of the ongoing adjustment to developmental and environmental factors. Weaver et al. showed that increasing licking and grooming of rat mothers reduced methylation of the glucocorticoid receptor (GR) promoter region in the hippocampus. Thus, rats that experienced high-quality maternal behavior exhibited increased GR expression, greater glucocorticoid feedback sensitivity, and a reduced response to stress later in life. The epigenetic alteration was noticeable in the first week after birth and persisted during adulthood [43–46]. Finally, during aging, there is a gradual loss or gain of methylation, depending on the tissue, cell, or organ. The interaction between aberrant methylation and age is recognized as a possible early step in carcinogenesis [46]. Gastric cancer cells often overexpress DNA methyl transferase enzymes, with hypermethylation of genes relevant to the etiology of gastric cancer, including human mut 1 homologue 1 (hHMLH 1) thrombospondin 1 (THBS-1), and e-cadherin. The methylation of oncogenes or tumor suppressor genes is mediated by dietary folate intake [45–47]. Folate, which is found in fresh fruit and vegetables, acts as a methyl donor for methylation. Folate deficiency is associated with hypermethylation of the p16 INK4a (CDKN2A) gene in human head and neck squamous cell carcinoma and in a rat model of hepatocellular carcinoma. Inheritance of methylation patterns is of great interest because it provides a mechanism by which acquired alteration in methylation could be inherited by offspring, as may be the case in the transgenerational effects of diethylstilbestrol (DES) exposure. As also observed in mice, the children and grandchildren of humans exposed to DES in utero exhibit increased rates of uterine sarcomas and adenocarcinomas, lymphomas, malignant reproductive tract tumors in both males and females. Li et al. [45] showed that DES exposure alters methylation patterns associated with the promoters of many estrogen-response genes that control reproductive organ development in both mice and humans. Ruden et al. [47] recently suggested that the transgenerational effects of DES are associated with altered DNA methylation, possibly mediated through modified WNT signaling, i.e., the pathway that is altered in patients with germline APC mutations. In addition, several genotoxic and environmental factors, including cadmium and several pesticides, have been shown to cause DNA strand breaks or fragmentation.

Bis phenol A (BPA) is a synthetic estrogen that is used as a plasticizer in polycarbonate plastic, dental sealants, and the lining of food cans. Both BPA and 4-nonylphenol (NP), a derivative of non-ionic surfactants, have been shown to activate estrogen receptor alpha (ER-A), induce estrogen-dependent gene expression, and stimulate growth in estrogen-responsive MCF7 breast cancer cells. Li et al. [45] suggested that increased NF-AT (nuclear factor of activated T-cells) concentrations in the nucleus up-regulate interleukin-4 transcription, causing the T-cell allergic response observed with BPA, NP, or octylphenol exposure. Therefore, the effects of environmental estrogens also include an increased allergic response.

Air Pollution

Air pollution consists of tiny ambient particles measuring <10–15 micron (PM_{10}) and arising from dust, smoke, or aerosol liquids produced by vehicles, factories, or burning wood. Air pollution can include residual oil fly ash (ROFA), an organic and inorganic mixture of silicates and metal salts containing vanadium, zinc, iron, and nickel, released during the combustion of low-grade oil. In vitro studies have shown that exposure to diesel soot and other PM_{10} particles activates pro-inflammatory genes in a process mediated by free radical/oxidative stress mechanisms. These, in turn, induce pro-inflammatory transcription factors, such as nuclear factors-κB (NF-κB) and activator protein 1 (AP-1), which promote increased histone acetyl transferase activity, histone acetylation, release of interleukin-8 (IL-8), a marker of inflammation, and, finally, expression of inflammatory genes. ROFA exposure stimulates a similar cascade of events. Samet et al. [48] showed that the vanadium component of ROFA can inhibit tyrosine phosphatases, causing phosphorylation of NF-κB and other proinflammatory transcription factors, including activating transcription factor 2 and c-Jun. Again, this leads to the expression of inflammatory genes, chronic inflammation, and, in some cases, cancer development.

Currently, there is great concern regarding traffic-related air pollution. Gauderman et al. [52] showed that children living or attending school close to major intersection develop impaired respiratory function during childhood that persisted for the rest their lives, irrespective of background pollution due to other sources. Thus, exposure to some, not yet identified pollutants during the "vulnerability window", i.e., in the first years (or weeks) of life, when the respiratory system is not yet fully developed, has lifetime adverse consequences. Moreover, not only fuel-related pollution (petrol, diesel exhaust, etc), but also inorganic (transitional metals, such as Fe, Pb, Cr, V, Zn) and organic compounds, e.g., found in tires or brake linings, are responsible for the adverse health effects [53, 54]. Consequently, the public and many government and European agencies have called for more stringent protection measures aimed at reducing both traffic-related and background pollution in metropolitan areas [55].

However, the adverse health effects of air pollution are difficult to dissect since the atmosphere contains about 18,000 different substances, each of which is present at very low concentration. Despite the well-known in vitro toxicity, mutagenicity, and carcinogenicity of many pollutants, documented by experiments in animal models, it must be stressed that in most of these studies, the exposure level to each pollutant, e.g., polycyclic aromatic hydrocarbons (PAHs) and TCDD, is higher than that occurring under actual conditions, in which PAHs are present at 10 parts per million (ppm), ozone at ppb (part per billion), and TCDD at ppt (part per trillion). Therefore the health damage caused by a single pollutant, even after long-term exposure, is likely to be very low. However, individuals are usually co-exposed to a broad range of pollutants that usually exert their dangerous effects by similar mechanisms or pathways, mainly involving the generation of reactive oxygen species (ROS). The effects of co-exposure to multiple pollutants are not only additive but may also enhance their individual effects. Accordingly, epithelial cell alterations are greatly enhanced by co-exposure to particulate material (PM), gaseous pollutants such as NOx, SOx, and ozone, and/or biogenic substances such as pollen, aeroallergens, and bacterial endotoxins. In particular, the various components of PM seem to have different specific biological effects: PM_{10} is more effective into "priming" cells to the subsequent activity of $PM_{2.5}$, which is more able to produce DNA adducts, whereas the ultrafine component of PM, PM_1, is responsible for damage to cell and mitochondrial membranes. Chronic exposure of experimental animals to a combination of ozone and nitrogen dioxide elicits inflammatory and fibrotic lesions in lung tissues that are greater than those produced by either toxicant alone. We recently suggested that ozone exposure has a deleterious added value, as a "sequential co-exposure." This means that, in addition to concomitant co-exposure, i.e., the contemporaneous activity of multiple toxicants, the specific toxicity of a pollutant must be considered. For example, ozone is particularly abundant during summer months because it results from the interaction of ultraviolet light (sunlight) with airborne volatile organic compounds (VOCs), especially oxides of nitrogen that are derived primarily from the combustion of fossil fuels. Ozone exposure is maximum when exposure to other pollutants is "usually lower", because the PM concentration is higher in winter. Therefore, ozone could impact the temporal window during which the repair process usually occurs, thus interfering with tissues repair mechanisms [56]. Indeed, pathological interactions among pollutants are both complex and unpredictable.

Adaptive Amplification/Mutation

When faced with death, cells adapt both individually and as a population. For example, in *Escherichia coli*, starvation of Lac- bacteria on lactose medium induces Lac+ revertants. The revertants exhibit either amplification (20- to 100-) of the lac- allele or a compensatory frame-shift mutation that randomly produces the lac+ allele. The revertants are apparently produced "de novo" in response to starvation, because they occur more rapidly and at higher frequencies than would be predicted by selection alone. This phenomenon is termed "adaptive amplification/mutation." *E. coli* provides empirical evidence for the ability of cells to enhance their survival in response to environmental pressures through genomic plasticity and adaptation. A major difficulty that affects cancer therapy is the progressive development of drug resistance, observed in a subset of patients. Thus, as in *E. coli*, tumor cells can respond to treatment by amplifying and /or mutating genes that promote their survival [41].

Conclusions

The increased life expectancy that has been achieved with dramatic improvements in the diagnosis and treatment of primary tumors has been accompanied by the occurrence of second or third solid tumors in some cancer patients. These multiple tumors are apparently not related to germline mutations of tumor suppressor genes.

Increased exposure to traffic-related air pollution in densely populated metropolitan areas and to a wide variety of genotoxic xenobiotics, introduced either by diet or by inhalation, together with spontaneous mutations related to aging, are likely responsible not only for the observed incidence of chronic inflammatory diseases but also of malignant tumors. Future research will better elucidate the mutual, highly complex relationships between inherited and environmental factors in the occurrence of malignancies. As stated in Koch's postulates, mechanistic relationships between a given pathogenetic agent and disease must be established before a causal relationship can be claimed. This task is made more difficult by the fact that malignant diseases are likely to be multi-factorial. Moreover, the phenotypic manifestations of the same germline mutation of a tumor suppressor gene are highly variable, even when patients belong to the same kindred. This is mainly due to superimposed epigenetic factors, which could be sex-based or environmentally related. Likewise, health damage from occupational exposure to known carcinogens, such as PAHs or even asbestos, greatly varies among individuals with the same exposure level and/or belonging to the same family because of individual susceptibility [50–52]. This includes not only inherited predisposition due to ethnic or individual differences in genetic polymorphisms for the genes encoding enzymes involved in xenobiotic metabolism, but also in "acquired predisposition," related to the effects of aging, concomitant chronic or metabolic disease, such as infections, immunodepression or diabetes, and variable exposure to environmental agents, beginning from fetal development and/or the first weeks of life. Elucidation of mechanistic, cause and effect relationships between a single genetic or environmental factor and the final outcome, i.e., a well characterized disease or malignancy, has not only medical significance but also important medicolegal implications, requiring a thorough understanding and cautious application of the biological findings.

References

1. Vasen HFA (2000) Clinical diagnosis and management of hereditary colorectal cancer syndromes. J Clin Oncol 18:81s-92s
2. Wu JS, Paul P, McGannon EA, Church JM (1998) APC genotype, polyp number, and surgical options in familial adenomatous polyposis. Ann Surg 227:57–62
3. Vasen HFA, Van der Luijt RB, Slors JFM et al (1996) Molecular genetic tests as a guide to surgical management of familial adenomatous polyposis. Lancet 348:433–435
4. Groden J, Thliveris A, Samowitz W et al (1991) Identification and characterization of the familial adenomatous polyposis coli gene. Cell 66:589–600
5. Bulow S, Bjork J, Christensen IJ et al (2004) Duodenal adenomatosis in familial adenomatous polyposis. The DAF Study Group. Gut 53:381–386
6. Giardiello FM, Petersen GM, Brensinger JD et al (1996) Hepatoblastoma and APC gene mutation in familial adenomatous polyposis. Gut 39:867–869
7. Cetta F, Montalto G, Petracci M (1997) Hepatoblastoma and APC gene mutation in familial adenomatous polyposis. Gut 41:417–420
8. Cetta F, Cetta D, Petracci M et al (1997) Childhood hepatocellular tumors in FAP. Gastroenterology 113:1051–1052
9. Cetta F, Mazzarella L, Bon G et al (2003) Genetic alterations in hepatoblastoma and hepatocellular carcinoma associated with familial adenomatous polyposis. Med Pediat Oncol 41:496–497
10. Curia MC, Zuckermann M, De Lellis L et al (2008) Sporadic childhood hepatoblastomas show activation of beta-catenin, mismatch repair defects and p53 mutations. Mod Pathol 1:7–14

11. Gruner BA, De Napoli TS, Andrews W et al (1998) Hepatocellular carcinoma in children associated with Gardner syndrome or familial adenomatous polyposis. J Pediatr Hematol Oncol 20:274–278
12. Giardiello FM, Offerhaus GJ, Lee DH et al (1993) Increased risk of thyroid and pancreatic carcinoma in familial adenomatous polyposis. Gut 34:1394–1396
13. Cetta F, Montalto G, Gori M et al (2000) Germline mutations of the APC gene in patients with familial adenomatous polyposis-associated thyroid carcinoma: results from a European cooperative study. J Clin Endocrinol Metab 85:286–292
14. Cetta F, Olschwang S, Petracci M et al (1998) Genetic alterations in thyroid carcinoma associated with familial adenomatous polyposis: clinical implications and suggestions for early detection. World J Surg 22:1231–1236
15. Cetta F, Curia MC, Montalto G et al (2001) Thyroid carcinoma usually occurs in patients with familial adenomatous polyposis in the absence of biallelic inactivation of the adenomatous polyposis coli gene. J Clin Endocrinol Metab 86:427–432
16. Cetta F, Chiappetta G, Melillo RM et al (1998) The ret/ptc1 oncogene is activated in familial adenomatous polyposis-associated thyroid papillary carcinomas. J Clin Endocrinol Metab 83:1003–1006
17. Cetta F, Pelizzo MR, Curia MC, Barbarisi A (1999) Genetics and clinicopathological findings in thyroid carcinomas associated with familial adenomatous polyposis. Am J Pathol 155:7–9
18. Cetta F, Brandi ML, Tonelli F et al (2003) Papillary thyroid carcinoma. Am J Pathol 27:1176–1177
19. Cetta F, Gori M, Baldi C et al (1999) The relationships between phenotypic expression in patients with familial adenomatous polyposis (FAP) and the site of mutations in the adenomatous polyposis coli (APC) gene. Ann Surg 229:445–446
20. Cetta F, Dhamo A, Malagnino G, Barellini L (2007) Germ-line and somatic mutations of the APC gene and/or beta-catenin gene in the occurrence of FAP associated thyroid carcinoma. World J Surg 3:1366–1367
21. Cetta F, Montalto G, Petracci M, Fusco A (1997) Thyroid cancer and the Chernobyl accident. Are long-term and long distance side effects of fall-out radiation greater than estimated? J Clin Endocrinol Metab 82:2015–2017
22. Turcot J, Despres JP, St Pierre F (1959) Malignant tumors of the central nervous system associated with familial polyposis of the colon: report of two cases. Dis Colon Rectum 2:465–468
23. Hamilton SR, Liu B, Parsons RE et al (1995) The molecular basis of Turcot's syndrome. New Engl J Med 332:839–847
24. Paraf F, Jothy S, Van Meir EG (1997) Brain tumor polyposis syndrome: two genetic diseases? J Clin Oncol15:2744–2758
25. Attard TM, Giglio P, Koppula S et al (2007) Brain tumors in individuals with familial adenomatous polyposis: a cancer registry experience and pooled case report analysis. Cancer 109:761–766
26. Caspari R, Olschwang S, Friedl W et al (1995) Familial adenomatous polyposis: desmoid tumours and lack of ophthalmic lesions (CHRPE) associated with APC mutations beyond codon 1444. Hum Mol Genet 4:337–340
27. Iwama T, Mishima Y, Okamoto N et al (1990) Association of congenital hypertrophy of the retinal pigment epithelium with familial adenomatous polyposis. Br J Surg 77:273–276
28. Soravia C, Berk T, Cohen Z (2000) Genetic testing and surgical decision making in hereditary colorectal cancer. Internat J Colorect Dis 15:21–28
29. Bertario L, Russo A, Sala P et al (2003) Multiple approach to the exploration of genotype–phenotype correlations in familial adenomatous polyposis. J Clin Oncol 21:1698–1707
30. Aceto G, Curia MC, Veschi S et al (2005) Mutations of APC and MYH in unrelated Italian patients with adenomatous polyposis coli. Hum Mutat 26:394–401

31. Sampietri K, Hadjistilianou TH, Mari F et al (2006) Mutational screening of the RB1 gene in Italian patients with Retinoblastoma reveals eleven novel mutations. J Hum Genet 51: 209–216.
32. Acquaviva A, Ciccolallo L, Rondelli R et al (2006) Mortality from second tumour among long-term survivors of retinoblastoma: a retrospective analysis of the Italian retinoblastoma registry. Oncogene 25:5350–5357
33. Kleinerman RA, Tucker MA, Abramson DH et al (2007) Risk of soft tissue sarcomas by individual subtype in survivors of hereditary retinoblastoma. J Natl Cancer Inst 99:24–31
34. Kleinerman RA, Tarone RE, Abramson DH et al (2000) Hereditary retinoblastoma and risk of lung cancer. J Natl Cancer Inst 92:2037–2039
35. Kleinerman RA, Stovall M, Tarone RE, Tucker MA (2005) Gene environment interactions in a cohort of irradiated retinoblastoma patients. Radiat Res 163:701–712
36. Kleinerman RA, Tucker MA, Tarone RE et al (2005) Risk of new cancers after radiotherapy in long-term survivors of retinoblastoma: an extended follow-up. J Clin Oncol 23:2272–2279
37. Tucker MA, D'Angio GJ, Boice JD Jr et al (1987) Bone sarcomas linked to radiotherapy and chemotherapy in children. N Engl J Med 317:588–593
38. Eng C, Li FP, Abramson DH et al (1993) Mortality from second tumors among long-term survivors of retinoblastoma. J Natl Cancer Inst 85:1121–1128
39. Fletcher O, Easton D, Anderson K et al (2004) Lifetime risks of common cancers among retinoblastoma survivors. J Natl Cancer Inst 96:357–363
40. Kaye FJ, Harbour JW (2004) For whom the bell tolls: susceptibility to common adult cancers in retinoblastoma survivors. J Natl Cancer Inst 96:342–343
41. Edwards TM, Myers JP (2007) Environmental exposures and gene regulation in disease etiology. Environ Health Perspect 115:1264–1270
42. Baccarelli A, Hirt C, Pesatori AC et al (2006) t(14;18) translocations in lymphocytes of healthy dioxin-exposedindividuals from Seveso, Italy. Carcinogenesis 27:2001–2007
43. Cheng RYS, Alvord WG, Powell D et al (2002) Increased serum corticosterone and glucose in offspring of chromium(III)-treated male mice. Environ Health Perspect 110:801–804
44. Lee MH, Kim E, Kim TS (2004) Exposure to 4-tert-octylphenol, an environmentally persistent alkylphenol, enhances interleukin- 4 production in T cells via NF-AT activation. Toxicol Appl Pharmacol 197:19–28
45. Li SF, Hursting SD, Davis BJ et al (2003) Environmental exposure, DNA methylation, and gene regulation – lessons from diethylstilbesterol-induced cancers. In: Epigenetics in cancer prevention: Early detection and risk assessment. New York Academy of Sciences, New York, pp 161–169
46. Richardson B (2003) Impact of aging on DNA methylation. Ageing Res Rev 2:245–261
47. Ruden DM, Xiao L, Garfinkel MD, Lu X (2005) HSP90 and environmental impacts on epigenetic states: a model for the transgenerational effects of diethylstilbestrol on uterine development and cancer. Hum Mol Genet 14:R149-R155
48. Samet JM, Silbajoris R, Huang T, Jaspers I (2002) Transcription factor activation following exposure of an intact lung preparation to metallic particulate matter. Environ Health Perspect 110:985–990
49. Carbone M, Emri S, Dogan AU et al (2007) A mesothelioma epidemic in Cappadocia: scientific developments and unexpected social outcomes. Nat Rev Cancer 7:147–154
50. Carbone M, Albelda SM, Broaddus VC et al (2007) Eighth international mesothelioma interest group. Oncogene 26:6959–6967
51. Carbone M, Rizzo P, Grimley PM et al (1997) Simian virus-40 large-T antigen binds p53 in human mesotheliomas. Nat Med 3:908–912
52. Gauderman WJ, Vara H, McConnell R et al (2007) Effect of exposure to traffic on lung development from 10 to 18 years of age: a cohort study. Lancet 369:571–577
53. Gualtieri M, Mantecca P, Cetta F, Camatini M (2008) Organic compounds in tire particle induce reactive oxygen species and heat-shock proteins in the human alveolar cell line A549. Environ Int 34:437–442

54. Cetta F, Dhamo A, Schiraldi G, Allegra L (2008) Metallic and organic emissions from brake lining and tires as major determinants of traffic related health damage. Environ Sci Technol 42:278–279
55. Cetta F, Dhamo A, Schiraldi G, Camatini M (2007) Re: particulate matter, science and European Union policy. Eur Respir J 30:805–806
56. Cetta F, Della Patrona S, Azzarà A et al (2008) Airway abnormalities induced by ozone exposure in the sheep. EAG Conference, Thessaloniki 2008. Abstract TO9A018P

Chapter 12
"Sporadic" Colorectal Tumors in Multiple Primary Malignancies

Concetta Dodaro, Enrico Russo, Giuseppe Spinosa, Luigi Ricciardelli, Andrea Renda

Introduction

Strategic innovations in the fight against cancer have resulted in improved diagnosis of multiple primary malignancies (MPM). In fact, early detection has translated into an increased reported incidence of MPM, due to the spread of screening programs and to increasingly sophisticated instrumental diagnostic surveys. The high sensitivity and specificity of modern diagnostic technologies are such that second primary malignant neoplasms can be identified in their early stages, during follow-up for the first primary malignant tumor and even if the symptomatology is vague or the findings incidental. Also, the combined approach (with or without a neoadjuvant) to cancer therapy has yielded better long-term survival. In turn, compared to 30 years ago, more patients are being diagnosed with a second primary tumor [1–4].

In developed countries, colorectal cancer is the most frequent neoplasm of the digestive system and the second cause of tumor-related death, in males (after lung tumor) and in females (after breast cancer).

In the USA., the age-adjusted incidence of colon tumor is 48.1 per 100,000 males and 37.8 per 100,000 females, while the annual percent change (APC) has decreased steadily, being 0.6 for males and –0.7 for females, within 95% confidence [5].

Every year in Italy, 25,000–30,000 new cases of colorectal carcinoma and 15,000–18,000 deaths are recorded. The overall incidence is of 30–50 new cases per year for every 100,000 inhabitants, with higher rates in central northern regions. The disease affects men and women with equal frequency, although rectal tumors have a higher prevalence in the former.

Biologically, the pathology that may lead to colorectal cancer does not have a high malignant potential, so, if detected at an early stage, correctly diagnosed, and treated, there is a good probability of long-term survival with complete eradication of the lesion/tumor. Therefore, nowadays, surgical technique combined with a radical oncological approach yields satisfactory results, in terms of survival, in the treatment of colorectal adenocarcinoma. Compared to patients treated radically and with adjuvant therapy for other solid neoplasms; the survival at 5 years is currently about 70% [6–8].

A. Renda (ed.), *Multiple Primary Malignancies.*
©Springer-Verlag Italia 2009

After skin and breast tumors, colorectal carcinoma is "historically" the malignancy most often associated with MPM. Among the many observed and reported associations discussed in the literature, only some of the tumors in these cases can be regarded as distinct clinical entities. Here we review some of the literature data in literature [9] (Tables 12.1–12.4).

Two classes of patients with colorectal adenocarcinomas are susceptible to developing MPM: (1) those whose tumors have a hereditary basis (discussed in another chapter) and (2) those whose tumors are sporadic (or definitely non-hereditary). It is the latter group that is the subject of this chapter.

Table 12.1 Multiple primary malignancies: frequency by (solid tumor) site (from [9])

Site	Number of primary cancers	MPM (%)
Lip and oral cavity	1,429	8.2
Esophagus	339	8.2
Thyroid	687	17.0
Lung	1,493	1.7
Colon/rectum	**1,441**	**10.6**
Cervix	44,440	5.2
Endometrium	1,192	8.6
Ovary	13,309	11.5
Skin	281	2.7
Prostate	919	8.2

Table 12.2 Multiple primary malignancies: metachronous tumors (from [9])

Index tumors	Number of cases	Metachronous tumor sites
Lip/oral cavity	4,493	Lung/larynx /esophagus / skin
Lung	42,439	Larynx/stomach
Breast	30,800	Oral cavity/ovary/lung/colon/urinary bladder /uterus/thyroid/bile ducts
Stomach	43,275	Lung/rectum/breast
Colon/rectum	**22,153**	**Lung/uterus/stomach/prostate/ovary/bile ducts**
Uterus	22,247	Oral cavity/breast /colon/rectum/urinary bladder/lung
Ovary	20,877	Brain/uterus/lung / urinary bladder /colon
Kidney/ureter/urinary bladder	13,111	Thyroid
Prostate	13,014	Stomach/lung /pancreas/urinary bladder
Skin	9,522	Testicle/brain lip/salivary gland/lung /prostate

Table 12.3 Second primary malignancies following colorectal cancers (SEER data)

Count	N	Percent
All sites	48,085	15.0
All sites excluding non-melonoma skin	47,950	15.0
All solid tumors	44,497	13.9
Digestive system	19,662	6.1
Colon and rectum	15,562	4.9
Colon excluding rectum	12,592	3.9
Male genital system	7,132	2.2
Prostate	7,058	2.2
Respiratory system	5,924	1.8
Lung, bronchus, trachea, mediastinum, and other respiratory organs	5,565	1.7
Lung and bronchus	5,554	1.7
Breast	3,945	1.2
Female breast	3,904	1.2
Urinary system	3,577	1.1
Rectum, rectosigmoid junction, anus, anal canal, anorectum	3,143	1.0
Rectum and rectosigmoid junction	2,970	0.9
All lymphatic and hematopoietic diseases	2,905	0.9
Sigmoid colon	2,896	0.9
Cecum	2,620	0.8
Urinary bladder	2,241	0.7
Ascending colon	2,075	0.6
Rectum	2,071	0.6
Transverse colon	2,003	0.6
Female genital system	1,908	0.6

N, Number of patients

Table 12.4 Percentage of MPM for different districts based on SEER data

Anatomic site	First tumor: number of patients	Number of patients with multiple tumors	Percent
Breast	394,033	53,804	13.7
Colon and rectum	320,686	48,085	15.0
Prostate	373,285	42,078	11.3
Urinary system	174,412	33,087	19.0
Lung and bronchus	358,034	19,033	5.3
Corpus and uterus, NOS	89,298	12,803	14.3
Skin excluding basal and squamous cell carcinomas	93,090	12,684	13.6
Oral cavity	49,783	10,687	21.5
Ovary	48,602	3,807	7.8
Thyroid	39,413	3,503	8.9
Stomach	54,794	2,723	5.0
Esophagus	25,340	1,265	5.0

Personal Experience

During surgical treatment carried out between 1980 and 2005, 121 patients had MPM (63 M and 58 F) involving a colorectal carcinoma (anus excepted) (Tables 12.5, 12.6). These patients represented 6.8% of the 1,784 patients with sporadic colorectal cancers who were hospitalized during the same period. Of these, 117 patients had two tumors; had two tumors, while a third neoplasm developed in four patients. In 47 patients, both neoplastic sites were colorectal:15 (32%) synchronous and 32 (68%) metachronous. Patient age at the first event ranged from 34 to 79 years (Table 12.5). None of these cases met the Amsterdam criteria nor were any hereditary syndromes detected in this series. The 15 synchronous neoplasms had the topography shown in Fig. 12.1. Nine of these tumors occurred in males (60%) and six in females (40%).

The 5-year survival for evaluable cases was of 58%. Of the 32 patients with metachronous tumors, 15 (47%) were male and 17 (53%) female, with an average diagnostic interval of 5 years and 9 months (24 maximum, minimum 1 year) and with tumor stage at diagnosis as reported in Table 12.5. The 5-year survival after diagnosis of the second tumor was 44%.

The second class (62% of 121 patients) of MPM involving colorectal cancer consisted of patients in whom colorectal carcinoma was part of a multi-tumoral syndrome. In this group of 74 patients (39 M and 35 F), the colorectal site was the initial one (index tumor) in 23 patients (31%), whereas in 48 (65%) the colorectal site was temporally second, and in three (4%) it was temporally third. Patient age of onset at diagnosis of the first neoplasm ranged from 29 to 71 years.

A hereditary predisposition was also not evident in this group of patients. With the exception of the synchronous cases, the average onset interval between the first and the second tumors (in 70 patients involving two locations) was 5 years and 8 months (with a maximum of 40 years and a minimum of 1 year). In four patients, the tumors were diagnosed synchronously or simultaneously. The tumor stage and the survival after the last neoplastic event are reported in Table 12.6. In Table 12.6 each patient has a single colorectal cancer (CRC) whose stage is reported in column 10. The tumors associated with colorectal cancer are listed in order of frequency in Table 12.7.

Considerations

Our experience is one of case histories experience, rather than statistical or registry-documented. Therefore, it is limited to the reports of an active general surgery team specifically dedicated to performing colorectal surgery [10-14]. Even so, there are several useful considerations.

12 "Sporadic" Colorectal Tumors in Multiple Primary Malignancies 183

Table 12.5 Synchronous[a] and metachronous colorectal tumors (1980–2005)

Patient	Number of synchronous tumors	Patient age	Sex	1st site	Stage	Interval to 2nd tumor (years)	2nd site	Stage	>5 years survival
1		60	F	Transverse colon	T2N0M0	3	Sigmoid	T3N1M0	No
2		49	M	Left colon	T3N0M0	7	Rectum	T2N0M0	Yes
3		34	M	Rectum	T3N1M0	24	Right Colon	T3N1M0	Alive (2 yrs)
4		59	F	Rectum	T2N0M0	8	Transverse	T3N0M0	Yes
5		52	M	Right colon	T3N1M0	5	Sigmoid	T3N0M0	No
6		42	F	Right colon	T2N1M0	3	Left colon	T2N1M1	No
7	1	72	M	**Sigmoid**	**T1N0M0**	**Synchronous**	**Rectum**	**T3N1M0**	**Yes**
8		60	F	Right colon	T2N1M0	5	Left colon	T3N1M1	No
9	2	48	M	**Right colon**	**T3N0M0**	**Synchronous**	**Rectum**	**T1N0M0**	**Unknown**
10		67	M	Transverse colon	T2N1M0	4	Rectum	T3N1M0	Unknown
11		60	F	Sigmoid	T2N0M0	9	Rectum	T3N1M1	No
12	3	47	M	**Sigmoid**	**T1N0M0**	**Synchronous**	**Rectum**	**T3N0M0**	**Yes**
13		59	F	Right colon	T3N1M0	3	Left colon	T3N0M0	No
14	4	76	F	**Right colon**	**T2N0M0**	**Synchronous**	**Right colon**	**T3N0M0**	**Yes**
15		49	M	Right colon	T3N0M0	14	Sigmoid	T1M0N0	Yes
16		55	M	Sigmoid	T3N0M0	3	Right colon	T3N1M1	No
17		50	M	Sigmoid	T2N1M0	7	Transverse	T3N0M0	Yes
18		45	F	Right colon	T2N0M0	4	Left colon	T3N1M0	Yes
19	5	37	M	**Sigmoid**	**T1NxM0**	**Synchronous**	**Rectum**	**T3N1M0**	**No**
20	6	54	F	**Right colon**	**T3N1M0**	**Synchronous**	**Rectum**	**T1N0M0**	**Yes**
21		32	F	Rectum	T2N0M0	17	Right colon	T2N1M0	Yes
22	7	65	M	**Sigmoid**	**T3N0M0**	**Synchronous**	**Rectum**	**T1N0M0**	**Yes**
23		50	F	Right colon	T3N0M0	2	Rectum	T1N0M0	Yes

continue →

continue **Table 12.5**

24	8	66	F	**Left colon**	**T4N1M1**	**Synchronous**	**Rectum**	**T3N1M1**	No
25		53	M	sigmoid	T2N0M0	5	Right colon	T3N1M0	No
26		44	F	Left colon	T2N0M0	3	Rectum	T1N0M0	Yes
27	**9**	**68**	**F**	**Right colon**	**T3N1M0**	**Synchronous**	**Left colon**	**T2N0M0**	**Unknown**
28		47	F	Rectum	T3N0M0	4	Transverse	T2N1M0	Yes
29		60	M	Sigmoid	T3N0M0	6	Right colon	T3N1M0	Unknown
30	**10**	**71**	**M**	**Left colon**	**T3N1M0**	**Synchronous**	**Rectum**	**T1N0M0**	**No**
31		35	M	Rectum	T3N1M0	2	Transverse	T3N1M1	No
32		59	F	Right colon	T2N1M0	5	Rectum	T2N0M0	Yes
33		67	M	Right colon	T2N0M0	4	Left colon	T2N0M0	Yes
34		64	F	Transverse	T3N0M0	5	Rectum	T2N0M0	Yes
35	**11**	**58**	**F**	**Sigmoid**	**T3N0M0**	**Synchronous**	**Rectum**	**T2N0M0**	**Yes**
36		61	F	Rectum	T3N0M0	7	Right Colon	T3N1M0	No
37	**12**	**55**	**M**	**Right colon**	**T3N1M0**	**Synchronous**	**Sigmoid**	**T2N0M0**	**Yes**
38		49	F	Right colon	T2N1M0	3	Left colon	T3N1M1	No
39		51	M	Right colon	T2N1M0	5	Rectum	T2N0M0	Yes
40	**13**	**68**	**M**	**Sigmoid**	**T3N0M0**	**Synchronous**	**Rectum**	**T1N0M0**	**Yes**
41		47	M	Rectum	T2N0M0	2	Transverse	T3N1M0	Yes
42	**14**	**60**	**M**	**Sigmoid**	**T1NxM0**	**Synchronous**	**Rectum**	**T3N1M0**	**No**
43		63	F	Right colon	T3N0M0	5	Left colon	T1N0M0	Yes
44	**15**	**79**	**M**	**Right colon**	**T3N1M0**	**Synchronous**	**Sigmoid**	**T3N0M0**	**Alive (3 years)**
45		70	F	Right colon	T3N0M0	4	Sigmoid	T2N0M0	Alive (3 years)
46		67	F	Left colon	T2N1M0	3	Rectum	T3N0M0	Alive (2 years)
47		62	M	Rectum	T3N1M0	3	Right Colon	T3N1M1	Alive (2 years)

[a]Cases involving synchronous tumors are noted in bold

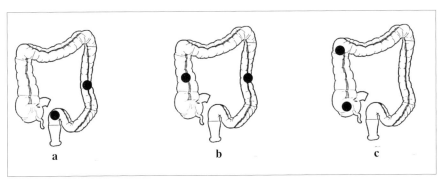

Fig. 12.1 Synchronous colorectal tumors in a series of 15 patients: 9 men (60%) 6 women (40%). Tumor sites: **a** left colon + rectum (9 patients, 60%; **b** right colon + left colon/rectum (5 patients, 33%); **c** right colon + right colon /1 patient, 7%)

Impact

The estimated incidence of sporadic colorectal cancer in MPM of 6.8% is too low. There are two possible reasons for this: (a) a previous neoplasm (skin, breast, or cervix) escaped anamnesis and (b) patients initially operated on by our team for colon cancer were later hospitalized for new neoplasms in another department or institution. Based on SEER data [5], the incidence is 12%, with 34,765 cases observed in 288,974 patients in the years 1973–2004.

Familiarity

Even though all cases of verified inheritance and of cancer following polyposis were excluded, we cannot rule out that some patients are carriers of genetic, germline alterations that result in MPM. Elsewhere in this volume, genetic alterations, unknown and/or at low penetrance, or "de novo" mutations, as the cause of MPM were discussed. It is possible that, in the near future, many "non-codified associations" will indeed turn out to have a hereditary genesis. Currently, the genetic-oncological model is based on Knudson's two-hit hypothesis", which states that a first predisposing germline (oncologically related) mutation is subsequently acted on by environmental factors, thus resulting in the onset of one or more tumors. Further experimental studies will no doubt lead to the identification of new genetic elements [15, 16].

For example research on melanoma in which microsatellite sequences were examined has yielded interesting results. Microsatellites are highly codifying, polymorphic, and repetitive DNA sequences that, although widely distributed in the human genome, are not uniformly dimensioned. Due to their ubiquity, identification by means of PCR, co-dominant Mendelian heredity, and extreme polymorphism, they serve as useful markers, even if their origin and function remain unclear. Microsatellite instability is demonstrated when the length of the

Table 12.6 Colorectal tumors involved in multiple primary malignancies[a] (1980–2005)

Patient n:	with 3 tumors	Patient age	Sex	Site of 1st tumor	Interval to 2nd tumor (years)	Site of 2nd tumor	Interval (years) to 3rd tumor	Site of 3rd tumor	CRC stage	>5 years survival
1		60	F	Endometrium	2	Rectum	–	–	T3N1M0	No
2		52	F	Right Colon	7	Endometrium	–	–	T3N1M0	Unknown
3		70	M	Prostate	3	Sigmoid	–	–	T2N0M0	No
4		65	F	Endometrium	Synchronous	Rectum	–	–	T3N0M0	Yes
5		57	M	Rectum	4	Liver (hepatocellular carcinoma)	–	–	T2N1M0	No
6	**(1)**	**42**	**F**	**Endometrium**	**5**	**Breast**	**8**	**Left colon**	T3N0M0	Yes
7		41	F	Breast	17	Rectum	–	–	T3N1M0	No
8		68	M	Prostate	3	Rectum	–	–	T4N1M1	No
9		45	F	Ovary	6	Right colon	–	–	T4N1M0	No
10		66	M	Stomach	2	Rectum	–	–	T2N0M0	Yes
11		64	M	Prostate	5	Rectum	–	–	T3N1M0	No
12		58	M	Prostate	4	Right colon	–	–	T2N1M0	Yes
13		42	F	Endometrium	40	Rectum	–	–	T3N1M0	Unknown
14		71	F	Cervix	1	Sigmoid	–	–	T2N0M0	Yes
15	**(2)**	**50**	**M**	**Iris**	**3**	**Bladder**	**6**	**Sigmoid**	T3N1M0	No
16		78	M	Prostate	3	Sigmoid	–	–	T3N1M0	No
17		40	F	Endometrium	1	Rectum	–	–	T3N0M0	Yes
18		55	M	Right Colon	7	Cardiac	–	–	T3N1M0	No
19		52	F	Cervix	10	Rectum	–	–	T1N0M0	Yes

continue →

12 "Sporadic" Colorectal Tumors in Multiple Primary Malignancies 187

continue **Table 12.6**

20		65	M	Prostate	7	Right colon	–	–	T3N1M0	No
21		41	F	Endometrium	15	Left colon	–	–	T3N0M0	Yes
22		66	F	Thyroid	7	Sigmoid	–	–	T3N0M0	Yes
23		51	M	Stomach	12	Rectum	–	–	T3N1M0	No
24		39	F	Ovary	1	Left colon	–	–	T3N1M0	No
25		45	F	Endometrium	9	Rectum	–	–	T2N0M0	Yes
26		50	M	Lung	10	Rectum	–	–	T3N1M0	No
27		68	F	Left Colon	5	Breast	–	–	T3N1M0	Yes
28		48	F	Endometrium	7	Sigmoid	–	–	T2M0N0	Yes
29		38	F	Cervix	3	Rectum	–	–	T3N1M0	Yes
30		68	M	Lung	2	Rectum	–	–	T3N0M0	No
31		63	F	Endometrium	5	Left colon	–	–	T2N1M0	Yes
32		60	M	Stomach	6	Rectum	–	–	T3N1M1	No
33	**(3)**	**34**	**M**	**Seminoma**	**24**	**Sigmoid**	**5**	**Cardiac**	**T3N0M0**	**No**
34		52	F	Right Colon	7	Endometrium	–	–	T2N0M0	Yes
35		60	M	Right Colon	2	Pleural mesothelioma	–	–	T3N1M0	No
36		51	F	Endometrium	6	Rectum	–	–	T1N0M0	Yes
37		57	M	Rectum	3	Liver cholangiocarcinoma	–	–	T3N1M0	No
38		24	M	Lymphoma	18	Right colon	–	–	T2N1M0	Yes
39		61	F	Right Colon	5	Lung	–	–	T3N1M0	No
40		67	M	Liver (hepatocellular carcinoma)	3	Rectum	–	–	T3N1M0	No

continue →

continue **Table 12.6**

41	70	M	Bladder	2	Rectum	–	T1N0M0	Yes
42	39	F	Lymphoma	7	Left colon	–	T3N1M0	No
43	59	M	Left colon	1	Kidney	–	T4N1M1	No
44	60	F	Right colon	7	Breast	–	T3N0M0	Yes
45	44	M	Left colon	6	Astrocytoma	–	T2N0M0	No
46	56	M	Liver (hepatocellular carcinoma)	Synchronous	Rectum	–	T3N1M0	N0
47	41	M	Lung	10	Rectum	–	T4N1M1	No
48	58	F	Sigmoid	4	Ovary	–	T2N1M0	Yes
49	51	M	Right colon	7	Lung	–	T3N1M0	Unknown
50	59	F	Left colon	3	Ovary	–	T3N1M0	Unknown
51	63	F	Breast	5	Right colon	–	T3N1M0	Yes
52	50	M	Rectum	Synchronous	Testicle	–	T1N0M0	Yes
53	47	F	Breast	5	Right colon	–	T3N0M0	Yes
54	62	M	Rectum	2	Stomach	–	T3N1M0	No
55	**52** (4)	**F**	**Breast**	**3**	**Leukemia**	**7**	**Left colon**	**T3N1M0**	**Yes**
56	59	M	Rectum	9	Lymphoma	–	T2N0M0	Yes
57	61	M	Rectum	5	Pancreas	–	T3N1M0	No
58	67	M	Sigmoid	6	Liver (hepatocellular carcinoma)	–	T3N1M0	Unknown
59	70	M	Prostate	5	Sigmoid	–	T3N0M0	Yes
60	55	F	Left colon	6	Breast	–	T3N0M0	Yes

continue →

continue **Table 12.6**

61	60	F	Thyroid	11	Sigmoid	–	–	T2N1M0	Yes
62	59	M	Sigmoid	4	Melanoma	–	–	T3N0M0	Yes
63	54	F	Leukemia	7	Right colon	–	–	T3N1M1	No
64	48	F	Ovary	3	Sigmoid	–	–	T2N0M0	Yes
65	29	F	Hodgkin	19	Right colon	–	–	T3N0M0	Yes
66	46	M	Stomach	5	Transverse colon	–	–	T4N1M1	No
67	49	F	Breast	9	Rectum	–	–	T1N0M0	Yes
68	53	F	Endometrium	10	Sigmoid	–	–	T3N1M0	Yes
69	61	M	Prostate	Synchronous	Left colon	–	–	T3N1M0	Alive 4 years
70	70	M	Right colon	6	Lung	–	–	T3N1M0	Alive 3 years
71	61	M	Kidney	7	Sigmoid	–	–	T3N0M0	Alive 3 years
72	69	M	Prostate	1	Left colon	–	–	T3N0M0	Alive 3 years
73	66	M	Bladder	3	Sigmoid	–	–	T2N0M0	Alive 2 years
74	50	M	Rectum	12	Pancreas	–	–	T1N0M0	No

[a] Triple sites in bold.

Table 12.7 Multiple primary malignancies and colorectal cancer: authors' experience

Colorectal-cancer-associated tumors	N	Percent
Uterus	16	20.5
Breast	9	11.5
Lung	6	7.7
Prostate	9	11.5
Stomach	7	8.9
Ovary	5	6.4
Liver	5	6.4
Pancreas	2	2.6
Testicle	2	2.6
Thyroid	2	2.6
Lymphoma	4	5.1
Bladder	3	3.8
Kidney	2	2.6
Leukemia	2	2.6
Astrocytoma-iris	2	2.6
Pleural mesothelioma	1	1.2
Melanoma	1	1.2
Total	78	100

microsatellite DNA sequence in a tumor differs from that of corresponding healthy tissue. Instability is determined by genetic tests, using PCR, and appears as alterations in the length of a particular sequence, as a result of insertions and/or deletions of a repetitive unit within the microsatellite DNA of the tumor. Many colorectal carcinomas show microsatellite instabilities, such that their analysis is an excellent functional and prognostic test. Microsatellite instability has been reported in sporadic colorectal adenocarcinomas and in hereditary non-polyposis colorectal cancer (HNPCC). It should also be noted that microsatellite instability would also be expected in sporadic and familiar breast cancer, although involving different microsatellites. A study by Catasus (1998) regarding microsatellite instability in endometrial carcinomas, either as the only cancer or in association with colorectal cancer in the same patient, found that microsatellite Bat 26 has an important role in colorectal carcinogenesis [17–21].

Synchronous Tumors

A reasonable percentage of MPMs involve simultaneous associations or multicentric neoplasms. In three of the five patients in our series who had the association left colon-rectum + right colon tumors, the histological aspect between the two sites differed, because the carcinomas at the cecal-ascending-colon-hepatic

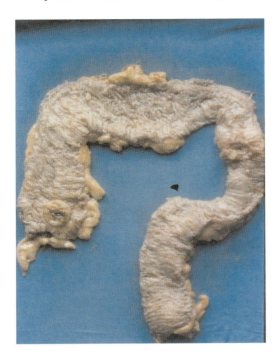

Fig. 12.2 Total colectomy for synchronous colorectal tumors

flexure site had mucinous characteristics. One of the remaining two patients had a left ulcerative colitis (Fig. 12.2). In terms of therapy, intervention has been modulated on the basis of topography and possible associated pathologies. Of the nine anterior resection-left hemicolectomy procedures, in one the tumorectomy was aimed at the low rectal site; four patients underwent total colectomies with ileo-rectal anastomosis; two had right hemicolectomies, in one case associated with local treatment (endoscopic) of rectosigmoid cancer.

Metachronous Tumors

The topographic distribution is reported in Table 12.3. In the 32 patients with survival at 5 years after the second neoplasm (66.7%) the tumor was detected during routine endoscopic follow-up of the first neoplasm. In two patients with T1 stage tumors, treatment of the metachronous neoplasms consisted of endoscopic exeresis; in the remaining patients, we proceeded surgically [22, 23].

Extracolonic Associations

In our experience, colorectal cancer represented the beginning of the MPM syndrome (index tumor) in 23 patients (21%) and in three patients was the third neoplasm. Associated tumors are reported in order of frequency in Table 12.7. There was a strong association between colorectal cancer and genital tumors, either male or female (breast, uterus, cervix, prostate, testicle). These tumors accounted for >50% of all associated tumors.

Over the long term, the outlook for patients with multi-centric tumors (synchronous and metachronous colorectal tumors) is less encouraging. For MPM patients with two tumors who were followed for 5 years, successful results were obtained in 51.6%, practically 10% lower than patients in the previous category (synchronous and metachronous tumors) although the standard of treatment (surgical and complementary) did not differ between the two groups.

The Endocrine Correlation

In MPMr, the "endocrine correlation" between the occurrence of tumors of the male and female genital organs and colorectal cancer has been suggested by data from several studies[24–26], which highlighted the following: First, the age of the onset is lower in women, and perhaps related, the subgroup of females with low childbirth rates are at higher risk. Second, hormone therapy reduces the risk of colorectal carcinoma. Third, recent immunohistochemical studies demonstrated alterations in the expression of sex hormone receptors (estrogens and progestogens) on colonic carcinomatous cells. We examined this finding in our own series and in literature reports in an attempt to determine whether there was a preferential association between colorectal adenocarcinoma and malignant neoplasms of genital organs, assuming that sex hormones also regulate the growth of colorectal cells. Estrogen receptors (ERs) and progestogen receptors (PRs) were indeed found on normal colonic tissue and on malignant neoplastic tissue. Many studies dealing with colorectal hormone receptors have been limited by the small number of cases; in others, the results have been inconclusive. Issa (1994) concluded that ER gene promoter regions are not present in colorectal tumors. Slattery (2000), in accordance with other studies, found that of 156 women with colorectal carcinoma, none had ER-positive tumors, and only one tumor was PR-positive. Neoptolemos (1993), by contrast, detected ERs and PRs in the malignant colonic mucosal cells and in the corresponding normal tissue. While ERs seem to be more characteristic of normal colonic mucosa than of carcinomatous tissue, their role in the latter might be to regulate PR synthesis.

A therapeutic role for tamoxifen (non-steroidal, anti-estrogenic) is supported by more certain data, as this drug has been widely used in the management of breast cancer since the 1960s. In women with breast cancer, adjuvant therapy with tamoxifen reduces the risk of disease relapse and increases survival. However, many studies have found that tamoxifen increases the risk of second malignant tumors in the gastrointestinal tract, especially colorectal tumors. In a meta-analysis of results of the Stockholm Trial (1995), the Southern Sweden Trial (1986), and The Danish Group for the Study of Breast Tumors (1998), a net increase of colorectal carcinomas was found in those patients who had taken tamoxifen (relative risk 1.9). Jordan (1995) also found a slight increase in colorectal carcinomas in patients treated with anti-estrogens. These results were not confirmed by the NSABP B-14 study (1985) or the Christie Hospital trial (1988), and other studies have emphasized that an increased risk of colorectal cancer following breast cancer is not related to tamoxifen therapy. Therefore, the link between tamoxifen and colorectal tumor requires further evaluations and, based on a review of the international scientific literature, the role of hormonal control of colorectal cells, either normal or neoplastic, is still very uncertain [27–31].

Conclusions

According to our experience, "sporadic" colorectal tumors are often more frequently associated with other neoplasms. Apart from those cases of certain hereditary genesis, multi-centric lesions that occur metachronously with colorectal tumors are relatively frequent. Regarding extracolonic sites, there appears to be a preferential association with tumors of the male and female genital tracts. An analysis of case histories offers etiopathogenic and clinical (follow-up) starting points that, in our opinion, deserve consideration in further studies.

References

1. Moertel C (1977) Multiple primary malignant neoplasms. Cancer 40:1786–1792
2. Parkin DM (2000) Global cancer statistics in the year 2000. Lancet Oncol 2:533–543
3. Dodaro C (1997) Colonic carcinoma associate to primari extracolic malignant tumors. Dig Surgery 10:105–106
4. Kan JY, Hsieh JS, Pan YS (2006) Clinical characteristics of patients with sporadic colorectal cancer and primary cancers of other organs. Kaoshing J Med Sci 22:547–553
5. Anonymous (2007) Surveillance, Epidemiology, and End Results (SEER) Program (www.seer.cancer.gov) SEER*Stat Database: Incidence – SEER 9 Regs Limited-Use, Nov 2006 Sub (1973–2004) – Linked To County Attributes – Total US, 1969–2004 Counties, National Cancer Institute, DCCPS, Surveillance Research Program, Cancer Statistics Branch, released April 2007, based on the November 2006 submission
6. Arnold MW, Young DM, Hitchcock CL et al (1998) Staging of colorectal cancer: biology vs. morphology. Dis Col Rect 41:1482–1487
7. Renda A, Iovino F, Capasso L et al (1998) Radioimmunoguided surgery in colorectal cancer: a 6 years experience with four different technical solutions. Sem Surg Oncology 15:226–230
8. Nastro P, Sodo M, Dodaro CA et al (2002) Intraoperative radiochromoguided mapping of sentinel lymph node in colon cancer. Tumori 88:352–353
9. Cangemi V (1990) I tumori maligni multipli primitivi. Chirurgia 3:461–4666
10. De Rosa M, Scarano MI, Panariello L et al (1999) Three submicroscopic deletions at the APC locus and their rapid detection by quantitative-PCR analysis. Eur J Hum Genet 7:695–703
11. De Rosa M, Scarano MI, Panariello L et al (2003) The mutation spectrum of the APC gene in FAP patients from southern Italy: detection of known and four novel mutations. Hum Mutat 21:655–656

12. Ueno M, Muto T, Oya M et al (2003) Multiple primary cancer: an experience at the Cancer Institute Hospital with special reference to colorectal cancer. Int J Clin Oncol 8:162–167
13. Wang HZ, Huang XF, Wang Y et al (2004) Clinical features, diagnosis, treatment and prognosis of multiple primary colorectal carcinoma. World J Gastroenterol 10: 2136–2139
14. Chiang JM, Yeh CY, Changchien CR et al (2004) Clinical features of second other-site primary cancers among sporadic colorectal cancer patients – a hospital-based study of 3,722 cases. Hepatogastroenterology 51:1341–1344
15. Suspiro A, Fidalgo P, Cravo M et al (1998) The Muir-Torre Syndrome: a rare variant of Hereditary nonpolyposis colorectal cancer associated with hMSH2 mutation. Am J Gastroenterol 93:1572–1574
16. Saegusa M, Hashimura M, Hara A, Okayasu I (1999) Loss of Expression of the gene deleted in colon carcinoma (DCC) is closey related to histologic differentiation and lymph node metastasis in endometrial carcinoma. Cancer 85:453–464
17. Serleth HJ, Kisken WA (1998) A Muir-Torre syndrome family. Am Surg 64:365–369
18. Chen HS, Sheen Chen SM (2000) Synchronous and early metachronous colorectal adenocarcinoma. Dis Colon Rectum 43:1093–1099
19. Derks S, Postma C, Carvalho B et al (2008) Integrated analysis of chromosomal, microsatellite and epigenetic instability in colorectal cancer identifies specific associations between promoter methylation of pivotal tumor suppressor and DNA repair genes and specific chromosomal alterations. Carcinogenesis 29:434–439
20. Catasus L, Machin P, Matias-Guiu X, Prat J (1998) Microsatellite instability in endometrial carcinomas: clinicopathologic correlations in a series of 42 cases. Hum Pathology 29:1160–1165
21. Neugut AI, Meadows AT, Robinson E (1999) Multiple primary cancer. Library of Congress Cataloging-in-Publication Data
22. Scaife CL, Rodriguez-Bigas MA (2003) Lynch syndrome: implications for the surgeon. Clin Colorectal Cancer 3:92–98
23. Togashi K, Konishi F, Ozawa A et al (2000) Predictive factors for detecting colorectal carcinomas in surveillance colonoscopy after colorectal cancer surgery. Dis Colon Rectum 43:S47-S53
24. Chen HS, Sheen Cen SM (2000) Synchronous and early metachronous adenocarcinoma. Dis Colon Rectum 43:1093–1099
25. Di Leo A, Linsalata M, Cavallini A et al (1992) Sex steroid hormone receptors, epidermal growth factor receptor and polyamines in human colorectal cancer. Dis Colon Rectum 35:305–309
26. Heron DE, Komarnicky LT, Hyslop T et al (2000) Bilateral breast carcinoma: risk factors and outcomes for patients with synchronous and metachronous disease. Cancer 88(12):2739–2750
27. Promegger R, Ensinger C, Steiner P et al (2004) Neuroendocrine tumors and second primary malignancy – a relationship with clinical impact? Anticancer Res 24:1049–1051
28. Fukagai T, Ishihara M, Funabashi K et al (1996) Multiple primary malignant neoplasms associated with genitourinary cancer. Hinyokika Kiko 42:181–185
29. Hendrickse CW, Jones CE, Donovan IA et al (1993) Oestrogen and progesterone receptors in colorectal cancer and human colonic cancer cell lines. Br J Surg 80:636–640
30. Slattery ML, Samowitz WS, Holden JA (2000) Estrogen and progesterone receptors in colon tumors. Am J Clin Pathol 113:364–368
31. Ribeiro G, Swindell R (1988) The Christie hospital adjuvant tamoxifen trial – status at 10 years. Br J Cancer. 57:601–603

Chapter 13
Multiple Primary Malignancies: "Non-codified" Associations

Alessandro Scotti, Alessandro Borrelli, Gioacchino Tedesco, Francesca Di Capua, Cristiano Cremone, Michele Giuseppe Iovino, Andrea Renda

Introduction

A retrospective analysis of the most important international statistics on non-hereditary multiple tumors has demonstrated neoplastic associations (of unknown pathology) in which the appearance of a neoplasm in a determinate organ increases the risk of developing a second tumor in a "predefined" organ. Here we examine the most frequent associations, starting from an "index tumor" arising in a particular organ, and analyze the site and type of second and third tumors. The goal is to identify potential new syndromes as yet referred to as "not codified." Since colorectal tumors are dealt with in a separate chapter, only those neoplasms frequently observed by the department of General Surgery are considered in the following.

Primary Malignancies: Post-esophageal Cancer

In recent years, the survival of patients with esophageal cancer has increased after esophagectomy. In fact, overall, the survival rate after 5 years is around 50%, according to a survey carried out in Japan that analyzed patients admitted to specialized centers for the treatment of such neoplasms [1, 2]. Updated imaging techniques have improved the early diagnose of esophageal tumors and the surgical techniques has evolved such that curative resections are more frequent. In addition, the use of combined strategies (neoadjuvant chemo or radiotherapy) has improved the prognosis.

Neoadjuvant chemotherapy increases the rate of R0 resections in patients with locally advanced neoplasms and in patients with malignancies at unfavorable sites, It also reduces the percentage of local or distant relapses and improves long term survival. Neoadjuvant radiotherapy reduces the neoplastic mass, controls local neoplastic growth, and reduces the risk of tumor spread following surgical manipulation [3]. Additional potential benefits from such methods are the pre-operative elimination of micrometastasis and the downstaging of lesions.

A. Renda (ed.), *Multiple Primary Malignancies.*
©Springer-Verlag Italia 2009

However, along with the increase in post-esophagectomy survival, the incidence of a second neoplasm [4, 5] has increased and has become an important prognostic factor in long term survival.

Statistical Experience

There have been several studies by Japanese authors that retrospectively examined patients treated for esophageal cancer. Kumagai et al. [6] examined 744 patients who underwent esophagectomy for cancer in the Department of Surgery of the Tokyo Medical and Dental University School of Medicine, from January 1985 to December 1998. Of these, 154 (20.7%) post-surgical esophageal carcinoma patients developed a second tumor and 11 (1.5%) a third tumor. Analysis of the histological type shows 143 squamous cells tumors, three undifferentiated cancer, two adenosquamous carcinomas, two melanomas and four tumors of other histologies. The characteristic of the patients with multiple malignant tumors after esophagectomy are reported in Table 13.1.

According to Kumagai's statistics, it can be deduced that the second tumor tends to strike mainly the men (93% of the cases) in the 55- to 70-year-old-age range, and in 37% of the cases the index tumor is a stage 1 neoplasm.

The site where a second tumor most frequently develops in post-surgical esophageal carcinoma patients is the head and neck region (42.4% of the cases), especially the pharynx and larynx (71.4%) followed in importance by the tongue, the buccal mucosa, and the nasal cavity. The stomach is the second most frequent site (32%), with gastric tumors usually appearing synchronously with esophageal carcinoma (70.6%). Other possible sites of a second malignancy are the colon (synchronous in 66% of the cases), lungs, breasts, urinary system, liver, gallbladder, prostate, and uterus.

Table 13.1 Second malignancies after esophagectomy in 154 patients (143 males, 11 females, ages 55–70): results of Kumagai et al. [6]

Stage of the index tumor	Multiple primary malignancies	
	n	%
0	1	0.6
1	57	37
2	33	21.4
3	38	24.7
4	25	16.2

n, Number of patients

Natsugoe et al. [7] retrospectively analyzed 652 cases comprising patients with squamous cell cancers of the esophagus who underwent surgery between 1980 and 1999 at the Kagoshima University Hospital (Table 13.2). In 157 of these patients (24.1%), a second tumor developed in another organ, 60 (38%) synchronously and 97 (62%) metachronously. The patients were subdivided into four different groups according to 5-year periods based on the date of the esophageal surgery. Analysis of these four groups showed that 21.2% of patients who underwent surgery for esophageal cancer between 1980 and 1984 developed a second tumor, 19.4% between 1985 and 1989, 21% between 1990 and 1994, and 33% between 1995 and 1999. The most frequently affected sites of the second tumor were the head and neck region and the stomach, followed by the colon, lung, liver, and urinary tract. From a clinicopathological point of view, these 157 patients who subsequently developed a second tumor initially had a better prognosis. In fact, at the time of diagnosis, these patients had tumors with a better TNM and therefore less invasion of the wall, less lymph node invasion, and fewer distant mestastases.

Regarding long-term survival, of the 60 patients with synchronous multiple tumors, 11 were alive in December 2004. Of the 49 who died, the cause of death was the esophageal tumor in 24, the development of other tumors in 11, non-neoplastic causes, such as lung infection or sudden death, in nine, and related to surgical causes in five. Of the 97 patients with metachronous multiple tumors, 21 were alive at December 2004 and 76 died. Of the latter, 18 deaths were due to the esophageal tumor, 32 to neoplasms developed in other organs, 23 to non-neoplastic causes, and three related to the surgery.

There were no significant statistical differences among patients with only esophageal cancer and those with primitive multiple tumors with respect to 5-year survival. Patients with metachronous tumors had a better prognosis than those with synchronous tumors.

Table 13.2 Incidence over time of second malignancies after esophageal cancer: results of Natsugoe et al. [7]

Group	Patients	Second tumor (%)
1 (1980–1984)	137	29 (21.2)
2 (1985–1989)	165	32 (19.4)
3 (1990–1994)	167	35 (21)
4 (1995–1999)	183	61 (33)

Matsubara et al. [8] analyzed the risk of developing a second malignant neoplasm after esophagectomy of squamous cell carcinoma of the thoracic esophagus. Their study population consisted of 753 patients who underwent surgery between 1985 and 2001 at the Cancer Institute Hospital of Tokyo. All the patients had a pre-surgical esophagogastroduodenoscopy and a CT scan of the head and neck and the chest. Curative oncological resection was possible in 679 of these patients; in this group, the risk of developing a second neoplasm was evaluated. Accordingly, a second tumor was detected in 254 (37%) of the esophagectomy patients. Most of those second tumors were in the head and neck region, followed by stomach, lung, residual esophagus, and colon-rectum. Thus, in the 679 patients who underwent surgery, the risk of developing a second malignancy in 5 or 10 years was 16 and 35%, respectively, with a net prevalence in males. The neoplastic risk for age- and sex-matched Japanese population is 6 and 13%, respectively.

Moreover, the risk of head, neck, stomach, and lung tumors was significantly higher in esophagectomy patients than in the general population.

The authors reviewed other risk factors, such as smoking and alcohol and found that the risk of a second neoplasm is less in non-smokers and non-consumers of alcohol.

Considerations

Today many patients surgically treated for esophageal cancer have a higher life expectancy due to progress in prevention, early diagnosis, and improved therapeutic options. Recent estimates of 5-year survival after esophageal cancer are around the 50%, according to a survey carried out by Japanese centers specialized in the treatment of these neoplasms.

Enhanced imaging techniques and new methods of diagnosis (CT-PET) have facilitated the early, pre-operative diagnosis of other neoplasms and their parallel treatment. An awareness of those patients at risk of developing a second tumor, the target organs of these tumors have improved screening and follow-up, with a diagnostic focus of second neoplasms.

Reports in the literature confirm the association between esophageal cancer and the development of a new neoplasm in another organ. The percentage of patients who develop a second tumor varies from around 21% (Kumagai) to above 30% (Matsubara).

The increased prevalence of second tumors in esophageal cancer patients, as reflected by the most recent statistics, is probably due to improved survival of esophagectomy patients, who now live long enough to develop a second neoplasm. In addition, post-esophagectomy screening of these patients has intensified, resulting in better detection of a second tumor (e.g., the research of Natsugoe et al. covering the period 1995–1999). The statistics cited show that men are more likely to have a second neoplasm and the organs most frequently involved by second malignant tumors, synchronous and metachronous, after esophageal carcinoma are those in the upper aerodigestive tract (head, neck, stomach, and lungs). Indeed, in >70% of the cases, the second tumor was located in the head and neck or stomach, thus implicating the same carcinogenetic factors as in the esophageal cancer. From an epidemiological point of view, neoplasms in the tongue, pharynx, and esophagus are well-known to be associated with the same environmental carcinogens, tobacco smoking and alcohol. In the examined population, around 85% of the patients with a tumor in the head and neck region associated with esophageal cancer were heavy smokers or drinkers.

From the molecular point of view, important genetic differences involving p53, FHIT, ADH2, and ALDH2, have been observed between patients who develop esophageal tumors and the healthy population [9]. The frequent correlation of esophageal tumors with tumors in the aerodigestive tract (pharynx, larynx, tongue, oral cavity, in order of frequency) is based on the presence of squamous epithelium in all of these areas, which is then targeted by the same carcinogenetic factors acting through the same mechanisms.

As also noted, the second most likely tumor in post-surgical esophageal cancer patients is stomach cancer, in over half of the cases it occurs synchronously. For this reason, esophageal cancer patients should undergo gastric imaging (CT, endoscopy) not only to diagnose a possible simultaneous tumor but also because the stomach is often used to rehabilitate digestive continuity (gastric tubulization) but may harbor a synchronous or metachronous tumor that was actually simultaneous but not diagnosed during surgery; this scenario could worsen the patient's prognosis (Table 13.3).

Table 13.3 Multiple primary malignancies (MPM) associated with esophageal carcinoma: summary

Author	Post-operative esophageal cancer patients (*n*)	MPM (%)	Age	Location of 2nd tumor
Kumagai	744	154 (20.7)	55–70	1. Head and neck 2. Stomach 3. Colon
Natsugoe	652	157 (24.1); 60 (38) synchronous, 97 (62) metachronous	>55	1. Head and neck 2. Stomach 3. Colon
Matsubara	679	254 (37)	≥60	1. Head and neck 2. Stomach 3. Lungs

n, Number of patients

However, gastric tubulization also has a "protective" advantage in avoiding the development of a second tumor, because with this technique the small gastric curve is eliminated in order to form a tubule that substitutes for the esophagus. It is exactly in this area of the stomach where most gastric metachronous carcinomas tend to localize; thus, the mucosal area most susceptible to developing a neoplasm is removed [10]. During post-esophagectomy follow up, the gastric tubule is systematically checked.

As far as prognosis is concerned, there are no important differences in terms of survival between patients with only the esophageal tumor and patients who subsequently develop a second tumor, since the latter generally occur in patients whose esophageal tumor is detected while still at an early stage, a higher possibility of cure and a longer life expectancy. Patients with a first esophageal tumor of stage III or IV have a worse prognosis, shorter life expectancy, and therefore a lower probability of developing a second tumor. Similarly, the prognosis of patients with primitive multiple tumors would be determined mostly by the stage of the index tumor stage, in this case, esophageal carcinoma.

Primary Malignancies: Post-gastric Cancer

In gastric carcinoma patients, the prevalence of second tumors varies according to the reported statistics ranges from 2.8 to 6.8% [11]. In Japan Yoshino et al. reported primitive multiple tumors associated with gastric carcinoma in 2.1% of the patients with apparent single gastric tumors. While little is known about the pathogenesis of second tumors in the stomach cancer patients, microsatellite instability and genetic mutations have been suggested as potential causes.

Statistical Experience

Park et al., from the Department of Surgery of Chonnam National University Hospital, South Korea [12] carried out a study from January 1986 to December 2000 that consisted of 2,509 patients with gastric carcinoma, 65 of whom (2.6%) had another primitive malignant associated tumor (Table 13.4). In this subgroup of patients, there were 37 men and 28 women, with an average age of 57.6 years.

A comparison of the patients with a second neoplasm with the rest of the study group showed a clear male prevalence (ratio 2:1) in the latter, while the difference in the second-neoplasm group were not statistically significant. Tumor localization was similar in both categories of patients, with neoplasms more frequently occurring at the third inferior level of the stomach. Poorly differentiated tumors were less common in patients who had developed another primitive tumor than in those in whom disease was limited to a gastric tumor, whereas tumor stage did not statistically differ between the two groups.

Of the 65 patients who had developed at least one other primitive malignant neoplasm, in 28 (43%) the second tumor involved the gastrointestinal tract,

Table 13.4 Site of second malignancies after gastric cancer: results of Park et al. [12]

Number of patients (%)	Site of second neoplasm
22 (33.8)	Colon-rectum
7 (10.8)	Hepatobiliary
6 (9.2)	Uterus
5 (7.6)	Breast
4 (6.2)	Esophagus
4 (6.2)	Urinary tract
2 (3.1)	Small bowel
15 (23.1)	Other sites

especially the colon (22 cases), distal esophagus (4) and ileum (2). Other locations were the liver and pancreas (7 patients), uterus (6 patients), breast (5 patients), kidneys, and urinary tract (4 patients). Five-year survival for patients with gastric tumors only was 51.6% and while for those with a second malignant tumor rate it was 50.7%, i.e., not significantly different.

Another statistically and epidemiologically interesting study is that of Ikeda et al. [13], who examined 1070 patients diagnosed with early gastric cancer [13] (Table 13.5). This form of gastric carcinoma seems to have increased among the Japanese population in the last 20 years and now constitutes 50% of all the stomach tumors diagnosed in Japan. A similar increment has been noted in western populations despite a progressive decrease in the incidence of advanced gastric cancer.

Table 13.5 Sites and time of occurrence of second malignancies after early gastric cancer (EGC): results of Ikeda et al. [13]

Site of second tumor	n	Time of occurrence (post-operative years after gastric cancer surgery)		
		≤5 years (n = 31)	≤10 years (n = 14)	>10 years (n = 9)
Lung	17	13	2	2
Colon-rectum	10	7	2	1
Esophagus	6	3	2	1
Breast	5	1	3	1
Residual stomach	5	0	1	4
Liver	4	2	20	0
Pancreas	2	1	1	0
Prostate	2	1	1	0
Other	3	3	0	0

n, Number of patients

In early gastric cancer (EGC), the lesion is confined to the mucosal and submucosal membrane, in contrast to advanced gastric cancer where the muscularis propria or even deeper layers are affected. A Japanese classification of EGC subdivides it into three principal types; polypoid (type I), superficial (type II), and excavated (type III). The superficial type is further subdivided in three subtypes raised (IIa), flat (IIb), and depressed (IIc). Patients with EGC have a high possibility of recovery after adequate resection, with a 5-year survival of around 90%.

The 1,070 patients of Ikeda et al. study were treated at the Department of Surgery of the National Kyushu Medical Centre from January 1979 to December 2002. Follow-up included hematochemical evaluation, abdominal CT, chest X-ray, echography, and endoscopy of the gastrointestinal tract every 3 months for the first year, with subsequent intervals of 6–12 months. Of the 131 patients who died during follow-up, deaths were caused by a revival of the illness or to the development of a second tumor while the remaining 72 deaths were due to other causes. In the study group, a second malignancy was detected in 54 (5%) while 30 (2.8%) suffered a relapse of the first tumor. The second primary tumor was, in most cases (17 of 54) located in the lung, followed by the colon-rectum (10 cases), esophagus (6), breast and residual stomach (5), liver (4), pancreas, and prostate (2). In 31 patients the second metachronous tumor appeared within first 5 years of the first surgery, while in nine it developed after 10 years (Table 13.5). From a clinicopathological point of view, old age and male sex were the factors most highly associated with the development of a second tumor.

These results have been confirmed in a smaller series (105 patients) in a study by the Italian group of Bozzetti et al., Gastrointestinal Surgery Department, National Cancer Institute of Milan [14] (Table 13.6).

The 105 study patients underwent surgery for EGC from 1973 to 1990, with a mean follow-up of 71 months, and were evaluated for the possibility of developing a second multiple malignant tumor. Five-year survival rate was 82% and there were 10 cases (9.5%) of a second neoplasm: 3 lung tumors, 2 cases of breast cancer, 2 bladder cancers, 1 esophageal cancer, 1 malignant melanoma,

Table 13.6 Sites of second malignancies after early gastric cancer: results of Bozzetti et al. [14]

Types of tumors	N
Breast cancer	2
Lung cancer	3
Bladder cancer	2
Esophageal cancer	1
Malignant melanoma	1
Non-Hodgkin lymphoma	1

N, Number of patients

and 1 non-Hodgkin lymphoma. The neoplasms were synchronous in three patients (two patients with lung tumors and 1 with an esophageal tumor), in the remaining 10 patients the tumors were metachronous.

Considerations

The data reported by Park et al. were obtained from a large number of gastric carcinoma patients (2509). In this population, the percentage of developing a second tumor was 2.6%, and mostly affected older men. The second tumor was predominantly located in the gastrointestinal tract (43%), mainly the colon, thus suggesting a carcinogenetic process similar to that for tumors of the colon. No statistically significant difference was noted between patients with disease limited to gastric cancer and patients who later developed a second neoplasm. The results confirmed those of Japanese authors regarding patients treated surgically for stomach cancer; in this group, the prevalence of a second neoplasm varied from 2.8 to 6.8%. According to the findings of Yoshino et al. [15], colon cancer was the neoplasm most highly associated with gastric cancer (26.6%), followed by cancer of the uterus (11.6%), esophagus (10.1%), breast (8.1%), and liver (6.8%).

Kim et al. [16] hypothesized that the high susceptibility of the lower gastrointestinal tract for developing a second neoplasm may be due to: (1) changes in the bacterial intestinal flora in response to modified gastric secretions, (2) overload of this section of the intestine, which can occur after gastrectomy, and (3) carcinogenetic processes similar to those active in colon cancer.

Several reports have shown that a second malignancy tends to develop in the initial stage of gastric cancer [17]. In these cases, in which the disease is detected early and the prognosis is usually good, there is enough time over the patient's life for a second tumor to develop, in contrast to the poor survival time of patients with advanced gastric cancer. While this assertion is not confirmed by the statistics of Park et al., it is entirely consistent with the findings of Ikeda et al. and Bozzetti et al. regarding EGC, Both groups reported that the incidence of second tumors in surgically treated EGC patients is clearly higher than in those patients with advanced gastric cancer.

Ikeda reported a 5% incidence of a second tumor, based on a series of 1,070 patients, while the Italian series was smaller (105 patients), with a 9.5% incidence of second neoplasms. In both cases, the most frequently affected organ was the lung: 17 cases out of 54 in the Japanese research, and three cases out of 10 in the Italian study. The second most-often targeted organ was the colon-rectum, 10 cases out of 54 in the Japanese statistics, followed by the esophagus and breast. In the Italian data, the breast was the second most frequently involved. All studies found that male sex and age >60 years old were the factors statistically most often associated with the development of a second neoplasm, while the tumor site, histological type, vascular and lymph-node involvement did not seem to influence the development of a second tumor.

The reasons for this increased susceptibility to the development of a second neoplasm in EGC patients are not still clear. Some authors [16] have hypothesized that, due to continuous nitrosification of their environment, the bacteria in the residual stomach form N-nitroso compounds, which subsequently play a carcinogenetic role on the target organs. Regardless of the reasons, post-surgical EGC patients should be carefully followed, with particular attention paid to the lung, colon-rectum, breast, and esophagus, especially during the first 5 years after surgery, as this is the period when, according to the statistics reported above, there is a higher possibility of developing a second tumor (Table 13.7). Given the favorable prognosis of the EGC, the second neoplasm becomes an important prognostic factor regarding long-term survival. Moreover, according to Ikeda et al.'s research, the risk of a second tumor is almost double that of tumoral recurrence (5% vs. 2.8%).

In patients with advanced gastric cancer, the risk of a second neoplasm is low enough (2.8–6.8%) that a strict association between the primary stomach tumor and the risk of second primary neoplasm can be excluded (Table 13.7).

Table 13.7 Multiple primary malignancies (*MPM*) associated with gastric cancer: summary

Tumor	Patients (n)	MPM (%)	Location (%)
Advanced gastric cancer	2,509	65 (2.6)	Colon-rectum (33.8%)
			Hepatobiliary (10.8)
Early gastric cancer	1,070 (Ikeda)	54 (5)	Lung (17/54)
			Colon-rectum (10/54)
	105 (Bozzetti)	10 (9.5%)	Lung (3/10)
			Breast (2/10)

n, Number of patients

Primary Malignancies: Post-pancreatic Cancer

Overall, patients with pancreatic cancer have an unfavorable outcome, with the exception of the IPMC (intraductal papillary mucinous carcinoma) form, in which long-term survival is good. IPMC is characterized by intraductal growth and intense mucosal secretion into the pancreatic ducts. Histologically, IPMC consists of different cell types with different characteristics, ranging from adenoma to invasive carcinoma. In the following, we analyze the incidence and characteristics of other (second) tumors in association (simultaneous, synchronous, metachronous) with IPMC [18–20].

Statistical Experience

From 1980 to 2004, 79 patients with IPMC, diagnosed by endoscopic retrograde cholangio-pancreatography (ERCP), were treated at Tokyo Metropolitan Komagone Hospital. Of the 79 patients in the study population, 79 were male and 25 female, with a mean age of 68.5 ±9.2 years.

Second malignancies were found, in association with pancreatic IPMC, in other sites in 24 (30.3%) patients [21]. The most frequently associated second tumors were gastric cancer and colorectal cancer, followed by pulmonary and esophageal cancer. The mean follow-up time was 3.2 ±0.5 years (range 0.2–20); the mean age was 71.9 ±8.2 years. Interestingly, there were no differences in terms of sex (Table 13.8).

Considerations

The incidence of a second malignant tumor (simultaneous, synchronous, metachronous) in association with pancreatic cancer is reported to be 7% [18], but we found that the incidence was much higher (30.3%). Similar results were obtained by Yamaguchi et al. [19], who reported an incidence of 27% of second malignancies in association with IPMC. Thus, the association between IPMC and the development of a primary malignant tumor in another site is not rare – a possibility that must be considered in the diagnostic and staging phases. Furthermore, during follow-up the probability of a second tumor in the most frequently associated organs must be seriously considered and investigated [21, 22].

Table 13.8 Tumors associated with intraductal papillary-mucinous carcinoma: results of Kamisawa [21]

Second tumor (*n*)	Simultaneous/synchronous	Metachronous
Gastric (8)	7	1
Colon-rectum (3)	3	0
Esophageal (1)	1	0
Pulmonary (4)	2	2
Pancreatic (3)	2	1
Breast (0)	0	0
Hepatocellular (2)	2	0
Uterine (0)	0	0
Pharyngeal (0)	0	0
Bile duct (1)	1	0
Prostatic (1)	1	0
Laryngeal (1)	0	1

Primary Malignancies: Post-gynecological Cancer

Ovarian cancer is the most important cause of death due to gynecological tumors. In a Canadian National Tumor Institute study, Dent et al. [23] evaluated 284 women with ovarian cancer: 29 women (11%) had a second tumor, 24 of which were solid and five hematologic.

Second tumor after ovarian cancer developed in 11 women with stage IA, two with stage IB, four with stage IIA, ten with stage IIB, and two with stage III disease. In accordance with previous studies, this analysis showed a relationship between chemotherapy and development of a second tumor, above all leukemia and bone marrow tumors. During a 13.5-year follow-up, the higher risk of developing a second tumor (RR = 1.55) may have been due to genetic factors.

The greater survival after invasive breast cancer is to the result of early diagnosis and improved postoperative treatment. However, several studies have shown that these women have a high incidence of a non- mammary second gynecological tumor.

Escobar of the Cleveland Clinic Foundation (Ohio) [24] studied 4126 women with ductal carcinoma, infiltrating or in situ; of these 125 (3%) developed a second neoplasia. In 63%, the second tumor was detected at stage I TNM stage for breast cancer; 93 patients (74%) developed a non-gynecological tumor (17 colorectal cancers, 18 lung cancers, 8 lymphomas, 11 pancreatic cancers, 5 thyroid cancer, and 34 other tumors). The 32 gynecological tumors involved the uterus or endometrium (12), cervix (3), ovaries (14), vagina or vulva (3). Of the 125 cancers, 49 (39%) were synchronous and 76 (61%) metachronous with respect to the breast cancer; 47 (62%) patients with metachronous cancer had received adjuvant radiotherapy.

This study demonstrates 3% of breast cancer patients may develop a second tumor in the first follow-up year. A second tumor is associated with a higher mortality, despite successful treatment of the first tumor, and likely occurs for genetic reasons (BRCA1/BRCA2) or after chemotherapy or radiotherapy.

The low radiation exposure and doses have largely eliminated second tumors in these patients, and a role for tamoxifen in second-tumor development has not been established.

Non-radiotherapy-induced second tumors include such as thyroid cancers or sarcoma. Takeda et al. [25], in a retrospective study of 1,044 women who had a gynecological tumor, concluded that breast cancer was the most likely second tumor after endometrial or ovarian cancer. Others studies have shown a relationship between these tumors such that the risk is well-recognized. In the following, hereditary BRCA1/BRCA2-related breast and ovarian cancers will not be discussed; instead, we examine only those neoplasms not related to genetic anomalies.

Neely underlined the high incidence of ovarian cancer (RR = 1.4) in 49,975 women with breast cancer, and noted a correlation with aging (>60 years), menopause, familial ovarian cancer, use of birth control pills.

An epidemiological study by Rozen et al. [26] showed that women who underwent surgery for breast, uterine, or ovarian cancer had a higher incidence of colorectal cancers, as determined through a screening program including: occult stool blood and colonoscopy. The study was carried out on 183 women with breast, uterine, or ovarian cancer and 252 healthy women. Tumors, neoplastic lesions, and adenomatous polyps were 2.5 more frequent in the cancer group. In the largest group, those women with a past breast cancer history, the correct relative risk because of a family history of gastrointestinal cancer was of 3.0 ($p = 0.03$). This pilot study confirmed the importance of regular screening of these patients, especially those with a positive family history for gastrointestinal cancer. The American Cancer Society recommends that in asymptomatic women, over 50 years old a sigmoidoscopy should be carried out every 3 or 5 years after two negative exams in a single year.

Molecular-based hypotheses to explain the development of a second tumor are numerous and controversially discussed. Menopausal women with a previous gynecological tumor have a higher risk of developing colorectal cancer. This was demonstrated in a study carried out by Corrao et al. [27] on the risk of tumor development in menopausal women who had been on hormonal replacement therapy. This long-term study highlighted that the hormonal replacement therapy is associated with a high-risk of breast cancer and a low risk of colorectal cancer; it instead recommended transdermal therapy as it carries a lower cancer risk than oral therapies.

Takano et al. [28] found microsatellite instability (MSI) together with altered mismatch repair genes (MMR) MLH1, MSH2 and MSH6 in 63 patients with endometrial sporadic cancers who subsequently developed colorectal and breast cancer. MMR gene alterations are involved in the carcinogenesis of colorectal and breast cancers. The presence of MSI in endometrial sporadic cancer may serve as a predictive risk marker of colorectal cancer.

A study by Werner, reported by the International Federation of Gynecology and Obstetrics (FIGO) [29], evaluated the risk of developing a second primitive tumor in 125 women with cervical carcinoma. Patients with stage I and II tumors treated with oncologically radical procedures and radiotherapy were included. During the 34-month follow-up metachronous (breast, lung, melanoma, non-Hodgkin lymphoma, and vulval tumors) as well as synchronous (bladder and thyroid) tumors were diagnosed. All second tumors were situated in non-irradiated sites. The highest incidence of metachronous tumors were those of the breast. This led to the conclusion that genetic anomalies are at the basis of a common etiology to develop a second tumor. Other authors consider that, beyond radiotherapy, human papillomavirus (HPV) infection and cigarette smoking are risk factors for the development of a second tumor in women previously treated for cervical cancer. Chaturvedi [30] noted that in long-term follow-up (40 years average) women who had not been treated with radiotherapy had the same risk of developing a second tumor as those who had. HPV is considered the main cause of cervical cancer, but in women already treated for this cancer viral infection plays an important etiological role in the development of a second tumor, most often in the vagina, vulva, anus, or the oropharynx.

Cigarette smoking acts is associated with second tumors of the pharynx, trachea, bronchi and lung, pancreas, and bladder.

Malignancies of the female genital sphere, while hormonally related, show very different and variable behaviors. As adjuvant and neo-adjuvant therapy, an etiological role for radiotherapy has been cited in some studies as the cause of second tumors, although in other studies conflicting results have been reported. Long-term follow-up is fundamental and should not be limited to the primary organ; instead all organs and organ systems have to be examined, with the aim of diagnosing a second neoplasm as early as possible, as they are the main cause of death. Most authors agree on the factor (HPV, cigarette etc.) that contributed to the development of the first neoplasm if the risk persists, it may lead to the development of a second tumor as well, In these cases, monitoring specific organs can lead to the identification of multiple primary tumors at a subclinical stage.

Conclusions

The data presented here offer strong support for systematic monitoring in patients at risk for a second tumor. Cost-benefit considerations are such that post-operative oncological screening must be aimed at those organs most frequently affected by a second malignancy. Several studies have demonstrated that a patient who developed a sporadic cancer has a 1.3-fold higher risk of developing a second malignancy compared to someone who has never had a tumor [21]. This suggests a role for molecular as well as many other factors, including the characteristics of the index tumor.

Moreover, a good prognosis is, at the same time, associated with a higher probability to develop a second neoplasm, as confirmed by the fact that patients with esophageal tumors detected at an early TNM stage have a greater likelihood of a second neoplasia. Similarly, EGC and IPMC of the pancreas, i.e., malignancies with a relatively good prognosis, are mainly correlated with the development of a second tumor. The relationship between better prognosis and the development of a second neoplasm seems to suggest a "predisposition" in some patients.

Chronic exposure to non-hereditary risk factors (tobacco smoking, alcohol, HPV) is not only implicated in the development of the first tumor bur in the second as well. In some cases, the latter can present with the same histological characteristics as the index tumor, even if it is located in a distant organ or in another body region.

In some cases the same therapies that cure the first tumor contribute or cause the development of the second one. According to one study [16], gastric resection, used to cure stomach cancer, can result in anatomical and physiopathological modifications that favor the development of colon cancer. It has also been observed that the use of hormone adjuvant therapies in the treatment of gynecological tumors can, in the long term, lead to a second neoplasia in distant organs.

The "non-codified" syndromes, or "neoplastic associations," discussed in this chapter are not genetically transmitted pathologies. Their incidence is relatively low, except in esophageal cancer, in which the risk of second-tumor development is 20–30%, and EGC, with a second-tumor risk of 5–10%. This low incidence perhaps explains why general screening programs have not been implemented. However, since the prognosis of multiple malignancies is significantly correlated with that of the "index tumor" when the latter has the same characteristics, we think it appropriate to orientate follow-up towards those organs where second malignancies more frequently occur, both at the initial staging phase, to exclude probable double or synchronous neoplasms, and in a second, long-term phase, to promptly identify the beginning of a metachronous tumor.

References

1. The Research Group for Population-based Cancer Registration in Japan (2002) Cancer incidence and incidence rates in Japan in 1997: estimates based on data from 12 population-based cancer registries. Jpn J Clin Oncol 32:318–322
2. Taeger D, Sun Y, Keil U et al (2000) A stand-alone Windows application for computing exact person-years, standardized mortality ratios and confidence intervals in epidemiological studies. Epidemiology 11:607–608
3. Bidoli P, Bajetta E, Stani SC et al (2002) Ten-year survival with chemotherapy and radiotherapy in patients with squamous cell carcinoma of the esophagus. Cancer 94:352–361
4. Kumagai Y, Kawano T, Nakajima Y et al (2001) Multiple primary cancers associated with esophageal carcinoma. Surg Today 31:872–876
5. Wind P, Roullet MH, Quinaux D et al (1999) Long-term results after esophagectomy for squamous cell carcinoma of the esophagus associated with head and neck cancer. Am J Surg 178:251–255
6. Kumagai Y, Kawano T, Nakajima Y et al (2001) Multiple primary cancers associated with esophageal carcinoma. Surg Today 31:872–876
7. Natsugoe S, Matsumoto M, Okumura H et al (2005) Multiple primary carcinomas with esophageal squamous cell cancer: clinicopathologic outcome. World J Surg 29:46–49
8. Matsubara T, Yamada K, Nakagawa A (2003) risk of second primary malignancy after esophagectomy for squamous cell carcinoma of the thoracic esophagus. J Clin Oncol 21:4336–4341
9. Yasuda M, Kuwano H, Watanabe M et al (2000) p53 expression in squamous dysplasia associated with carcinoma of the oesophagus evidence for field carcinogenesis. Br J Cancer 83:1033–1038
10. Matsubara T, Ueda M, Uchida C et al (2000) Modified stomach roll for safer reconstruction after subtotal esophagectomy. J Surg Oncol 75:214–216
11. Lundegardh G, Hansson LE, Nyren O et al (1991) The risk of gastrointestinal and other primary malignant disease following gastric cancer. Acta Oncol 30:1–6
12. Park YK, Kim DY, Joo JK et al (2005) Clinicopathological features of gastric carcinoma patients with other primary carcinomas. Langenbecks Arch Surg 390:300–305
13. Ikeda Y, Saku M, Kishihara F, Maehara Y (2005) Effective follow-up for recurrence or a second primary cancer in patients with early gastric cancer. Br J Surg 92:235–239
14. Bozzetti F, Bonfanti G, Mariani L et al (2000) Early gastric cancer: unrecognized indicator of multiple malignancies. World J Surg 24:583–587
15. Yoshino K, Asanuma F, Hanatani Y et al (1985) Multiple primary cancers in the stomach and other organs: frequency and the effects on prognosis. Jpn J Clin Oncol 15:183–190

16. Kim SH, Min JS, Whang KC (1984) Multiple primary malignant tumors. J Korean Stat Soc 26:314–319
17. Ikeda Y, Saku M, Kawanaka H et al (2003) Features of second primary cancer in patients with gastric cancer. Oncology 65:113–117
18. Sugiyama M, Atomi Y (1999) Extrapancreatic neoplasm occur with unusual frequency in patient with intraductal papillary mucinous tumors of the pancreas. Am J Gastroenterol 94:470–473
19. Yamaguchi K, Yohohata K, Noshiro H et al (2000) Mucinous cystic neoplasm of the pancreas intraductal papillary-mucinous tumor of the pancreas. Eur J Surg 166:141–148
20. Eguchi H, Ishikawa O, Ohigashi H et al (2006) Patients with pancreatic intraductal papillary mucinous neoplasm are at high risk of colorectal cancer development. Surgery 139(6):749–754
21. Kamisawa T, Tu Y, Egawa N, Nakajima H (2005) Malignancies associated with intraductal papillary mucinous neoplasm of the pancreas. World J Gastroenterol 11(36):5688–5690
22. Eriguchi N, Aoyagi S, Hara M et al (2000) Synchronous or metachronous double cancer of the pancreas and other organs: report on 12 cases. Surg Today 30:718–721
23. Dent SF, Klaassen D, Pater JL et al (2000) Second primary malignancies following the treatment of early stage ovarian cancer: update of a study by the National Cancer Institute of Canada-Clinical Trials Group (NCIC-CTG). Ann Oncol 11:65–68
24. Escobar PF, Patrick R, Rybickiy L et al (2006) Primary gynecological neoplasms and clinical outcomes in patients diagnosed with breast carcinoma. Int J Gynecol Cancer 16(Suppl 1):118–122
25. Takeda T, Sagae S, Koizumi M et al (1995) Multiple primary malignancies in patients with gynecologic cancer. Int J Gynecol Cancer 5:34–39
26. Rozen P, Fireman Z, Figer A, Ron E (1986) Colorectal tumor screening in women with a past history of breast, uterine, or ovarian malignancies. Cancer 57(6):1235–1239
27. Corrao G, Zambon A, Conti V et al (2007) Menopause hormone replacement therapy and cancer risk: an Italian record linkage investigation. Ann Oncol 19(1):150–155
28. Takano K, Ichikawa Y, Ueno E et al (2005) Microsatellite instability and expression of mismatch repair genes in sporadic endometrial cancer coexisting with colorectal or breast cancer. Oncol Rep 13(1):11–16
29. Werner-Wasik M, Schmid CH, Bornstein LE, Madoc-Jones H (1995) Increased risk of second malignant neoplasms outside radiation fields in patients with cervical carcinoma. Cancer 75(9):2281–2285
30. Chaturvedi AK, Engels EA, Gilbert ES et al (2007) Second cancers among 104,760 survivors of cervical cancer: evaluation of long-term risk. J Natl Cancer Inst 99(21):1634–1643

Chapter 14
Laboratory for Patients at Risk of Multiple Primary Malignancies

Marcello Caggiano, Angela Mariano, Massimiliano Zuccaro, Sergio Spiezia, Marco Clemente, Vincenzo Macchia

Introduction

Biomarkers are a useful laboratory diagnostic approach for the non-invasive early detection of disease and recurrent disease. An ideal tumor marker is a protein or protein fragment that can be easily detected in the patient's blood or urine, but is not detectable in healthy people. The first of such biomarkers to be used in laboratory testing was carcinoembryonic antigen (CEA), introduced in 1965. Other biomarkers currently in use are CA 19-9 (gastrointestinal tumors), CA125 (ovarian cancer), Ca 15-3 (breast cancer). However, while the levels are very low in healthy people they become substantially elevated only when a considerable amount of cancer is present. Moreover, these markers are for the most part not specific for a single tumor. Women with breast cancer or gynecological disease may have elevated CEA and CA 125. Another cancer biomarker, and perhaps the best known one, is prostate-specific antigen (PSA), which allows for the early detection of prostate disease. The serum PSA test is used in screening programs for prostate cancer and has brought about a dramatic increase in early detection of the disease. Nonetheless, for most cancers biomarkers with high specificity and sensibility are lacking, which limits our ability to screen the majority of tumors. PSA, for example, is very sensitive but has low specificity. It remains the only tumor biomarker certified by the US Food and Drug Administration for widespread screening, which is carried out along with digital rectal examination. Technological advances in genomic and proteomics have produced candidate markers with screening potential. Most biomarkers are used in follow-up evaluation; these include CA125, which is present in a subset of ovarian cancers. CA125 is also elevated in endometriosis and some other benign conditions, CEA is a marker of colon cancer but its specificity and sensitivity are too low to recommend its use as a screening marker although is measured in follow-up examinations. In addition, CEA levels influence the surgical strategy in patients who have previously had colorectal resection or neoplasia.

In multiple primary malignancies (MPM), biomarkers have several advantages as screening too as they reveal the association of the tumors and can aid the clinician in determining the optimal therapeutic approach, either non-invasive or invasive (surgical, other). The newest biomarkers are based on gene arrays and proteomic technologies; others can simply be measured in the urine, including bladder tumor antigen. Thus, multiple biomarkers and/or signature protein/gene profiles can be used to identify a particular cancer. Further developments in identifying protein biomarkers together with progress in genetic and cytological markers will provide a tool of satisfactory predictive value, thus overcoming the limitations posed by low sensitivity and specificity. In the following, we describe a rational use of biomarkers in the detection and follow-up of MPM.

Multiple Endocrine Neoplasia 1

This hereditary syndrome is transmitted in an autosomal dominant manner and is caused by an inactivating mutation of the MEN 1 gene, which manifests as primary hyperparathyroidism, islet cell tumors, and pituitary adenomas. Patients can also present with cutaneous manifestation and other neoplastic manifestation, including carcinoids, thyroid tumors, adrenal adenomas, lipomas, pheochromocytomas, and meningiomas.

Tumoral markers provide an important test for diagnosis and follow-up (gastrin, pancreatic peptide, prolactin, IGF-1). The newest, chromogranin is a polypeptidic group that increases in the blood of patients with endocrine neoplasias, including hyperparathyroidism and tumors of pancreatic islet cells. Neuron-specific enolase (NSE) is increased in pancreatic islet cells tumor. Other biomarkers expected to aid in the diagnosis of MEN 1 are S-100, 7-B2, neurotensin, and the alpha subunit of human chorionic gonadotrophin (hCG).

Multiple Endocrine Neoplasia 2

This autosomal dominant disease is characterized by the presence of medullary thyroid carcinoma (MTC), primary hyperparathyroidism, and pheochromocytoma. These often clinically occult cancers are difficult to accurately diagnose and treat, although minimal elevations of plasma calcitonin (CT) can be measured by a specific immunoassay. Because MTC occurs in nearly 100% of patients with MEN IIa and MEN IIb and is usually the first abnormality expressed, diagnosis of these diseases in kindred at risk is accomplished by screening for the presence of the thyroid tumor. Measurement of the peptide pentagastrin has proved to be more potent than the standard 4-ho calcium infusion in stimulating CT secretion from MTC cells. Many authors [1] recommend that family members at risk for the development of MTC undergo annual calcium pentagastrin stimulation testing, beginning as early as age 5 and continuing until age of 40–45. The diagnosis of pheochromocytoma in MEN IIa and MEN IIb patients can be made biochemically, by measuring urinary excretion of catecholamine and catecholamine metabolites. Since Ishikawa and Hanada demonstrated elevated plasma levels of CEA in patients with MTC, several investigators have evaluated this glycoprotein as an additional tumor marker. Basal plasma CEA levels are rarely increased in patients with early MTC, and they do not increase after calcium or pentagastrin stimulation. However, in some patients serial measurements of plasma CEA levels may provide a better index of tumor burden than plasma calcitonin levels. In addition, measurements of this marker may be useful in following patients with metastatic disease [1].

Lynch Syndrome (Hereditary Non-polyposis Colorectal Cancer)

Lynch syndrome is best understood as a hereditary predisposition to malignancy characterized by an autosomal dominant inheritance, early onset of malignancy with a predilection for the proximal colon, multiple colorectal cancers, the absence of premonitory lesions (e.g., adenoma) and the occurrence of cancer in certain extracolonic sites, notably endometrium and ovary. The management of laboratory values [2] in this pathology includes serum CA 125 levels, an increase of which has been associated with epithelial ovarian cancer. Elevated serum CA 125 levels (≥35 units per ml.) were detected in 50–96% of patients with non-mucinous epithelial ovarian carcinoma confined to the pelvis. CEA, hCG, and tissue polypeptide antigen (TPA) have also been used to predict disease extent or presence in patients with epithelial ovarian cancer. Serum levels of neither CEA nor HCG have any utility as tumor markers in ovarian carcinoma, whereas the utility of TPA and serum levels of CA125 in monitoring ovarian cancer has been confirmed. The use of monoclonal antibodies directed toward cancer antigens, such as TAG 72,3 and CA 15-3 in combination, improved sensitivity over that of CA 125 alone.

Von Hippel Lindau Disease

This is an autosomal-dominant inherited familial cancer syndrome caused by mutations in the VHL tumor suppressor gene. VHL disease is characterized by marked phenotypic variability but the most common tumors are hemangioblastomas of the retina and central nervous system and clear-cell renal cell carcinoma. Endocrine tumors, most commonly pheochromocytoma and non-secretory pancreatic islet cell cancers, demonstrate marked interfamilial variations in frequency and are significant causes of morbidity and, sometimes, mortality. DNA polymorphism analysis can identify individuals likely to carry the VHL disease gene among asymptomatic members of disease families. This technique serves to focus attention on those individuals who require periodic medical examination and may help to alleviate the morbidity and mortality associated with this disease. High urinary concentrations of catecholamines, metanephrine, and plasma chromogranin A are suggestive of pheochromocytoma [3].

Hereditary Breast-Ovarian Cancer

Early age of onset of breast cancer (often before age 50), a family history of both breast and ovarian cancer, bilateral cancers (developing in both breasts or both ovaries, independently), and the development of both breast and ovarian cancer are typical features of HBOC. Again, there is an autosomal dominant pattern of inheritance and an increased incidence of tumors of other specific organs, such as the prostate. Other predisposing factors include: family history of male breast cancer and Ashkenazi Jewish ancestry. DNA linkage studies identified the first gene associated with breast cancer, BRCA1, located on chromosome 17. Mutations in BRCA1 are transmitted in an autosomal dominant pattern. Both copies of a tumor suppressor gene must be altered or mutated before a person develops cancer. In HBOC, the first mutation is inherited from either the mother or the father and is therefore present in all cells of the body. This is called a germline mutation. Whether a person who has a germline mutation will develop cancer and where the cancer(s) will develop depends upon where (which cell type) the second mutation occurs. What causes these additional mutations to be acquired is unknown, but chemical, physical, or biological environmental exposures, or chance errors in cell replication have been suggested. Heterozygous ataxia telangiectasia mutated (ATM) gene mutations have also been associated with increased risk for breast cancer and potentially for other cancers as well.

Few data are available on the circadian rhythmicity in cancer patients. Since monitoring individuals for HBOC usually implies the follow-up of blood concentrations of a number of biological variables, it would be of value to examine the circadian variations of serum cortisol and tumor marker antigens. We carried out a study of 33 cancer patients (13 breast cancer patients and 20 ovarian cancer patients) [4]. The profiles of serum cortisol were documented, since this hormone is considered to be a strong marker of circadian rhythms. The results showed that eight out of 13 breast cancer patients and 15 out of 20 ovarian cancer patients had deeply altered cortisol circadian patterns. The modifications were either high levels over a 24-h period, and/or erratic peaks and troughs, and/or flattened profiles. Within 24 h, variations of tumor marker antigens as large as 70% were observed but no typical individual circadian patterns could be identified, neither could a relationship between cortisol subgroups and concentration of tumor marker antigens at 8 h be observed. The question thus arises as to the origin of the cortisol circardian alterations, whether they are related to a cause or a consequence of the disease, and their possible influence on therapeutic strategies.

Serum CA 125 is the most useful marker, as its level is elevated in the majority of HBOC patients. In one study, serum CA 15-3 levels were elevated >100 U/ml in 89% of patients. Also important is measurement of serum PSA because of the risk of these patients to develop prostatic neoplasias.

Peutz-Jegher Syndrome

Here, hamartomatous polyps of the gastrointestinal tract (stomach, small bowel, colon) are associated with mucocutaneous pigmentation (lips, oral mucosa, fingers, forearm, toes, umbilical area). Although there is said to be no relation between this syndrome and the development of cancer, River et al. [5] reported that is a series of 51 patients, ten (19.6 %) had polyps in which carcinomatous changes were detected. Thus, all patients with Peutz-Jegher syndrome should be considered at risk of developing neoplasias and therefore undergo biochemical screening.

Similarly, there is also a higher incidence of pancreatic cancer in those with Peutz-Jeghers syndrome. Latchford [6] suggested that screening strategies should be reviewed. CEA levels and CA 19.9 are the most useful markers. Although benign polyps may result in slight elevations of serum CEA, a fivefold increase is consistent with the development of carcinoma. Measurement of serum CEA levels in a patient who presents with a suspicious polypoid lesion is recommended by some clinicians. If an elevated level is confirmed on repeat assay, the patient should undergo thorough imaging evaluation. A new method is the use of radiolabeled antibody to CEA and external scintigraphy to detect the exact location and extent of the tumor. In some reports, radioimmunolocalization appears promising, and labeled monoclonal antibodies to tumor antigens are being developed to image and treat these tumors. In one study, systemic preoperative imaging of patients with In-labeled anti-CEA monoclonal antibody detected 69% of primary tumors [6].

MPM: "Not Codified" Syndromes

Improvements in cancer therapy and early diagnosis have allowed many patients with a first tumor to have a normal life expectancy. However, some of these patients will develop a second primary neoplasia. Therapeutic success in treating the second tumor clearly depends on its early diagnosis.

Esophageal Tumors

Patients who have had an esophageal tumor seem to be an increased risk of developing a second primary neoplasia in the head and neck (42.4%, of which 71.4% occur in the respiratory tract), stomach (32%), lung, and colon. To date, there are no biomarkers that allow the detection of either upper respiratory tract or epidermal tumors. The use of serum M2-pyruvate kinase for the detection of early gastric cancer remains unclear. The detection of lung neoplasia by measuring biomarkers in sputa, serum, and exhaled breath is being explored, as is the measurements of cytokines, CYFRA 21-1, ProGRP, and circulating cell free DNA. Only NSE and chromogranin A have been confirmed for the early detection and diagnosis of neuroendocrine lung neoplasias. Elevated CEA levels may also be indicative, as for neoplasias of the gastrointestinal tract. Despite their low sensitivity, the concentration of biomarkers should be measured every 3 months, especially in male, elderly patients, smokers, and those with a history of alcohol abuse. In these patients these tests should be carried out in association with follow-up imaging procedures.

Gastric Tumors

Although the degree of association between gastric tumors and other neoplasias varies in literature reports, a relationship has been established. For example, one study found a 26% increase in colorectal tumors, a 10% increase in esophageal tumors, 8% for breast cancer, and 6% for tumors of involving the live. Other associations are pancreatic cancer and subsequent prostate cancer (1%), and endometrial cancer (6–11%), and lung and urinary tract tumors (8 and 3%, respectively) [7]. The 5-year survival of these patients with a second primary tumor is high and is the same as in those patients with only one gastric neoplasia. This is due to frequent follow-up with gastroscopy and CT scan. Laboratory diagnosis has only a marginal role, and the measurement of colorectal cancer markers is not widespread because of their low specificity. Instead, given the high number of gastrointestinal neoplasias, serum CEA levels, especially in male patients with gastric neoplasia in the distal part of the stomach, should be assayed every 6 months.

Colorectal Cancer

Colorectal cancer is the third most common neoplasia in industrial countries. The development of a new primary colorectal neoplasia is strongly associated with a previous tumor of the colon, prostate cancer, and ovarian cancer (endocrinologically based). Currently, screening for colon cancer by fecal occult blood testing still misses many early cases, up to almost 85%. Therefore, research is being directed at the identification of genetic markers or peptides that accurately detect colorectal cancer [8–11]. Among these, microsatellite instability, which results in mutations in DNA mismatch repair genes (such as MLH1, MSH6 or MSH6) is associated with the prognosis of colorectal cancer. However, like other markers of colorectal cancer marker, the specificity of microsatellite instability is low such that it is not widely used. Moreover, screening for colon cancer is notorious for its poor compliance even though measurement of serum CEA is a milestone in the post-operative follow-up of colorectal cancer patients [12].

In screening for prostate cancer, PSA does not predict disease outcome in newly diagnosed patients and cannot by itself determine the course of treatment

[13]. Recent interest in the author's laboratory and by other researchers has focused on identifying biomarkers that distinguish tumors with the capacity to metastasize, such as thymosin beta-15, which is elevated in metastatic prostate cancer and in combination with PSA can predict the recurrence of prostate cancer with more sensitivity and specificity than PSA alone. Other useful biomarkers are CA 125, which has been tested as a diagnostic and prognostic marker in ovarian cancer but its use is limited by its low specificity and low selectivity. The overexpression of cyclin D1 is related to a more aggressive tumor phenotype and poor prognosis. While expression is not limited to ovarian cancer, it is advisable to measure CD1 serum levels in patients at risk. Serum concentrations of C-terminal telopeptide of type I collagen (ICTP) and tumor-associated trypsin inhibitor have also been measured with respect to the use of these proteins as biomarkers. More advanced techniques have been applied to compare serum protein profiles in different stages of ovarian cancer. Despite the intense efforts carried out thus far, there is still no reliable biomarker strategy that allows improved early detection of this disease. In a follow-up post treatment program for colorectal patients, the only helpful measurements are those of serum PSA or CA 125, together with CEA levels in a standard follow-up program.

Sporadic Breast and Ovarian Cancer

The "non-codified" association between breast and ovarian cancer has long been well known. The occurrence of both neoplasias is thought to have a common endocrinological etiology. Several recent studies have identified proteins that contribute to the detection of breast cancer, such as familial BRCA1 and BRCA2 mutations. A sensitive assay to identify biomarkers that can accurately diagnose the onset of breast cancer using non-invasively collected clinical specimens would be ideal for the early detection of this disease. The earlier and more accurately the diagnostic biomarker can predict disease onset, the more valuable it becomes. Other potential biomarkers include osteopontin, which is a transformation-associated protein. High levels of osteopontin have been detected in patients with cancers of the prostate, breast, and lung. Expression of the HER 2 oncogene in tissue or serum is the most commonly used predictive biomarkers in breast cancer and is significantly related to positive lymph nodes, poor nuclear grade, lack of steroid receptors, and high proliferative activity. CA 125 has been tested as a diagnostic and prognostic marker in ovarian cancer, but it has several limitations including low specificity and low selectivity [14]. Increases in ICTP and tumor-associated trypsin inhibitor have also been studied for their diagnostic and prognostic value. In the future, autoantibodies and abnormal tumor-specific DNA methylation found in cell-free plasma DNA may provide the best opportunity for constructing multiplexed and highly redundant tests that are specific and sensitive enough to be used for early detection of breast cancer [15, 16]. Technologies developed for breast cancer detection will no doubt be useful for other types of cancer [17] (Table 14.1).

Table 14.1 Markers useful in clinical practice

Index tumor	Association	Available markers	Level of information
Esophageal	Gastric	CEA	+/−
Gastric	Lung	NSE	+/−
		Chromogranin A	+/−
	Gastric	M2 PK	Unknown
	Gastrointestinal	M2 PK	+
Breast	Breast	BRCA study	++
	Ovarian	CA 125	+++
	Gastrointestinal	CEA	+
Ovarian	Gynecological	CA 125	+++
	Breast	Osteopontin	+/−
	Gastrointestinal	CEA	+
Colon	Gastrointestinal (colon)	CEA	++
	Prostate	PSA	++
	Pancreas	CA 19-9	+/−
Prostate	Prostate	PSA	+++
	GI	CEA	+
	Lung	NSE	+/−

Technology: Present and Future

Recent advances in genomic and proteomic technologies, including gene array, serial analysis of gene expression (SAGE), and improved 2D PAGE and new mass spectrometric techniques, coupled with bioinformatics tools offer great promise in meeting the demand for new biomarkers that are both sensitive and specific [18]. Genomic approaches have involved the genes encoding ki 6 and prothymosin alpha, which have been previous been identified as prognostic markers of breast cancer. To date, the most significant biomarkers that have emerged from microarray analysis include estrogen/progesterone receptor protein expression, HER 2 alterations, 17 q23 genomic amplifications, and cyclooxygenase-2 protein expression, all of which are suggestive of breast cancer; insulin like growth factor (IGF)-binding protein 2 protein as a marker of prostate cancer; vimentin expression for kidney cancer; and myc na A1 B1 expression for hepatocellular carcinoma. Proteomic approaches aid in the discovery of new biomarkers discovery [19, 20]. The major limitation of 2D PAGE technology is its inability to detect low-abundance proteins and the difficulty of its application to high-throughput assays. Mass spectrometry can be used to quantify the difference in expression of individual proteins under two different conditions, by calculating the ratio of intensities of corresponding peaks containing heavy and light amino acids [21]. This technology has been effectively used in the validation of serum prostate-specific membrane antigen. A proteomic pattern that distinguished different stages of ovarian cancer was identified by this technology. However, problems regarding reproducibility and reduced sensitivity for high molecular weight proteins remain. Immunochemistry is a validated approach but it depends on biopsy samples that are collected using invasive techniques and it misses adjacent, potentially more aggressive tumor cell populations. Enzyme-linked immunoassorbent assay is widely accepted as a clinical tool and is very sensitive. Chip technology has led to a surge in the development of protein-based chips. Glass or plastic chips can be printed with an array of molecules, such as antibodies, that can capture proteins. Ideally, a protein chip containing a panel of antibodies would be able to predict a cancer state by a simple serum or urine test.

The success of any new method depends on it being simple, inexpensive, robust, and reliable. The future of cancer prognosis may rely on a small panel of six to ten markers that allow accurate molecular to indicate the likelihood of metastatic involvement, new neoplasias, and optimal treatment (rapid systemic therapy/surgery). High-throughput technology platforms will support microarray chip technology as well as 2D gel and mass spectrometry; however, they are not easily applicable to the clinical setting and require well-equipped laboratories and well-trained personnel [21, 22]. Simple, rapid, and sensitive microarray-based protein chip, label-free detection systems and antibody-based protein chip systems will advance the discovery of biomarkers and bring their use into clinical practice. We are approaching a time when the use of proper biomarkers will help detect cancer, monitor and manage progression of the disease, and improve its treatment.

References

1. Torre GC, Varaldo E, Bottaro P (2004) State of the art in the diagnosis and therapy of the MEN1 and MEN2 syndromes. G Chir 25(4):109–115
2. Boland CR (2007) Evaluation and management of Lynch syndrome. Clin Adv Hematol Oncol 5(11):851–873
3. Shuin T, Yamasaki I, Tamura K et al (2006) Von Hippel Lindau disease: molecular pathological basis, clinical criteria, genetic testing, clinical features of tumors and treatment. Jpn J Clin Oncol 36(6):337–343
4. Touitou Y, Bogdan A, Lévi F et al (1996) Disruption of the circadian patterns of serum cortisol in breast and ovarian cancer patients: relationship with tumor marker antigens. Br J Cancer 74(8):1248–1252
5. River L, Silverstein J, Tope JW (1976) Benign neoplasm of the small intestine: a critical comprehensive review with reports of 20 new cases. Int Abstr Surg 102:1
6. Latchford A, Greenhalf W, Vitone LJ et al (2006) Peutz-Jeghers syndrome and screening for pancreatic cancer. Br J Surg 93(12):1446–1455

7. Kumar Y, Tapuria N, Kirmani N, Davidson BR (2007) Tumour M2-pyruvate kinase: a gastrointestinal cancer marker. Eur J Gastroenterol Hepatol 19(3):265–276
8. Ouyang DL, Chen JJ, Getzenberg RH, Schoen RE (2005) Noninvasive testing for colorectal cancer: a review. Am J Gastroenterol 100(6):1393–1403
9. Alessandro R, Belluco C, Kohn EC (2005) Proteomic approaches in colon cancer: promising tools for new cancer markers and drug target discovery. Clin Colorectal Cancer 4(6):396–402
10. Bendardaf R, Lamlum H, Pyrhönen S (2004) Prognostic and predictive molecular markers in colorectal carcinoma. Anticancer Res 24(4):2519–2530
11. De Noo ME, Tollenaar RA, Deelder AM, Bouwman LH (2006) Current status and prospects of clinical proteomics studies on detection of colorectal cancer: hopes and fears. World J Gastroenterol 12(41):6594–6601
12. Duffy MJ, van Dalen A, Haglund C et al (2007) Tumour markers in colorectal cancer: European Group on Tumour Markers (EGTM) guidelines for clinical use. Eur J Cancer 43(9):1348–1360
13. Gray MA (2005) Clinical use of serum prostate-specific antigen: a review. Clin Lab 51(3–4):127–133
14. Bast RC Jr, Badgwell D, Lu Z et al (2005) New tumor markers: CA125 and beyond. Int J Gynecol Cancer 15(Suppl 3):274–281
15. Gadducci A, Cosio S, Carpi A et al (2004) Serum tumor markers in the management of ovarian, endometrial and cervical cancer. Biomed Pharmacother 58(1):24–38
16. Gadducci A, Cosio S, Zola P et al (2007) Surveillance procedures for patients treated for epithelial ovarian cancer: a review of the literature. Int J Gynecol Cancer 17(1):21–31
17. Lumachi F, Basso SM (2004) Serum tumor markers in patients with breast cancer. Exper Rev Anticancer Ther 4(5):921–931
18. Anderson JE, Hansen LL, Mooren FC et al (2006) Methods and biomarkers for the diagnosis and prognosis of cancer and other diseases: towards personalized medicine. Drug Resist Updat 9(4–5):198–210
19. Cho-Chung YS (2006) Autoantibody biomarkers in the detection of cancer. Biochim Biophys Acta 1762(6):587–591
20. Srivastava S (2006) Molecular screening of cancer: the future is here. Mol Diagn Ther 10(4):221–230
21. Wiesner A (2004) Detection of tumor markers with ProteinChip technology. Curr Pharm Biotechnol 5(1):45–67
22. Chatterjee SK, Zetter BR (2005) Cancer biomarkers: knowing the present and predicting the future. Oncology 37–50

Chapter 15

Multiple Primary Malignancies: Role of Advanced Endoscopy To Identify Synchronous and Metachronous Tumors of the Digestive Tract

Giuseppe Galloro, Luca Magno, Giorgio Diamantis, Antonio Pastore, Simona Ruggiero, Salvatore Gargiulo, Marcello Caggiano

Introduction

The development of new endoscopy systems represents a significant advance in the diagnosis of tumors. The prognosis for patients is strictly dependent on the early detection of malignant lesions, because early lesions of the digestive tract can be removed endoscopically by several techniques (e.g., polypectomy, endoscopic mucosal resection, submucosal endoscopic dissection).

Within the limits of multiple primitive malignancies (MPM), there are several associations involving gastrointestinal tumors, both synchronous and metachronous (esophagus-stomach, stomach-colon, colon-colon etc). Advanced endoscopy is the method of choice for the early diagnosis, treatment, and follow-up of these tumor associations, and complete cure is possible in many cases. It is important to detect not only the more common polypoid type of malignant lesions associated with a primary tumor but also flat and depressed neoplasias. Nowadays, endoscopy can be performed with new and powerful endoscopes whose optic features provide an improved resolution that reveals a wealth of surface detail.

Chromoendoscopy

Chromoendoscopy is an endoscopic examination involving the use of dyes [1]. Information that cannot be obtained or a structure that is poorly visualized by conventional endoscopy is well-defined by the addition of a dye, resulting in accurate lesion detection and precise qualitative diagnosis. The technique allows the detection of small non-polypoid lesions (as defined by the Paris classification [2]), which are very often missed by standard endoscopy, and confirms both the surface structure and the nature of the lesion's edges in detail point of view, about .

For many years, the Eastern and Western endoscopic and histologic classifications of early digestive tumors have diverged greatly. Many endoscopists, par-

A. Renda (ed.), *Multiple Primary Malignancies.*
©Springer-Verlag Italia 2009

ticularly those in the West, considered the Japanese classification, with its numerous divisions for the esophagus, stomach, and colon, to be too complex for practical use. Western endoscopists tend to base treatment decisions largely on the size and location of the tumor and on the histology of biopsy specimens. By contrast, Japanese endoscopists have found that the endoscopic classification of a lesion can be an important determinant of when endoscopic therapy is needed.

Another source of differences regarding the value of endoscopic classification of superficial neoplastic lesions arises from East/West differences in the pathological classification of intramucosal neoplasias. The recent Vienna classification [4] has, to some extent, resolved this conflict in its use of the terminology of dysplasia, adenoma, early cancer, and advanced cancer. Following the consensus reached in Vienna, an international group of endoscopists, surgeons, and pathologists gathered in Paris for an intensive workshop designed to explore the utility and clinical relevance of the Japanese endoscopic classification of superficial neoplastic lesions of the gastrointestinal tract. The result of the Paris symposium was the complete convergence of western and eastern views and thus a new common international classification of digestive superficial neoplastic lesions (extremely close to the Japanese one), as shown in Fig. 15.1. According to the Paris classification, there are three major types of superficial neoplastic lesions of the digestive tract as well as several subtypes (Table 15.1).

To improve the quality of diagnosis, the primary step is to identify the presence of an area of the mucosa that is slightly discolored (paler or redder), an irregular microvascular network, or a slight elevation or depression. The second

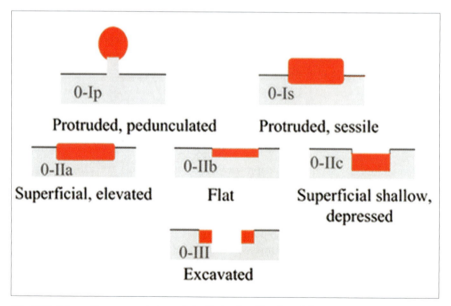

Fig 15.1 Schematic representation of the Paris classification: 0 I protruded or polypoid (Ip and Is), 0 II non-polypoid (II a, IIb, and II c), 0 III non-polypoid and excavated (III)

15 MPM: Role of Advanced Endoscopy To Identify Tumors of the Digestive Tract

Table 1. Paris classification of superficial neoplastic lesions of the digestive tract

Type 0 I protruded or polypoid	01 p (pedunculated)
	01 s (sessile)
Type 0 II or non-polypoid	02 a (superficial, elevated)
	02 b (flat)
	02 c (superficial, depressed)
Type 0 III or excavated	

diagnostic step is based on the use of chromoendoscopy to obtain a meticulous description of the lesion. This method is generally performed using one of the following three dyes.

Indigo Carmine

In the so-called contrast method, the sprayed dye accumulates in concave areas and thus demonstrates unevenness. Usually, 0.1–1% indigo carmine solution is employed. Even lesions with apparently flat surfaces are often minimally depressed and/or elevated. All such depressed lesions should be noted (Fig. 15.2). Another purpose of the contrast method using indigo carmine is to make innominate grooves distinct. The absence of these grooves in flat or depressed lesions is helpful in differentiating neoplastic from non-neoplastic lesions.

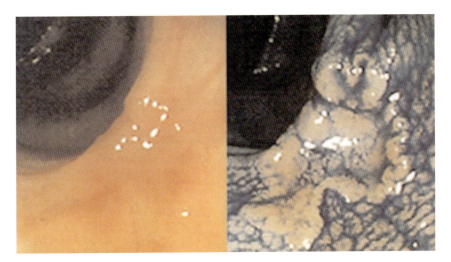

Fig. 15.2 Indigo carmine stain

Methylene Blue

Methylene blue solution (0.5–1%) is taken up and therefore stains the epithelium whereas glandular orifices (pits) are not stained. This feature is used together with magnification to distinguish these different structures.

Cresyl Violet

The lesion is completely washed with water, cleared of adhering mucus, and then sprayed with 0.2–0.4% cresyl violet solution to stain the glandular pits. This technique is used when the pit pattern is examined with magnifying endoscopes (Fig. 15.3).

Magnifying Endoscopy

A histologic diagnosis, including the depth of the lesion, is predicted on the basis of endoscopically obtained data regarding macroscopic morphology, size, color, surface characteristics, evenness, and severity of the mucosal depression. The diagnosis may be followed by biopsy, strip biopsy, polypectomy, surgery, or follow-up observation. To be considered reliable, the endoscopic diagnosis should agree with the histologic diagnosis. The goal of magnifying endoscopy is an accurate qualitative diagnosis based on a study of the pit pattern, i.e., the superficial orifices of the glandular crypts on the digestive mucosal surface [5, 6]. This is achieved by stereomicroscopic analysis of the pit pattern of a large number of digestive-tract lesions.

Magnifying endoscopic observation consists of three steps: (1) differentiation between neoplastic and non-neoplastic lesions; (2) differentiation between adenomas and cancers, including submucosal cancers; and (3) confirmation of the presence or absence of residual tumor after endoscopic treatment.

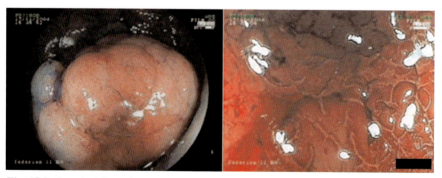

Fig. 15.3 Cresyl violet stain

In the esophagus, we use the Endo [7] classification (Fig. 15.4), with the pit patterns described in Table 15.2.

In the stomach, there are many classifications with no convergence of the endoscopic picture. For this reason, in the study of early non-protruding neoplastic lesions, some authors follow a classification based on the microvascular rather than the pit pattern. This classification, proposed by Yao [8], describes the following endoscopic pictures (Table 15.3).

An irregular microvascular pattern visible by magnified endoscopy can be a very useful marker for differentiating between gastritis and carcinoma.

In the colon-rectum, we use the Kudo [9] classification (Fig. 15.5), which describes the pit patterns listed in Table 15.4.

Based on these classification systems, clinicians can now establish more objectively than ever an endoscopic qualitative diagnosis of early gastrointestinal lesions.

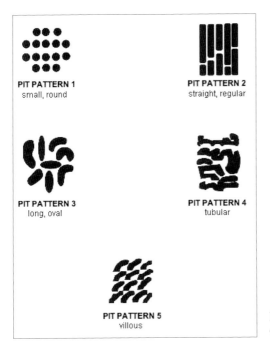

Fig. 15.4 Endo classification of esophageal pit pattern

Table 15.2 Endo classification of esophageal pit patterns (adapted from [7])

Type I	Rounded, regular, and small pits of relatively uniform size and shape
Type II	Long straight lines, of relatively uniform size and shape
Type III	Long oval and curved pits, larger than those of type I
Type IV	Tubular pits, complicated and twisted in a branched or gyrus-like structure
Type V	Villous pits with flat, finger-like projections

Table 15.3 Microvascular classification of gastric lesions

Normal mucosa with normal vascular submucosal pattern, regular and homogeneous distribution of submucosal vessels

Loss of the normal subepithelial capillary network pattern

Proliferation of microvessels that are irregular in both shape and distribution (irregular microvascular pattern)

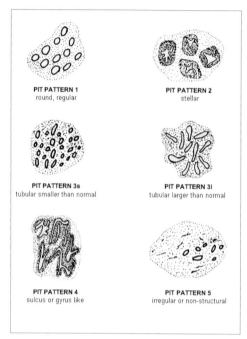

Fig. 15.5 Kudo classification of colorectal pit pattern

Table 4. Kudo classification of pit patterns in the colon-rectum (adapted from [4])

Type I	Normal, rounded, and regular pits 0.02 ± 0.07 mm in size. This is the typical pit of normal mucosa. Shape and size can vary from site to site
Type II	Relatively large pits with a star-like shape 0.02 ± 0.09 mm in size. This is the basic pit pattern of hyperplastic mucosa
Type III s	Tubular or rounded pits that are smaller than normal (0.01 ± 0.03 mm). This is the typical pit pattern of depressed tumors
Type III l	Tubular or rounded pits that are larger than normal (0.03 ± 0.09 mm). This is the typical pit pattern of protruded adenomas
Type IV	Sulcus, branched, or gyrus-like pattern. The pits are 0.2 ± 0.7 mm in size
Type V	Irregular or non-structured surface. This is the basic pattern of submucosal and invasive cancer

Computed Virtual Chromoendoscopy

In this technique, the defined mucosal surface and submucosal capillary vessels are visualized by adjusting the spectroscopic characteristics of the video-endoscopic system using a frame-sequential projection method [10]. Two different types of computed virtual chromoendoscopy systems are available nowaday: the narrow-band imaging system (NBI), developed by the Olympus Medical Systems, and Fuji intelligent color enhancement (FICE), developed by Fujinon Corporation

Video endoscope imaging requires several steps that are based on the frame-sequential image pickup method. Briefly, the light source unit consists of a xenon lamp and a rotation disk with three optical filters. The rotation disk and the monochrome charge-coupled device are synchronized and sequentially generate images [10] in three optical filter bands. By use of all three band images, a single color endoscopic image is synthesized by the video processor. The final image on the monitor is therefore heavily dependent on the spectral features of the optical filters.

In NBI, the three optical filters provide red-blue-green sequential illumination and narrow the bandwidth of the spectral transmittance. The central wavelengths of the three filters are 500, 445, and 415 nm, and each has a bandwidth of 30 nm. These properties of NBI provide limited penetration of light to the mucosal surface and enhanced visualization of the capillary vessels and their fine structure on the surface layer. It was reported that magnifying endoscopic observation of the microvascular architecture of superficial esophageal carcinoma is useful in determining the depth of invasion.

The intrapapillary capillary loops in the normal esophageal mucosa are seen with magnifying endoscopy. In cancerous lesions, computed virtual chromoendoscopy revealed characteristic changes of the intrapapillary capillary loops in the superficial mucosa according to the depth of tumor invasion [11]. Similarly, qualitative diagnosis of a colorectal tumor with a type V pit pattern was obtained using the features of the capillaries, including the vessel diameters, irregularity, and capillary network.

In FICE, the contrast of the mucosal surface is enhanced without the use of dyes. This technology was invented by Yoichi Miyake (Faculty of Engineering, Chiba University, Japan) and introduced by Fujinon. Like NBI, FICE technology is based on the selection of spectral transmittance with a dedicated wavelength. In contrast to NBI, in which the bandwidth of the spectral transmittance is narrowed by optical filters [11], FICE imaging is based on a new spectral estimation technique that obviates the need for optical filters. Instead, an ordinary endoscopic image captured by a video endoscope is sent to a spectral estimation matrix processing circuit in the EPX-4400 digital processor, which estimates the various pixilated spectra of the image. Since the spectra of the pixels are known, imaging can be implemented using a single wavelength. Such single-wavelenght images are randomly selected, and assigned to red, green and blue respectively to build and display a CVC-enhanced color image (Figs. 15.6, 15.7). The digital processing system is able to immediately switch between an ordinary image and

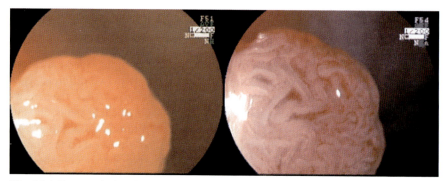

Fig. 15.6 Computed virtual chromoendoscopy: FICE system

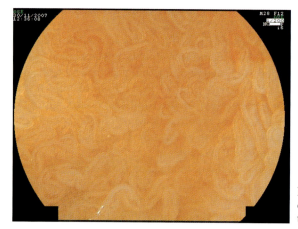

Fig. 15.7 Computed virtual chromoendoscopy: FICE system

a FICE image by the simple push of a button on the endoscope. It is also possible to select the most suitable wavelengths for examination because of the system's variable setting functions (with up to six settings).

The purpose of introducing optical electronics into video endoscopes is to improve the accuracy of diagnosis through image processing and digital technology. We have described the FICE system here, which involves the use of spectral estimation technology to visualize the target in narrowed red, green, and blue bands of the spectrum. Preliminary clinical tests suggest that the properties of FICE are not only of theoretical value but can make a real difference in the clinical setting [12]. Compared with the *conventional* system narrowing the bandwidth and cutting off the longer wavelengths via FICE improves the contrast of capillary patterns and the boundary between different types of tissue, which could improve the diagnosis of early neoplasia. The endoscopists can decide which is the area of interest and can remove the lesion in a targeted fashion without prior biopsy [12].

Confocal Laser Endoscopy

The closest step toward virtual histology is confocal laser endoscopy. Blue light excitation is used and the fluorescence light from endogenous or exogenous fluorophores as well as reflected light from distinct tissues is used to perform images of the colonic mucosa. Moreover, the images can enlarged 1000-fold, thus revealing cellular structures as well [13]. A future trend might be immune-related confocal laser endoscopy, in which specific tumor-related antibodies are coupled with fluorescent dyes and used to label neoplastic areas. This concept may be extended to enhance the contrast between tumor and normal tissue in endoscopic imaging in order to unmask synchronous malignant lesions. Thus, endoscopy is no longer boring routine, it develops into a complex and exciting field of clinical research with new visible details to be discovered [13].

Conclusions

These data show the big potential of advanced endoscopic techniques as a staging tool in the management of patients with suspected digestive dysplasia or early cancer. This kind of endoscopy increases the detection rate of diminutive or flat lesions in digestive tract and enhances the diagnosis and characterization of some mucosal lesions.

For all these reasons, its role in routine surveillance of patients with previoulsy diagnosed primary malignancies (expecially in digestive tract) is very important and remains pivotal for reliably and accuracy.

References

1. Apel M., Jakobs R, Schilling D et al (2006) Accuracy of high-resolution chromoendoscopy in prediction of histologic findings in diminutive lesions of the rectosigmoid. Gastrointest Endosc 63:824–828
2. Anonymous (2003) The Paris endoscopic classification of superficial neoplastic lesions. Gastrointest Endosc 35:S3-S27
3. Johanson JF, Schmitt C, Deas TM (2000) Quality and outcomes assessment in gastrointestinal endoscopy. Gastrointest Endosc 52:827–830
4. Schlemper RJ, Riddell RH, Kato Y et al (2000) The Vienna classification of gastrointestinal epithelial neoplasia. Gut 47:251–255
5. Yao K, Oishi T(2001) Microgastroscopic findings of mucosal microvascular architecture as visualized by magnifying endoscopy. Dig Endosc 13(Suppl):S27-S33
6. Yagi K, Aruga Y, Nakamura A (2005) Magnifying endoscopy for diagnosis of gastric cancer. Stomach Intestine 40:791–799
7. Endo T, Awakawa T, Takahashi H et al (2002) Classification of Barrett's epithelium by magnifying endoscopy. Gastrointest Endosc 55:641–647
8. Yao K, Oishi T, Matsui T et al (2002) Novel magnified endoscopic findings of microvascular architecture in intramucosal gastric cancer. Gastrointest Endosc 56:279–284
9. Kudo S, Tamura S, Nakajima T (1996) Diagnosis of colorectal tumorous lesions by magnifying endoscopy. Gastrointest Endosc 44:8–14

10. Pohl J, May A, Rabenstein T (2007) Computed virtual chromoendoscopy vs. conventional chromoendoscopy with acetic acid for detection of neoplasia in barrett's esophagus: a prospective randomized crossover study. Gastrointest Endosc 65(5):AB348
11. Messmann H, Probst A (2007) Narrow band imaging in Barrett's esophagus – where are we standing? Gastrointest Endosc 65:47–49
12. Burgos H, Porras M, Brenes F, Izquierdo E (2007) Fujinon FICE electronic chromovideoendoscopy helps differentiate the type of metaplasia in patients with chronic atrophic gastritis. Gastrointest Endosc 65:AB353
13. Yoshida S, Tanaka S, Hirata M et al (2007) Optical biopsy of GI lesions by reflectance-type laser-scanning confocal microscopy. Gastrointest Endosc 66:144–149

Chapter 16
Diagnostic Imaging Techniques for Synchronous Multiple Tumors

Vincenzo Tammaro, Sergio Spiezia, Salvatore D'Angelo, Simone Maurea, Giovanna Ciolli, Marco Salvatore

Introduction

According to the literature, 1.2–3.5% of cancer patients are unexpectedly affected by a new synchronous neoplasia (multiple primary malignancies, MPM), detected during a diagnostic or therapeutic phase. In fact, patients already successfully treated for a neoplasia have at least a two-fold possibility of developing a further cancer compared to an age-matched individual never been affected by a neoplastic disease [1]. Over the last several years, world-wide scientific research has been conducted aimed at understanding the cause of this increased risk.

The results of this research have shown that the so-called index tumor, with which the other tumors are often associated, are commonly located in the lungs, esophagus, head and neck, genital-urinary tract, gastrointestinal system and the skin [2]. Furthermore, the new tumor usually affects anatomically unfavorable tissues, such as those of the pancreas. It is therefore evident that an early diagnosis of these lesions is very important. To this end, diagnosis or staging will inevitably require the use of one or several imaging methods.

At present, imaging methods normally used in early diagnoses produce morphological data, which are very accurate but are nonetheless limited with respect to the location and analysis of neoplastic lesions. They are therefore not appropriate for accurate staging, especially when there are multiple and independent lesions. Moreover, while standard cancer screening and staging programs exist for every organ, this is not true for the assessment of MPM. Therefore, the aim of this chapter is to analyze the options for detecting the occurrence of synchronous neoplasias and to distinguish such tumors from metastases.

Organ-related Imaging

To identify synchronous lesions in relationship to an index tumor, it is first necessary to understand the uses and limitations of the main imaging methods.

Pulmonary neoplasias and, in general, those of the breathing apparatus, are analyzed primarily by chest X-ray and bronchoscopy. According to a 2002 survey conducted by Wax [3] with the aim of discovering potential synchronous lesions, traditional chest X-ray has an accuracy of 70%, the accuracy of computed tomography (CT) of the chest is 90% but that of bronchoscopy only 50%. Positron emission tomography (PET)-CT has 100% sensitivity, with a predictive value of 80%. We can therefore deduce that PET-CT will identify pulmonary lesions linked to neoplasia in nearly every case [3]. This is confirmed by our experience, in which PET-CT allowed us to identify pulmonary lesions in patients undergoing examination for other tumors (Fig. 16.1).

When the index tumor is localized to the upper digestive system (esophagus and stomach), the current medical guidelines prescribe endoscope examinations and CT to identify the stage. The first examination for liver and pancreas is ultrasonography (with or without contrast medium) followed by CT and/or nuclear magnetic resonance (NMR). Endoscopic retrograde cholangio-pancreatography (ERCP) is used for bile duct lesions. Correct tumor staging always requires that these procedures are integrated with diagnostic total-body imaging techniques.

Lesions of the colon and rectum are evaluated by a quite different approach. Computed tomography colonography (CTC) is currently used alongside traditional colonoscopy, which still offers not only the advantage of direct observation of suspected lesions but also their possible histological classification, with subsequent confirmation by biopsy. CTC is not an invasive technique, nor does it require any sedation. It is considered safe as the percentage of iatrogenic lesions is low (0.04% colon perforation) [4]. Its limitations are the same as those

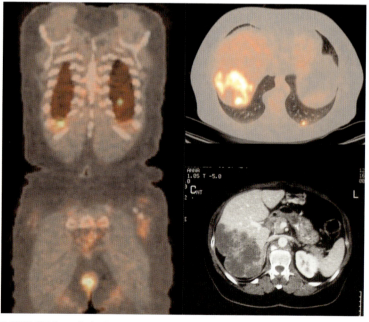

Fig. 16.1 PET-CT: hepatic lesion associated to a pulmonary index tumor

of the other imaging methods, i.e., the possibility of a false-positive result (e.g., traces of stool erroneously considered to be polyps) and, obviously, the impossibility of obtaining a biopsy or removing identified polyps [5]. For this reason, CTC is used especially in patients with an incomplete colonoscopy because it is not meant to replace conventional optic-tube colonoscopy, but rather to provide an alternative when a traditional colonoscopy is not possible. It is worth noting that the literature data show that CTC allows the identification of additional lesions, including MPM (Table 16.1).

An epidemiological review carried out by Xiong [6] compared 17 studies conduced by different authors [7–9] who analyzed the extra-colonic anomalies seen on CTC in 3,488 patients. Of these, 40% had at least one additional lesion; in 2.7%, extra-colonic tumors were identified (0.9% of which N0M0); in 14%, additional diagnostic examinations were needed because the lesions found at CTC were not previously known; and 0.9% of patients received prompt treatments (Table 16.1). In research carried out by Fenlon [10], 10.3% of 29 patients with occlusive distal cancer who could not be examined by endoscope methods were found to also have a proximal synchronous cancer. In another study [11], CTC identified synchronous cancers not seen by classical colonoscopy in three (10%) patients out of 29, as well as corroborating colon cancer in 10 patients in this series. Joo Hee Kim found that, among 75 patients with occlusive colon cancer, CTC identified six synchronous tumors (9%), three of them proximal to the occluded side of the colon and three located distally (Table 16.2). In that series, the accuracy of CTC was 96%, the sensitivity 83%, and the specificity 98% [12].

Table 16.1 Extracolonic lesions detected at virtual colonoscopy

Author	Number of patients	Age (range)	Further information	Patient Total	Other examination
Hellstrom (2004)	111	66 (19–86)	94	232	26
Pickhardt (2003)	1,233	57,8 (40–79)	223	223	none
Ginnerup (2003)	75	61 (33–78)	49	68	8
Gluecker (2003)	681	64 (41–80)	469	858	110
Munikrishnan (2003)	80	68 (29–83)	25	25	none
Edwards (2001)	100	65 (55–75)	15	15	6
Miao YM (2000)	201	71 (55–91)	24	25	none
Morrin (1999)	40	62 (22–96)	5	5	none
Dachman (1998)	44	58 (41–58)	26	32	none

Table 16.2 Cancer discovered at CT examination

Author	Number of patients	Colon and rectal cancer	Synchronous cancer[a]
Fenlon HM (1999)	29	29	3
Neri E (2002)	29	10	3
Joo Hee Kim (2002)	75	75	6
Hellstrom M (2004)	111	10	?

[a]Synchronous tumors found at CTC not seen by normal colonoscopy

An interesting recent clinical application is the integration of PET-CT [13], in which virtual colonoscopy is combined with standard PET-CT to produce three-dimensional image reconstructions called PET-CT colonography. The procedure requires about 30 min and yields accurate identification and classification of colonic lesions, depending on the amount of radiotracer used.

Nonetheless, as for other organs, correct cancer staging of tumors of the colon and rectum requires total-body imaging. The use of CTC in diagnostic phase could allow the early detection of associated lesions, and could be followed by imaging studies able to identify MPM.

Total-Body Imaging Techniques

As noted above, to identify a further primary tumor it is essential to carry out total-body imaging, most commonly by CT-TB, ^{18}FDG-PET, TB NMR, PET-CT. In the following we discuss their sensitivity and specificity in the diagnosis of synchronous and simultaneous MPM.

Presently, the most widespread method, and the one recommended by several medical guidelines for cancer staging, is contrast-medium CT, as it allows total-body evaluation within an extremely short time frame. Both the primary tumor and associated tumors in adjacent and/or distant organs are visualized [14] (Fig. 16.2).

CT is commonly used to discover metastasis, whereas other lesions, located outside the frequent sites of metastasis, are often not seen by CT. Multidetector-row CT (MDCT) represents the further evolution of this method [15]. Through volumetric acquisition, it provides a three-dimensional reconstruction of the tissues and organs of interest (Fig. 16.3). Nonetheless, while contrast-agent-mediated imaging allows good lesion to tissue contrast, it does not distinguish between benign and malignant lesions or, in cases of the latter, between MPM and metastasis [15, 16]. The certification of the lesion could be achieved only through CT-guided biopsy sampling.

Furthermore, despite the interesting perspective that is achieved by high-quality three-dimensional MDCT imaging and its utility in the correct assessment of tumor extension, this method focuses on a certain organ and cannot be used in the

16 Diagnostic Imaging Techniques for Synchronous Multiple Tumors 235

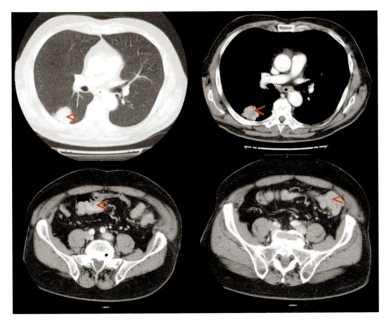

Fig. 16.2 MPM identified by total body contrast-medium CT

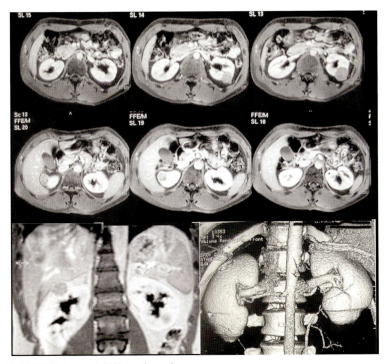

Fig. 16.3 MDCT image of bilateral renal cancer

detection of synchronous tumors [15, 16]. According to the international literature, CT sensitivity in discovering further tumors is only around 50% and therefore, this method cannot be considered when MPM, especially synchronous tumors, is suspected [17].

Techniques that non-invasively yield in vivo information on cellular metabolism, such as positron emission tomography (PET), can be used in early cancer assessment based on the increased uptake of radioactive tracer [18]. These molecular imaging techniques play important roles in diagnosis as well as tumor staging, because the molecular changes in in-vivo tissue metabolism anticipate the morphological modifications of cancer lesions [17]. In addition, tumor classification and the identification of tumor extent are possible [19].

In clinical practice and in for the study of cancers, the most commonly used radiotracer is ^{18}F-labeled fluorodeoxyglucose (FDG). FDG is actively taken up by cells via glucose transporters, phosphorylated but not metabolized; the compound therefore remains trapped within the cell, where it can be detected by PET tomography. Cancer lesions accumulate higher concentrations of radiotracer than normal tissue and are therefore recognizable as area of increased radioactive intensity, which can be quantified and followed over time [13]. The coronary, sagittal, and transaxial sections obtained in total-body imaging by PET tomography have a spatial resolution of about 5 mm [13]. The literature has broadly demonstrated the improved diagnostic accuracy of ^{18}FDG-PET and its better detection of early stages of many types of cancers compared to conventional imaging methods, especially contrast-agent-mediated CT. The additional diagnostic information provided by ^{18}F-FDG PET resulted in changes in the treatment of patients in more than 30% of the cases analyzed [20]. In a series of 366 esophageal cancer patients, analyzed by ^{18}FDG-PET, ten (2.7%) were found to have a second, synchronous malignant tumor localized as follows: two in the right colon, five in the kidney, one in the lung, one in the thyroid, and one in the oral cavity [21].

The limitation of ^{18}FDG-PET lies in its low spatial resolution, especially for body regions with considerable anatomical complexity (head-neck, mediastinum, pelvic floor) [22], where it may be difficult to localize neoplastic lesions or to distinguish between physiological and pathological concentrations of radioactive tracer (muscle tissues or hyperactive circumscribed areas in the intestinal lumen) [23, 24]. In addition, there is no qualitative distinction between inflammatory and neoplastic tissue [24, 25] and it is often difficult to assess those organs that tend to concentrate large amounts of FDG (e.g., thyroid, bladder) [26]. Thus, PET is not the optimal method to identify MPM, even if in our case study it identified synchronous tumors in some patients. It has therefore become increasingly apparent that PET-generated metabolic images must be assessed with reference to the anatomical images provided by CT or NMR [22, 24, 27–29]. However, image fusion is often difficult or impossible, as CT or NMR examinations are not always available, or they may have been performed at different times, or may not be appropriate for an effective comparison. Even if optimal images are available, complex software is required for image fusion, which creates numerous technical problems and long processing times [17].

This problem in clinical practice has prompted the manufacture of hybrid imaging devices consisting of a patient bed, a high quality PET scanner, and MDCT device [27, 30–33]. These so-called PET-CT scanners therefore combine the morphofunctional images of PET with the anatomical images provided by CT. These device offers the advantage of an accurate correspondence between areas of physiological and pathological radioactive tracer collection and anatomical landmarks – an essential feature in the correct interpretation of PET images – and thus reduce the number of false positives, yielding increased diagnostic and staging accuracy [34–36] (Fig. 16.4). A comparison of PET and PET-CT has shown that PET-CT provides additional information regarding location and interpretation of lesions with increased metabolism, especially for body regions of anatomical complexity and when the normal anatomy has been changed by surgery and/or radiation therapy [30, 33, 37, 38]. The overall sensitivity, specificity and diagnostic accuracy of PET-CT with respect to global TNM; staging is respectively, 80, 93 and 94% [33].

Of particular interest is the use of iodinated or barium-containing contrast materials during PET-CT in the visualization of the bowel loops, particularly those of the small bowel, and the vascular structures [17]. In a study of 14 patients with colorectal cancer examined by PET-CT [13], three otherwise-overlooked metastases, one synchronous colorectal cancer, and three synchronous MPM (thyroid, hepatocarcinoma, breast) were detected. Similar results were reported in a series of 547 patients in whom PET-CT revealed seven clinically unexpected metastases and 14 benign lesions; 4.8% of the lesions had not been highlighted by previous investigations. The reported sensitivity of PET-CT in the detection of MPM was 91% (31 out 34) and the specificity 69% (31 out 45) [28].

Several kinds of tumors are not FDG-amenable, such as renal cell carcinoma, prostate cancer, and gastric lesions, particularly small ones, in which the tracer concentration is limited (such as early gastric cancer), deep liver lesions, and low-grade soft-tissue malignancies. In the absence of pronounced morphological changes, this may lead to false-negatives in early-stage disease [36]. Furthermore, the high cost of PET-CT, its limited availability, restricted to a few specialized centers [35], and the European Union guidelines limiting the amount of radiation allowed for each first-stage diagnostic session restrict its use for secondary prevention or mass screening [36].

A review of the international literature and our own experience both suggested that PET-CT is particularly suitable for the detection of MPM. The other main indications of PET-CT are summarized in Table 16.3 [17]. PET-CT is a relatively recent method and will no doubt undergo further technological development, with increases in spatial resolution, diagnostic accuracy, and examination time. In addition, new radiotracers are being investigated, such as 18-fluoro-deoxy-L-thymidine, which is able to indicate changes in cell metabolism and growing tumors, or ^{11}C-choline, in the study of prostate carcinoma [17].

Another method commonly used in the diagnosis of neoplasms is NMR, a technique that has become extremely sophisticated. In total-body NMR, parallel

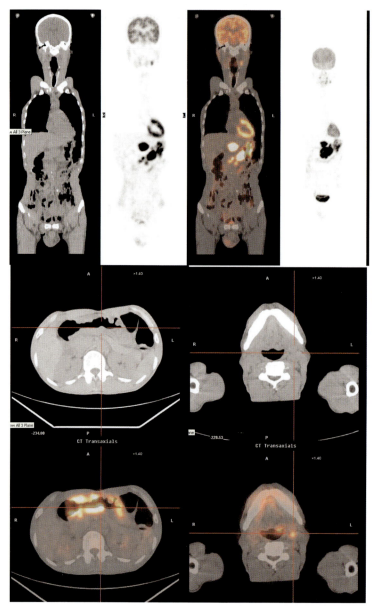

Fig. 16.4 PET-CT image of MPM

imaging is possible due to the multiple independent radiofrequency receiver coils of high intensity (>1.5 Tesla) and a rolling platform. This allows multiple scans without the need to move the patient and an improved acquisition time [33, 36]. In the recently introduced whole-body scanners, a system of multiple phased-array coils covering the entire body allows scans to be acquired in all three dimensions, with a longitudinal extent of 205 cm and a detailed anatomi-

Table 16.3 Clinical indication for PET-CT

- Staging of cancer in anatomically complex body regions
- Staging of tumors when assessment of possible lymph node; involvement is particularly important
- Assessing doubtful and inconclusive CT findings regarding relapse
- Tumors with indications for radical radiotherapy

cal representation [17]. Moreover, the introduction of specific acquisition protocols, with sequences specific for the various organs, has further decreased acquisition time and minimized the image distortions produced by respiratory movements and intestinal peristalsis.

TB-NMR is of interest in the study of abdominal organs, especially the liver (>3 mm lesions), bones (>2mm lesions). In the neurological field, spectroscopic sequences can be associated, so that it is possible to analyze the concentration of various metabolites. The technique is able to distinguish malignant from benign neoplastic lesions with a diagnostic accuracy of 93% [13, 33, 39–41] (Table 16.4). A comparison of the sensitivity and specificity of TB-NMR vs. PET-CT in diagnosis of neoplasms is shown in Table 16.5 [13, 33, 40].

Magnetic resonance imaging (MRI), with its excellent tissue contrast, high spatial resolution, and detailed morphological information is excellent for tumor screening [13, 36]. Its use has been limited mainly by the duration of the examination (relatively long) and the difficulty to simultaneously scan several anatomic as both the patient and the coils must be repositioned [36]. It is also unable to characterize kidney and lung injuries. However, the introduction of new diagnostic protocols has increased the sensitivity to >90% for lung injuries between 4 and 10 mm and to 100% for lesions >10 mm [31, 36, 40–42]. There has been considerable progress in MRI examinations of other organs due to the introduction of specific sequences; for example, MR colonography can detect intestinal lesions >10 mm, i.e., similar to the results obtained with CT colonography [42–44]. The same can be stated for the examination of other organs. With the use of specific protocols, the same excellent sensitivity for cerebral, liver, and bone lesions can be achieved for other organs (kidneys, prostate, etc.) [45–47]. Despite recent technological developments, it is not yet possible to distinguish with certainty between primary and recurrent lesions. MRI does distinguish vascular from other types of lesions. While spectroscopic sequences may indicate the presence and concentration of certain substances, the classification of the lesion can only be definitively achieved only through biopsy.

Finally, while the high effective radiation dose (about 25 mSv) of PET-CT makes it inadequate for secondary prevention, whole-body MRI, with its lack of ionizing radiation, is highly attractive for this purpose [17].

Although TB-NMR seems promising for the detection of MPM, we have no evidence at this time to confirm these claims. We have therefore used the data reported in the literature to compare PET-CT and TB-NMR in the identification

Table 16.4 Other lesions found at TB-NMR

Author	Number of patients	Index tumor	Other lesions
Eustace	25	Various	6 (24%) metastasis visceral and 1 (4%) cerebral metastasis
Walzer	17	Breast cancer	3 (17.6%) liver metastasis and 3 (17.6%) cerebral metastasis
Engelhard	22	Breast cancer	4 (18%) metastasis liver and/or lung
Ghanem	129	Various	32 (24.8%) metastasis visceral and 5 (3.,8%) cerebral metastasis

Table 16.5 Comparison between TB-NMR and PET-CT

Author	Patient nr	Index tumor	Cerebral	Lung	Liver	Bone marrow
Antoch	98	Various	–	23 vs. 25	13 vs. 12	11 vs. 8
Lauenstein	51	Various (not lung)	8 vs. 7	17 vs. 17	18 vs. 16	24 vs. 21
Schlemmer	68	Various (not lung)	8 vs. 7	12 vs. 15	22 vs. 19	28 vs. 12
Schmidt	38	Various (not lung)	6 vs. 0	37 vs. 36	71 vs. 62	76 vs. 50
Muller-Horwat	41	Melanoma	20 vs. 18	16 vs. 19	13 vs. 5	28 vs. 12

Lesions discovered at TB-NMR and PET-CT (*N*)

of MPM [33, 40, 42], in particular synchronous MPM, while taking into account the limits set by European Union legislation. According to the EU, mammography is the only radiological investigation approved as a mass screening tool [42]. The data obtained from various series seem to encourage a more widespread use of TB-NMR, especially in the detection of synchronous MPM. A breakthrough development might be the recent application of fused virtual PET-NMR images, which should further increase the diagnostic ability of this method. At present, however, the number of cases is not yet numerically significant, and the data are more accidental rather than the results of careful research.

It is therefore clear that in the absence of an ideal imaging method; the clinical approach must be tailored to suit each case. Once a neoplasia has been identified, the index tumor should serve as a starting point in considering possible neoplastic associations and thus the appropriate imaging technique, i.e., the one that provides the greatest sensitivity and specificity (Tables 16.6 and 16.7).

Not all patients with suspected cancers are candidates for a total-body survey. The indication for this type of examination should be made in accordance with the clinical findings (Table 16.8). Indeed, correct staging includes an examination of those organs under diagnostic suspicion and serves as the basis for establishing the need for total-body imaging [36]. In this case, a choice between PET-CT and TB-NMR can be made as to which offers the best opportunity to detect additional lesions and therefore also synchronous MPM (Tables 16.7 and 16.8).

The recent introduction of CTC, which obviates the need for a barium enema, may offer an alternative method to detect colorectal lesions. A positive finding should be confirmed and further explored by PET-CT and/or TB-NMR. In the near future, diagnostic guidelines for colonic lesions could very consist of colonoscopy, CTC-PET-CT/TB NMR. However, systematic research on the diagnosis of additional lesions would certainly increase their discovery, but raises ethical problems as well as a significant increase in costs [7].

Table 16.6 Total body imaging

	Sensitivity (%)	Specificity (%)
TB-CT	55	80
TB-NMR	90	95
[18]FDG PET	84	88
PET-CT	93	95

Table 16.7 Organ-specific accuracy of several imaging methods[a]

Anatomic region	Imaging technique			
	CT	TB-NMR	FDG PET	PET-CT
Lung	**46**	**82**	**62**	**89**
	86	*94*	*98*	*94*
Liver	n.a.	**93**	n.a.	**86**
	95			*96*
Pancreas	**85**		**92**	**97**
	67	*n.a.*	*85*	*76*

n.a. Data not available from our radiologic institute
[a]Sensitivity reported in bold type and specificity in italics

Table 16.8 Clinical indications for diagnostic total-body imaging

- High incidence of familial tumor-related death
- Early diagnosis
- Confirmation of the diagnosis
- Therapeutic strategy decisions
- Clinical doubt for MPM

Conclusions

At the moment there is no universal diagnostic technique with overall oncologic accuracy, neither are there diagnostic guidelines to identify synchronous MPM. As such, the diagnostic approach must be adapted on a case by case basis. The difficulties in comparing different cases lie in the different diagnostic protocols used at the various centers and the nature of the particular disease [17, 33, 36].

A more rational approach is needed for those patients in whom MPM is clinically suspected, especially in the case of lesions of the colon. CTC, especially when combined with CT-PET may be the strategy of choice to identify additional lesions in these patients.

Even if it is not possible to distinguish with certainty between primary and recurrent lesions, familiarity with the MPM regarding their anatomic locations (as opposed to that of the index tumor) and frequency of associations is essential. The technical characteristics of today's diagnostic imaging techniques, in particular those that allow whole-body image acquisition, such as CT, MRI, and PET-CT, make them ideal diagnostic tools for the study of MPM.

PET-CT is currently the most advanced method of metabolic imaging. In the detection of MPM, it has a sensitivity of 93%, specificity of 95%, and a global diagnostic accuracy of 94%. It also offers the highest diagnostic accuracy in identifying tumor stage. In about 20% of cases, improved recognition of anatomical landmarks guides the correct interpretation of lesions; this feature is particularly useful in the detection of synchronous MPM.

An interesting alternative is represented by TB-NMR, which offers good global sensitivity; its use is also currently favored by current legislation. The introduction of PET-NMR will hopefully represent the future gold standard imaging procedure for many different diseases, among them probably also synchronous MPM.

References

1. The Research Group for Population-based Cancer Registration in Japan (2002) Cancer incidence and incidence rates in Japan in 1997: estimates based on data from 12 population-based cancer registries. Jpn J Clin Oncol 32:318–322

2. Kumagai Y, Kawano T, Nakajima Y et al (2001) Multiple primary cancers associated with esophageal carcinoma. Surg Today 31:872–876
3. Wax MK, Myers LL, Gabalski EC et al (2002) Positron emission tomography in the evaluation of synchronous lung lesions in patients with untreated head and neck cancer. Arch Otolaryngol Head Neck Surg 128:703–707
4. Bar-Meir E (2004) Assessment of the risk of perforation at CT colongraphy. Presented at the 90th Scientific Assembly and Annual Meeting of Radiological Society of North America, Chicago, November 26–December 3, 2004
5. Heiken JP, Peterson CM, Menias CO et al (2005) Virtual colonoscopy for colorectal cancer screening: current status. Cancer Imaging 5:S133-S139
6. Xiong T, Richardson M, Woodroffe R et al (2005) Incidental lesions found on CT colongraphy: their nature and frequency. Br J Radiol 78:22–29
7. Hellstrom M, Svensson MH, Lasson A (2004) Extracolonic and incidental findings on CT colonography (virtual colono-scopy). AJR Am J Roentgenol 182:631–638
8. Hara AK (2000) Incidental extracolonic findings at CT colonography. Radiology 215:353–357
9. Pickhardt PJ (2003) Computed tomographic virtual colonoscopy to screen for colorectal neoplasia in asymptomatic adults. N Engl J Med 349:2191–200
10. Fenlon HM (1999) Occlusive colon carcinoma: virtual colonoscopy in the preoperative evaluation of the proximal colon. Radiology 210:423–428
11. Neri E, Giusti P, Bartolla L et al (2002) Colorectal cancer: role of CT colonography in pre-operative evaluation after incomplete colonoscopy. Radiology 223:615–619
12. Kim JH, Kim WH, Kim TI et al (2007) Incomplete colonoscopy in patients with occlusive colorectal cancer: usefulness of CT colonography according to tumor location. Yonsei Med J 48(6):934–941
13. Veit P, Kuehle C, Beyer T et al (2006) Whole body positron tomography/computed tomography (PET/CT) tumor staging with integrated PET/CT colonography: technical feasibility and first experiences in patients with colorectal cancer. Gut 55:68–73
14. Kalender WA (1995) Thin-section three-dimensional spiral CT: is isotopic imaging possible? Radiology 197:578–580
15. Ueda T, Mori K, Minami M et al (2006) Trends in oncological CT imaging: clinical application of multi detector-row CT and 3D-CT imaging. Int J Clin Oncol 11:268–277
16. Ros PR, Ji H (2002) Special focus session: multisection (multidetector) CT: application in the abdomen. Radiographics 22:697–700
17. Fanti S, Franchi R, Battista G et al (2005) PET e PET-CT. Stato dell'arte e prospettive future. Radiol Med (Torino) 110:1–15
18. Phelps ME (2000) Positron emission tomography provides molecular imaging of biological processed. PNAS 97:9226–9233
19. Van Rees BP, Cleton-Jansen AM, Cense HA et al (2000) Molecular evidence of field cancerization in a patient with 7 tumors of the aerodigestive tract. Hum Pathol 31:269–271
20. Gambhir SS et al (2001) A tabulated summary of the FDG PET literature. J Nucl Med 42(suppl):1S-93S
21. van Westreenen HL, Westerterp M, Jager PL (2005) Synchronous primary neoplasms detected on FDG PET in staging of patients with esophageal cancer. J Nucl Med 46:1321–1325
22. Wahl RL (2004) Why nearly all PET of abdominal and pelvic cancers will be performed as PET/CT. J Nucl Med 45(suppl):82S-95S
23. Bicik I, Bauerfeind P, Breitbach T et al (1997) Inflammatory bowel disease activity measured by positron-emission tomography. Lancet 350:262
24. Kamel EM, Thumshirn M, Truninger K et al (2004) Significance of incidental 18F-FDG accumulations in the gastrointestinal tract in PET/CT: correlation with endoscopic and histopathology results. J Nucl Med 45(11): 1804–1810
25. Kresnik E, Gallowitsch HJ, Mikosch P et al (2002) (18)F-FDG positron emission tomography in the early diagnosis of enterocolitis: preliminary results. Eur J Nucl Med MD Imaging 29:1389–1392

26. van Westreenen HL, Heeren PA, Jager PL et al (2003) Pitfalls of positive findings in staging esophageal cancer with F18-fluoro-deoxyglucose positron emission tomography. Ann Surg Oncol 10:1100–1105
27. Costa DL, Visvikis D, Crosdale I et al (2003) Positron emission and computed X-ray tomography: a coming together. Nucl Med Commun 24:351–358
28. Choi JY, Lee KS, Kwon OJ et al (2005) Improved detection of second primary cancer using integrated 18F fluorodeoxyglucose positron emission tomography and computed tomography for initial tumor staging. J Clin Oncol 23(30): 7654–7659
29. Schmidt GP, Haug AR, Schoenberg SO, Reiser MF (2006) Whole-body MRI and PET-CT in the management of cancer patients. Eur Radiol 16:1216–1225
30. Cohade C, Osman M, Leal J, Wahl RL (2003) Direct comparison of (18)F-FDG PET an PET/CT in patients with colorectal carcinoma. J Nucl Med 44:1797–1803
31. Beyer T, Townsend DW, Blodgett TM (2002) Dual-modality PET/CT tomography for clinical oncology. Am J Nucl Med 46:24–34
32. Bar-Shalom R, Yefremov N, Guralnik L et al (2003) Clinical performance of PET/CT in evaluation of cancer: additional value for diagnostic imaging and patient management. J Nucl Med 44:1200–1209
33. Antoch G, Freudenberg LS, Beyer T et al (2004) To enhance or not to enhance? 18F-FDG and CT contrast agents in dual modality 18F-FDG PET/CT. J Nucl Med 45(suppl 1):S56-S65
34. Townsend DW, Beyer T (2002) A combined PET/CT scanner: the path to true image fusion. Br J Radiol 75(suppl):S24-S30
35. Czermin Y (ed) (2004) PET/CT: imaging function and structure. J Nucl Med 45(suppl):1S-103S
36. Schmidt GP, Baur-Melnyk A, Herzog P et al (2005) High-resolution whole-body magnetic resonance image tumor staging with the use of parallel imaging versus dual-modality positron emission tomography-computed tomography: experience on a 32-channel system. Invest Radiol 40:743–753
37. Langenhoff BS, Oyen WJ, Jager GJ et al (2002) Efficacy of fluorine-18-deoxyglucose positron emission tomography in detecting tumor recurrence after local ablative therapy for liver metastases: a prospective study. J Clin Oncol 20:4453–4458
38. Vogel WV, Wiering B, Corstens FH et al (2005) Colorectal cancer: the role of PET/CT in recurrence. Cancer Imaging 5:S143-S148
39. Lauenstein TC, Goehde SC, Herborn CU et al (2004) Whole-body MR imaging: evaluation of patients for metastases. Radiology 233:139–148
40. Schlemmer HP, Schaefer J, Pfannenberg C et al (2005) Fast whole-body assessment of metastatic disease using a novel magnetic resonance imaging system: initial experiences. Invest Radiol 40:64–71
41. Schaefer JF, Vollmar J, Schick F et al (2005) Detection of pulmonary nodules with breath-hold magnetic resonance imaging in comparision with computed tomography. Roto Fortschr Geb Rontgenstr Neuen Bildgeb Verfahr 177:41–49
42. Ajaj W, Pelster G, Treichel U et al (2003) Dark lumen magnetic resonance colonography: comparision with conventional colonoscopy for the detection of colorectal pathology. Gut 52:1738–1743
43. Schroeder T, Ruehm SG, Debatin JF et al (2005) Detection of pulmonary nodules using a 2D HASTE MR sequence comparison with MDCT. AJR Am J Roentgen 185:979–984
44. Luboldt W, Bauerfeind P, Wildermuth S et al (2000) Colonic masses: detection with MR colonography. Radiology 216:383–388
45. Schaefer JF, Schlemmer HP (2006) Total-body MR-imaging in oncology. Eur Radiol 16:2000–2015
46. Willinek WA, Gieseke J, von Falkenhausen M et al (2003) Sensitivity-encoding for fast MR imaging of the brain in patients with stroke. Radiology 228:669–675
47. Cercignani M, Horsfield MA, Agosta F, Filippi M (2003) Sensitivity-encoded diffusion tensor MR imaging of the cervical cord. AJNR Am J Neuroradiol 24:1254–1256

Chapter 17
"DNA-Guided" Therapy

Nicola Carlomagno, Luigi Pelosio, Akbar Jamshidi, Francesca Duraturo, Paola Izzo, Andrea Renda

Introduction

Rapid progress in understanding the biomolecular basis of disease has brought new concepts to the diagnosis and treatment of some hereditary tumors. After the genes causing the syndromes were identified, the first step was the adoption of predictive genetic tests to identify within affected families those subjects considered to be carriers of the mutations, and then to enroll them in intensive surveillance program and perhaps even to offer prophylactic therapy. Over the years, and particularly following the detection of many types of alterations in the genes responsible for hereditary tumors, it has become possible to correlate genotype, as determined by genetic testing, with the heterogeneous forms of phenotypic expression and clinical manifestations, and thus to provide patients with prognostic information.

Genetic therapy, or the possibility of radically treating or arresting the progress of a tumor on the basis of surgical genetic engineering, is around the corner. A genetically guided clinical approach is already a reality, with precise genetic analysis increasingly requested in order to determine the most appropriate treatment for hereditary syndromes, such as the decision between radical surgery for the involved organs and more conservative surgery with close follow-up. Further genetic discoveries will likely allow the selection of patients greatly at risk for a particular tumor, including those likely to be operated on several times during their lifetime.

Screening

In all inherited syndromes, accurate screening of patients and their families is essential to early diagnosis and treatment.

Previously, all members of families affected by familial adenomatous polyposis (FAP) underwent endoscopy every 1–2 years, starting from the age of 10–12 years. However, this approach required frequent colonoscopies and enormous psychophysical stress. The observation of the precocious occurrence of some extra-colonic manifestations (ECMs), even before colonic polyps developed, led to their use as clinical markers to identify family members at high risk. Some of these markers turned out to be very common in the general population (dental anomalies) or relatively infrequent (14–81%) in FAP-affected patients (osteomas). By contrast, good results were obtained with ophthalmoscopic examination to identify patients with congenital hypertrophy of pigmented epithelium of the retina (CHRPE) (present in 0.03% of the healthy population) (Fig. 17.1).

With the identification of deletions in chromosome 5 [1, 2] and then of the APC gene, the genetics of FAP were quickly elucidated. This allowed DNA testing in combination with clinical screening (endoscope, ophthalmoscope), resulting in the ability to diagnose FAP with high specificity (95%) and accuracy (98%) [3]. In patients with multiple polyposis, especially those with malignant degeneration or synchronous tumors associated with classic FAP or attenuated FAP (AFAP), but with no mutations in the APC gene, mutations of the MYH gene are investigated [4].

For FAP, current screening consists of a peripheral venous blood sample for molecular analysis and an ophthalmoscopic examination, both of which are already possible in children and neonates. In positive subjects, an endoscope

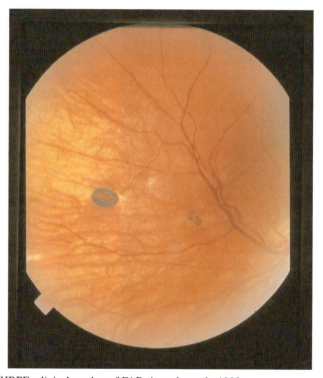

Fig. 17.1 CHRPE: clinical marker of FAP since the early 1990s

exam to confirm the diagnosis is obtained at 15 years and repeated annually until polyps develop, up to age 45 in families with "late onset" disease. If gene mutations are not found, a colonoscopy is nonetheless recommended at 18, 25, and 35 years, to allow for the possibility of a false negative test (regions of the gene not analyzed, limits and/or technical errors of laboratory), mosaicism, or de novo mutations. Patients who at molecular exam are definitively determined to not be carriers of genetic anomalies are spared endoscopic screening.

Unlike in FAP, there are no clinical markers to identify families with hereditary non-polyposis colorectal cancer (HNPCC); thus, instead, based on Lynch's description the clinical characteristics of the disease were systematically searched. Diagnostic criteria were defined a group of researchers joint in Amsterdam in 1990, but they turned out to be overly restrictive in that few families completely fulfilled all of them and they were subsequently modified [5–8] (Table 17.1).

Table 17.1 HNPCC: clinical criteria for diagnosis and mutational analysis

Amsterdam I[a]	1991	Three or more first-degree relatives with CRC; 2 generations affected; one family member <50 years, exclude FAP
Bethesda	1997	Patients with 2 HNPCC-related cancers (colorectal and extracolonic, synchronous as well as metachronous); one first-degree relative withHNPCC
Amsterdam II	1998	Same as Amsterdam I but CRC can be replaced by extracolonic (endometrium, small bowel, urinary tract) cancers
Revised Bethesda[b]	2003	CRC <50 years, multiple CRC- or HNPCC-related cancers, CRC + MSI <60 years, CRC- or HNPCC-related cancers in at least one family member <50 years, adenoma <40 years, CRC- or HNPCC-related cancers in at least two first- or second-degree relatives at any age
Revised Amsterdam	2004	Small nuclear family: 2 first-degree relatives with CRC; 2 generations affected; one family member <50 years. Families with 2 first-degree relatives with CRC and a 3rd one with CRC or endometrial cancer at early age. Young age at onset (<40 years) with no family history

FAP, Familial adenomatous polyposis; *CRC*, colorectal cancer; *HNPCC*, hereditary non-polyposis colorectal cancer; *MSI*, microsatellite instability
[a]All criteria must be met
[b]Any criterion can be met

Recognition of the hereditary aspect is the first step in approaching an inherited neoplastic syndrome, as outlined by Peterson [9]. A scrupulous medical history is mandatory for a correct diagnosis of HNPCC, distinguishing it from simple familial colorectal cancer (CRC).

Preparation and experience on the part of the physician are decisive for selecting individuals who should undergo molecular analysis. After a survey of different medical specialists, Batra [10] highlighted that 79% of 258 gastroenterologists were able to identify HNPCC, but only 34% were knowledgeable about the genetic tests and 16% about screening programs. These data are even more significant if we consider that gastroenterologists are better informed than general practitioners about CRC [11].

Once the mutation in the family has been identified, members can be screened at an early age to identify carriers. Effective genetic screening reduces the number of patients who will need to be examined endoscopically by 50%. This results in relevant economic and psychological benefits and doubles the efficacy of the examination. In CRC patients under age 50 who are positive for the Amsterdam I or II criteria, mutations in MSH2 or MLH1 genes are searched for directly. Patients who do not satisfy these characteristics but whose disease is described by less restrictive ones (Bethesda II), microsatellite instability (MSI) or immunohistochemistry (IHC) of MSH2 and MLH1 can be examined; if the result is positive, then mutations in MSH2 or MLH can be searched for, whereas MSI- and IHC-negative subjects do not require other genetic tests. Clinical surveillance is based on an annual colonoscopy beginning at age 20–25 [12]. Considering the natural history of HNPCC, which has an earlier onset and a faster adenoma-carcinoma progression than the sporadic form, some clinicians feel that the endoscopy should be every 12–24 months in patients with an ascertained mutation.

Screening efficacy has been confirmed by the reduction of cancer-related deaths rates. Jarvinen [13] compared two groups of subjects at risk of HNPCC over a 10-year period. Members of the first underwent periodic endoscopic screening, while those in the second were not followed with any surveillance. This latter group had a higher incidence of cancer (4.5% vs. 11.9%)m presumably owing to the endoscopic polypectomies in the screened group. The incidence of early-stage tumors and cancer-related deaths were also significantly decreased as a result of screening. In another study, comprising 114 HNPCC at-risk families, 35 cases of cancer were diagnosed but only one, discovered at a maximum interval of 2 years from the last endoscopy, was at advanced stage [14].

The high risk of premature death in individuals at risk of multiple endocrine neoplasia (MEN)1 justifies periodic genetic screening [15]. Mutational analysis of the MEN-1 gene is carried out on patients in whom there is clinical suspicion of disease. This approach reassures patient and their families while avoiding frequent and expensive periodic clinical checks of family members who lack the mutations. The aim of screening is to discover anomalies in pre-symptomatic stages. Early recognition of genetic alteration can lead to early diagnosis and consequently to a reduction in morbidity and mortality [16–18].

In MEN2, medullary thyroid cancer (MTC) is the first clinical manifestation and the main cause of death. Rapid identification is fundamental, mainly because of the tendency for metastases in very young patients [19]. Before the arrival of genetic testing, in the 1970s, MEN2A could be diagnosed with biochemical testing, such as the calcium test or the pentagastrin stimulation test to demonstrate the presence of MTC [19]. Although these tests are sensitive and specific, when performed annually they are expensive, laborious, and associated with troublesome side effects such that some members of affected families refuse repeated screening [20].

Genetics have opened up a new era in the prevention and treatment of MEN2. In some patients, this means prophylactic thyroidectomy, before clinical manifestation of the illness, based on the results of predictive DNA tests and after close study of the at-risk family's genealogical trees as well as the collection of DNA from sick and healthy members of the family for genotyping. The recent identification of the germline mutation of the proto-oncogene RET in patients with MEN2A, MEN2B, and familial MTC (FMTC), has confirmed the DNA test as the best method for screening at-risk family members, because it can be carried out at any age and requires only a single sample of peripheral blood [19, 20].

Women with a BRCA1 or BRCA2 germline mutation are at increased risk of breast and ovarian cancer compared with the general population. If the genetic alteration is not already known, obtaining an accurate clinical and familial history is the first step in identifying those at risk by molecular analysis. Detection of a germline BRCA mutation is more likely in families with: (a) breast cancer diagnosed at age <50 years in two or more related women, or in one woman but with ovarian cancer in one or more related women; (b) ovarian cancer in two or more relatives; (c) male breast cancer with any family history of breast and/or ovarian cancer [21].

Botkin et al. [22] identified BRCA mutation carriers, non-carriers, and individuals of unknown mutation status to determine the impact of test results. Follow-up included genetic testing of men and women, and mammography, breast self-exam, clinical breast exam, mastectomy, oophorectomy, transvaginal ultrasound, and CA125 screening for women. Of those fully informed of the opportunity for testing, 55% of the women and 52% of the men pursued genetic testing. With respect to mammography for women 40 years and older, 82% of mutation carriers obtained a mammogram in each year following testing compared to 72% of non-carrier women the first year and 67% the second year. The use of mammography increased significantly over baseline for both mutation carriers and non-carriers. Younger carrier women also significantly took advantage of mammography. Overall, 29% of the carrier women did not obtain a single mammogram by 2 years post-testing. At 2 years, 83% of the carrier women and 74% of the non-carriers reported adherence to recommendations for breast self-exam and over 80% of carrier women had obtained a clinical breast examination each year following testing. For all women age 25 and over, carriers and non carriers significantly increased their use of mammography from baseline at both 1 year ($p < 0.01$) and 2 years ($p < 0.01$) post-testing.

Current screening recommendations for breast cancer prevention consists of monthly breast self-examination beginning at 18 years of age, a clinical examination every 6 months, and yearly mammogram beginning at age 25. For ovarian cancer, annual or semi-annual transvaginal ultrasonography and CA 125 levels beginning at age 25–35 years are recommended; however, these screening procedures are limited in their ability to detect ovarian cancer at a curable stage [21–25].

Therapy

The therapeutic approach to FAP is particularly complex and demanding, because it entails prophylaxis and treatment of colonic adenomas, CRC and potentially lethal ECMs. Therapy must be modulated regarding: (a) colectomy (type of anastomoses, reconstruction, i.e., ileorectal anastomosis or ileal pouch-anal anastomosis, age at surgery), (b) treatment of ECMs, (c) possible complementary therapy and/or chemoprevention.

The adenoma-carcinoma progression is the most important event of FAP. Fortunately, it can be prevented by prophylactic colectomy (Fig. 17.2) in relatively young at-risk individuals, with good functional and oncological results. Although non-steroidal anti-inflammatory drugs may have some benefic effect on colonic adenomas, prophylactic surgery of the colon is still the only curative treatment for polyposis [26]. Nonetheless, the young age of the colectomy

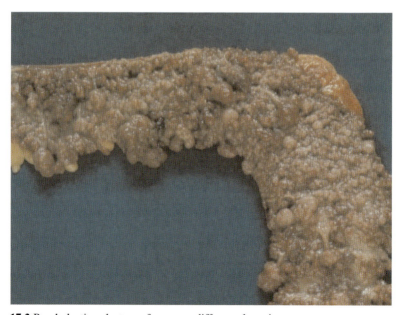

Fig. 17.2 Prophylactic colectomy for severe diffuse polyposis

patients (15–25 years) points out how surgery seriously affects the quality of life, education, and social relationships. The first problem that must be confronted is reconstruction after total colectomy. The two most common procedures – the proctocolectomy with ileo-anal anastomosis and interposition reservoir (IPAA) and total colectomy with ileo-rectal anastomosis (IRA) – are universally accepted, as total proctocolectomy with definitive ileostomies confined only to few patients. The choice between IPAA and IRA depends on a careful analysis of the main inauspicious events: the possible functional failure of IPAA or the risk of rectal stump cancer after IRA. IPAA is, from an oncological perspective, more promising but it carries a high risk of morbidity and worse functional results; if the procedure is not successful, surgeons must resort to a definitive ileostomy. However, IRA exposes patients to the risk of rectal-stump cancer, which exponentially increases in the years following prophylactic colectomy [27] despite careful endoscope control, as documented in the St. Marks experience, which reported the development of cancer less than 6 months after the last negative rectoscopy [28]. In the context of MPM, rectal stump cancer is clearly a metachronous tumor. Mutational analysis can have an important role in the decision at what age patients should undergo prophylactic surgery. Colectomy must be anticipated in families with a history of early disease onset but can be delayed in late-onset disease, albeit with a significantly high risk that these patients will develop ECMs, such as desmoids. Mutations in the first four exons, characteristic of AFAP, or in the region of exon 15, associated with a high risk of desmoids, requires a more cautious approach, postponing surgery until patients are at least 20 years of age.

Genotypic/phenotypic correlation can be useful in the choice between IRA or IPAA while taking into account other clinical criteria [27]. Some deletions are known to predispose patients to cancer and are therefore contraindications for IRA. Vasen [26] highlighted that, in the follow-up of 87 patients who underwent IRA, the need for a second operation rate was significantly higher in those with mutations after codon 1250. Church [29] reported that proctectomy was mostly performed in patients with alterations between codons 1309 and 1328.

Even though surgery is currently the most effective treatment for hereditary familiar tumors, recent studies have drawn attention to chemoprevention (oral supplements of Ca+, vitamin C, FANS, Cox2-inhibitors) [30, 31]. This mode of therapy is dealt with extensively in another chapter of this monograph. Briefly, over 20 years ago, Waddel [32] first described the action of sulindac in reducing the number and dimensions of colic adenomas in patients with FAP, as confirmed by Giardiello's perspective study [33]. In some randomized trials, interesting results were reported with sulindac and Celecoxib; such that, in 2001, the FDA approved the Cox2 course for FAP, with follow-up by endoscopic surveillance. However, Giardiello [34] recently downplayed the benefits of sulindac. Likewise, for desmoids and polyps of the upper gastrointestinal tract, several chemoprevention schemes have been proposed but with varying results.

Based on these observations, it becomes clear how molecular analysis can be effectively inserted in chemoprevention programs, in that the administration of these drugs would be limited to patients with ascertained mutations, with the goal being to prevent the occurrence of polyps and postpone colectomy.

In AFAP-affected patients with few adenomas, endoscopic polypectomy could be followed by the administration of Cox2 and endoscopic surveillance, as for patients with HNPCC, [35], even if Cox2 gene expression is less in patients with defective MMR and MSI genes than in patients with FAP and sporadic cancer [36, 37].

Also for FAP caused by mutations in MYH, which has a later onset than classic FAP (50.6 years, range 35–69), screening and polypectomy are not sufficient to prevent cancer; rather, prophylactic surgery is indispensable even if surgery is postponed [4].

In HNPCC, the role of surgery is not only limited to CRC exeresis, but also to the prevention and treatment of metachronous CRC or extra-colonic cancer. In patients with CRC and ascertained mutations, total colectomy is the most suitable operation because of the high incidence of synchronous and metachronous tumors [9]. In the past, there were many reports of patients who underwent two or three operations during their lifetime. In the presence of genetic alteration without CRC the role of prophylactic surgery can be considered. While for other hereditary syndromes (FAP, MEN2) it has been universally affirmed, in HNPCC it is a valid therapeutic option; after careful evaluation and detailed information, patients may decide either to undergo prophylactic surgery or to be rigorously followed [9]. However, the optimal age for surgery remains to be defined. Immediate prophylactic surgery may have greater benefits than intense endoscopic surveillance program and is often preferred by patients who particularly motivated and well informed on the clinical history of the disease. We advise colectomy over endoscopic surveillance because of the possibility that sessile adenomas, frequent in HNPCC, can escape endoscopic detection. The choice for surgery is particularly useful for cancer-phobic persons or those unable to comply with a surveillance program.

Unfortunately, neither prevention nor prophylactic treatment is available for the tumors in MEN1. Treatment is generally limited to surgery but only at the moment of clinical diagnosis [15].

In MEN2, MTC develops in all affected patients and is the only constant malignant component of the syndrome. Thus, independent of age, all such patients are candidates for total thyroidectomy (TT) as soon as a mutation of the RET gene is identified. The evidence suggests that this approach is curative or preventive for MTC in almost all cases, assuring the longest survival and the best quality of life [38]. Cohen and Moley recommended prophylactic TT for all carriers with identified mutations of c-RET [39]. Interesting data were obtained after reports of microscopic MTC [40] and nodal involvement [41] in pediatric patients. Microscopic MTC was also discovered in a metastatic stage during the first year of life [42–46]. The higher accuracy of DNA analysis compared to biochemical screening was demonstrated in one study, which found that after DNA+ patients underwent TT it was still possible to detect small breeding grounds of MTC despite normal levels of plasmatic calcitonin in 56.1% and microscopic MTC, hyperplasia of C cells, or both in 62.2% [20].

The problems of prophylactic surgery for MTC are the optimal age for surgery, the necessity of lymphadenectomy, and the possible need for radiotherapy. In these decisions, the information obtained from mutational analysis can be relevant in that it allows subjects with different risk levels to be identified such that the therapeutic approach can be personalized, as summarized in Table 17.2 [47]. Regarding prophylactic lymphadenectomy, there is no consensus, either with respect to possible additional morbidity or to the different clinical expressions of the disease and the significant differences in nodal involvement among patients. Surgeons and internists have different opinions on prophylactic lymphadenectomy. The former prefer to perform it at same time as TT, since potential difficulties can be met in the central department of the neck in cases of re-intervention. Internists, by contrast, fear the additional morbidity caused by hyperparathyroidism (HPT) and/or recurrent nerve lesions. Some authors advise lymphadenectomy only in cases of a positive CT scan after stimulation tests [47].

The problem of nodal diffusion is relevant considering that the finding of microscopic MTC within the first year of life in this setting is common, and even metastases have been described [47]. In less aggressive forms, nodal involvement has been verified in all cases except those involving mutations at codons 790 and 791 [47]; however, in all the three groups indicated in Table 17.2, if there is evidence of lateral nodal involvement, a more aggressive dissection is needed [19].

In MEN2B, central lymphadenectomy is a well-accepted approach and should be wide ranging if metastases are clearly identified [46].

In the literature there are few data and little support for the use of radioiodine to treat residual thyroid tissue. [47].

In HBOC, chemoprevention, mastectomy and prophylactic hysteroadnexectomy are current and still unresolved problems. Since screening procedures are limited in their ability to identify ovarian cancer at a curable stage, prophylactic bilateral salpingo-ophporectomy (BSO) is recommended once child-bearing is complete. Similar to Botkin's results [22], Lerman et al. [48] documented a relatively low use of CA 125 testing and transvaginal ultrasound, with only 21 and 15% of patients, respectively, reporting use of these measures within 1 year

Table 17.2 Risk of medullary thyroid cancer (MTC) stratified in three categories according to the mutations in the c-RET gene (from [48])

c-RET mutations (codons)	Risk (level)	Total thyroidectomy (patient age)
883, 918, 922	Very high (3)	<6 months + central node dissection
611, 618, 620 or 634	High (2)	<5 years ± central node dissection
609, 768, 790, 791, 804 e 891	Less aggressive (1)	5–10 years or periodic pentagastrin test and thyroidectomy at first alteration of test results

of diagnosis, while prophylactic surgery was clearly preferred over early detection measures to reduce the risk of ovarian cancer. Recent studies provided evidence for this recommendation, as prophylactic BSO was found to reduce the risk of ovarian cancer in women with a BRCA mutation by >95%. In addition, prophylactic BSO in premenopausal mutation carriers has been shown to reduce the risk of breast cancer by approximately 50% [23]. Bilateral prophylactic oophorectomy reduces the risk of coelomic epithelial cancer and breast cancer in women with BRCA1 or BRCA2 mutations [49, 50] (Table 17.3). Furthermore at the time of BSO, occult carcinomas were detected in 2.3–8.6% of patients [49, 51].

Because of the great risk of cancer for carriers of BRCA1 and BRCA2 mutations, the inevitable question of bilateral prophylactic mastectomy (BPM) has been posed. To summarize the results obtained thus far, BPM probably reduces the incidence of cancer by up to 80–90% in women at high ris. However, those who receive an annual mammography have an 80% survival. In light of a penetrance rate of 50–60%, the probability of death from breast cancer for mutation carriers is close to 10% if women do not undergo preventive mastectomy [52].

The 1997 Consensus Statement for BRCA1/2 carriers by the Cancer Genetics Studies Consortium [53] stated that no recommendation for BPM could be made because of the lack of evidence supporting the benefit conferred by the procedure. Since that time, there have been other retrospective and prospective studies that showed a high degree of risk reduction with mastectomy [54–57]. Recent data from Rebbeck et al. [49] are encouraging, showing that BPM reduces the risk of breast cancer in women with BRCA1/2 mutations by approximately 90%: 1.9% of 105 women and in 184/378 (48.7%) of matched controls who did not have the procedure, with a mean follow-up of 6.4 years. BPM reduced the risk of breast cancer by approximately 95% in women with prior or concurrent BSO and by approximately 90% in those with intact ovaries.

Botkin [22] demonstrated a marked difference in the women's use of mastectomy and oophorectomy as risk-reducing measures for cancer. In a study of

Table 17.3 Ovarian and breast cancer prevention: prophylactic oophorectomy (PO) vs. controls (from [50])

	PO	Controls
Ovarian cancer at the time of the procedure (%)	2.3[a]	19.9
Papillary serous peritoneal carcinoma (%)[c]	0.8[b]	
Breast cancer (%)[d]	21.2	42.3

[a] 100% stage I
[b] 3.8 and 8.6 years after bilateral prophylactic oophorectomy
[c] Hazard ratio 0.04; 95% confidence interval 0.01–0.16
[d] Hazard ratio 0.47; 95% confidence interval 0.29–0.77

BRCA1/2 testing in US women, Lerman [48] found that only 3 and 13% of carriers had, respectively, undergone BPM and BSO at 1 year after testing. A study of a Dutch population by Meijers-Heijboer et al. [56] yielded different results: 55 and 60% of unaffected female carriers had, respectively, opted for BPM and BSO by 2 years post-testing. Kauf prospectively followed 170 BRCA1 or BRCA2 mutation carriers age 35 years or older who had not had BSO, 58% of whom later chose risk-reducing BSO [50].

The reason for the different responses of women to mastectomy is unclear. Certainly cultural differences are likely to be highly influential. Julian-Reynier [58] documented a significant variation between cultures on attitudes toward cancer prevention strategies.

Surveillance for Second Tumors

In each of the codified syndromes, treatment of the first manifestation, the so-called index tumor, must be followed by clinical, laboratory, and instrumental surveillance. This is particularly demanding because of the huge spectrum of potential lesions, the multiple anatomic regions involved, and the long latency between onset of the tumors. It is therefore extremely important to take into account the clinical and, when available, genetic information in order to avoid useless exams and unnecessary patient stress. A detailed knowledge of the characteristics of each syndrome is indispensable, including the percentages of occurrence of possible MPM and the ability to identify at risk subjects for close follow-up. In this regard, the genotype-phenotype correlation can be very informative, as it often has a relevant role in predicting MPM.

Due to its many clinical manifestations, the follow-up of FAP [59] is very expensive and demanding. Endoscopy must include evaluation of the rectal stump (after IRA) and the ileo-anal pouch; the early diagnosis of ECM may require very sophisticated investigations. A precise genotype-phenotype correlation allows those exams targeted to the manifestations of genetic defects (e.g., desmoids, intestinal polyps) to be reserved for patients at high risk, with the additional benefit of economic savings.

Rectal stump cancer, as mentioned above, is a metachronous tumor. The degree of post-IRA endoscopic surveillance for this tumor can be determined by the type of genetic mutation. The tests must be particularly thorough in patients with alterations other than in codon 1250, due to the increased risk of cancer.

Esophagogastroduodenoscopy (EGDS) is obligatory for surveillance of the upper gastrointestinal tract starting in patients age 30 years, with an annual examination in positive cases or every 3–5 years in the absence of polyps. Suspected lesions can be endoscopically removed by laser or electrocoagulation.

Some patients (young women operated on at an early age, carriers of at-risk mutations) require very rigorous surveillance for desmoids, and therapy must be based on a multimodal approach, one that considers the clinical-biological characteristics of their disease state. Surgery, when feasible, is the treatment of choice, with radio- and medical therapy complementary or serving as alternatives if surgery is not possible or exeresis was unsuccessful. The results are generally good in parietal desmoids. In those particularly aggressive and refractory to other treatments, polychemotherapy with different combinations of antiblastic agents has been suggested but without encouraging results. Although genotyping can foresee the occurrence of desmoids, effective preventive measures are still lacking. Postponing colectomy may be a valid precaution, considering that surgical trauma is an important risk factor.

For other FAP-related MPM, such as thyroid cancer and hepatoblastoma we refer to the chapter by Cetta, which describes his extensive experience in treating these patients at the University of Siena.

In HNPCC, as for FAP, colectomy is followed by "ortho- and heterotopic" surveillance. The first addresses the high rates of metachronous CRC and rectal stump cancer after IRA, the second is aimed at the detection of extra-colonic neoplasms.

Today there is no general agreement as to the frequency or the modulation of post-surgical diagnostic procedures. Experience guided by long-term follow-up data is missing. Endoscopy is advised at intervals within 2 years [60] in patients at risk for post-IRA rectal-stump cancer. Rodriguez-Bigas [61] reported eight cases of rectal stump cancer in 71 patients followed on average for 10 years after total colectomy. In 75% of them, the last endoscope was performed less than 6–24 months before cancer diagnosis.

Oncological surveillance finalized at the early diagnosis of extra-colonic tumors (stomach, genito-urinary) follows the guidelines reported in the literature. According to the International Collaborative Group on HNPCC for tumor prevention in individuals at risk in HNPCC families surveillance should start from the age of 30–35 and carried out annually for the urinary tract (urine analysis and an urinary ultrasound,) genital sphere (pelvic and/or transvaginal echography and determination of CA125) and stomach (EGDS) [62, 63]. For women with ascertained mutations, examinations should start at age 25 years and must be performed yearly [64, 65].

Oncological markers, systematically measured repeatedly, can be a useful indicator of recurrence.

Prophylactic hysteroadnexctomy can be suggested in menopausal women or in women who do not wish further pregnancies. Schmeler compared prophylactic surgery with surveillance programs and obtained different results (Table 17.4) [66].

In MEN2A, genetic information is also useful to determine the risk of pheochromocytoma (PHEO) and hyperparathyroidism (HPT), and thus when to start clinical, laboratory, and instrumental surveillance and to decide how often it should be performed. The genotype-phenotype correlation can dictate different approaches according to the genetic alteration. Mutational analyses are recommended for all patients with a family history or in whom there is clinical suspicion of PHEO [67].

Annual determinations of fractionated urinary and free plasma metane-

Table 17.4 HNPCC: surgical prevention vs. surveillance (from [67])

	Endometrial cancer	Ovarian cancer
Cancer occurring during follow-up	0% vs. 33% controls	0% vs. 5% controls
Age at prophylaxis (median)	41	41
Age at cancer diagnosis (median)	46 (range 30–69)	42 (range 31–48)
Diagnosis <35 years	4 (6%)	2 (17%)
Incidental diagnosis	0	3

phrines and catecholamines are strongly recommended beginning as early as age 5 or 10 years or at the time of thyroidectomy for patients at high risk of pheochromocytoma (mutations at codons 609, 611, 618, 620, 630, 634, 790, V804L, 883, 918, or 922), but can be started later and done less frequently in other cases (609, 768, val804met, and 891) [19, 47].

Serum parathyroid hormone PTH and calcium, preferably ionized calcium, are measured yearly (patients with a mutation at codon 634) or every 2–3 years or more frequently if there is a family history of HPT (mutation at codon 609, 611, 618, 620, 790, and 791), while they can be omitted in patients with certain mutations (768, val804met, and 891, 883, 918, or 922). [47]. Some authors maintain that instrumental surveillance should be done every 3–5 years in patients 15 years old and older, even in the absence of biochemical alterations [47]. There is no unanimous consensus regarding the best instrumental investigation, but the majority use CT.

In patients with HBOC, the lifetime population risk for ovarian cancer is 1 in 75, while a BRCA1 gene carrier has a 1 in 2 risk of developing the disease and a BRCA2 gene carrier 1 in 5. Different studies have looked at the various modalities for early detection of ovarian cancer, including pelvic ultrasound scanning and serum screening for tumor markers. A major problem is that there is no clearly recognized pre-malignant stage to target. None of the available methods have been shown to detect disease at an earlier stage overall compared to ovarian cancer presenting with symptoms, although adequately powered studies are lacking at present [21–25, 68]. Current screening recommendations include annual or semi-annual transvaginal ultrasonography and CA 125 level beginning at age 25–35 years. However, these procedures are not able to discover ovarian cancer at a curable stage [24, 25].

The decision to undergo prophylactic BSO depends on a woman's level of concern about developing ovarian cancer, the perceived consequences of prophylactic surgery, and the role of subsequent hormonal replacement. Risk-reducing BSO is more frequently employed, particularly when childbearing is completed and the woman is approaching menopause. When performed laparoscopically, the acute morbidity of the procedure is modest, although the quality-of-life consequences and long-term health risks of premature estrogen deprivation have not been defined [21]. After BSO, the possibility of a primary peritoneal carcinomatosis still remains in 2–11% of patients [69].

The risk of prostate cancer among men with predisposing mutations (BRCA1 and BRCA2) is high and pancreatic cancer may occur in BRCA2 mutation carriers [70]. Individuals at risk should also undergo screening for these malignancies. While it is reasonable to initiate testing slightly earlier than in the general population, there is no clear evidence that there is a predilection for these cancers to occur at a young age [68].

Our Experience

In the context of our scientific interest in hereditary colorectal cancer (FAP and HNPCC), we reviewed our experience in treating FAP and HNPCC patients, with particular attention paid to: (a) DNA-guided therapy for FAP, (b) the occurrence and treatment of FAP-related MPM, and (c) the occurrence and treatment of HNPCC-related MPM.

"DNA-guided" Therapy

Between 1973 and 2007, 52 FAP patients were treated. The age range was 15–63 years, with a male-female ratio of 0.9. Three patients presented with cancer at the time of diagnosis. All were operated on.

We divided our series into three groups with respect to the two main events that contributed to modifying the surgical approach in FAP: the introduction of IPAA in the 1980s and genetic analysis in the 1990s (Fig. 17.3). Proctocolectomy with definitive ileostomy were all carried out during the first referral period, before the arrival of molecular diagnosis. Alongside clinical and instrumental data, genetics have assumed a relevant role in the choice of IRA vs. IPAA. Between 1994 and 2007, the surgical choice was influenced by molecular analysis: 22 patients (ages 16–45 years, M:F ratio =2) underwent surgical procedures that were based on the results of their genetic tests. The orientation was mainly directed at IRA in AFAP and at IPAA in severe forms (mutations at codons 1250-1444). (Fig. 17.4).

Occurrence and Treatment of FAP-related MPM

During follow-up, further therapy was necessary in 45 of the patients (23 IRA, 21 IPAA, 1 non restorative proctocolectomy. After IRA, only two patients underwent proctectomy with definitive ileostomy for rectal stump cancer. Only one pouch was removed for pelvic abscess.

The following extra-colic tumors were diagnosed: ileal carcinoma (1), thy-

17 "DNA-Guided" Therapy

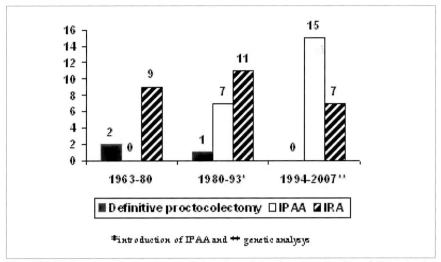

Fig. 17.3 FAP series: changes in surgical options following the adoption of IPAA in the 1980s (*) and mutational analysis in the 1990s (**)

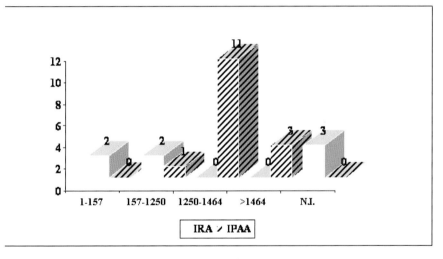

Fig. 17.4 DNA-guided surgery in FAP: our experience

roid Hurtle's cell adenoma (1), desmoids (5), osteomas (4), upper gastrointestinal tract polyps (9). Two of the four patients with osteomas were operated on. Six desmoids occurred in five patients (with a recurrence in one case). All five were female, age 17–42 years (average 25 years). In each of the five cases, genetic tests revealed a mutation in the APC region at codon 1444. The patients were members of two nuclear families whose history of FAP with desmoids was 3/5 (Fig. 17.5) and 2/2. Five of the desmoids were parietal (1 relapse) and one

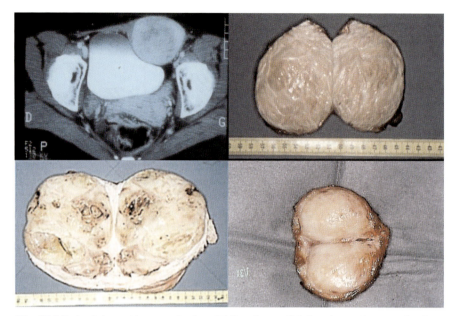

Fig. 17.5 Parietal desmoid tumors in three FAP patients, all belonging at the same family

intra-abdominal and all occurred following colectomy. The main symptoms were: abdominal pain, swelling (wall desmoids) and diffuse pain, weight loss, and occlusive crises (one intra-abdominal). The therapy was surgical with the removal of lesions in 83.3% of the cases (treatment of the parietal form was always surgical with exeresis). In the patient with intra-abdominal occlusion, the mass was unresectable. Neither post-operative morbidity nor mortality occurred, and there was just one relapse 2 years after surgery.

One patient underwent a total thyroidectomy for Hurtle's cell adenoma and an ileal resection for carcinoma. No patient with upper gastrointestinal polyps was operated on and neither periampullary carcinoma, nor hepatoblastoma, nor other rare extra-colonic tumors have been observed.

Occurrence and Treatment of HNPCC-related MPM

Our experience with HNPCC is based on 24 surgically treated CRC patients (4 with simultaneous CRC) (Fig. 17.6). In subjects with mutated MMR genes but healthy at endoscopy, no preventive colectomies were done, while two patients at menopausal age received counseling and subsequently opted for prophylactic hysteroadnexectomy at the same time as colectomy for CRC.

17 "DNA-Guided" Therapy

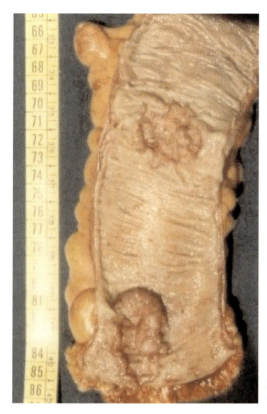

Fig. 17.6 Two simultaneous colonic cancers in a HNPCC patient

The following MPM were detected: five metachronous CRC (all patients had already been operated on before mutational analysis) (Fig. 17.7). All extracolonic tumors arose after CRC and all were ovarian cancers (one peritoneal carcinomatosis) that required hysteroadnexectomy.

Conclusions

The clinical implications of genetics in codified syndromes have in many cases significantly influenced and recently modified the surgical approach (Table 17.5). Identification of affected patients at a young age and in pre-clinical stages was the first clinical application of molecular analysis. In some pathologies (FAP, MTC), genetic screening programs have led to a relevant reduction of advanced cancers and significant prognostic improvement. The psycho-emotional benefits have been important, as a good percentage of family members have been freed from invasive and stressful diagnostic investigations. Moreover, the overall benefits of the economic savings are significant, as useless diagnostic exams for patients without genomic alterations can be avoided.

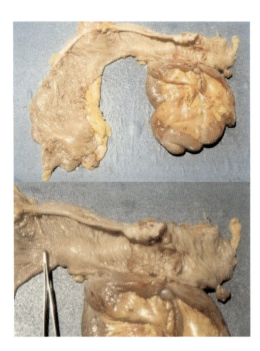

Fig. 17.7 HNPCC: en bloc resection for metachronous adenocarcinoma infiltrating the small bowel

Prophylactic surgery (the removal of an organ before malignant transformation or with cancer in situ) has a relevant role for those diseases with biomolecular alterations. Preventive colectomy and thyroidectomy for FAP and MEN2 represent the prototype of DNA-guided surgery. For HBOC and HNPCC, there is no consensus, and prophylactic surgery therefore remains a valid option in selected cases (e.g., patients with cancer phobia or who refuse periodic clinical observations).

The association of tumors in several organs requires rigorous patient surveillance. The physician's knowledge of specific genetic mutations can be applied to design patient-specific therapy and follow-up. As our knowledge of biomolecular mechanisms continues to improve, chemoprevention to inhibit and/or limit neoplastic proliferation will become an increasingly realistic therapeutic option.

Table 17.5 Clinical implications of genetics in hereditary neoplastic syndromes: epi-crisis

Syndrome	Screening	Prophylactic surgery	MPM surveillance
FAP	+	+	+
HNPCC	+	±	+
MEN1	+	−	±
MEN 2	+	+	+
HBOC	+	±	+

References

1. Bodmer WF, Bailey CJ, Bodmer J et al (1987) Localization of the gene for familial adenomatous polyposis on chromosome 5. Nature 328:614–16
2. Groden J, Thliveris A, Samowitz W (1991) Identification of the gene for familial adenomatous coli gene. Cell 66:589–600
3. Renda A, Izzo P, Carlomagno N et al (1997) Implicazioni cliniche delle conoscenze molecolari nei tumori eredofamiliari del colon-retto. Atti 99° Congresso Nazionale Società Italiana di Chirurgia. Pozzi, Rome
4. Leite JS, Isidro G, Martins M et al (2005) Is prophylactic colectomy indicated in patients with MYH-associated polyposis? Colorectal Dis 7:327–331
5. Vasen HFA (1991) The international collaborative Group on Hereditary non-polyposis colorectal cancer. Dis Col Rectum 34:425–425
6. Rodriguez-Bigas MA, Boland CR, Hamilton SR et al (1997) A National Cancer Institute workshop on hereditary nonpolyposis colorectal cancer syndrome: meeting highlights and Bethesda guidelines. J Natl Cancer Inst 89:1758–1762
7. Umar A, Boland CR, Terdiman JP et al (2004) Revised Bethesda Guidelines for hereditary nonpolyposis colorectal cancer (Lynch syndrome) and microsatellite instability. J Natl Cancer Inst 96(4):261–268
8. Vasen HF, Watson P, Mecklin JP, Lynch HAT (1999) New clinical criteria for hereditary non-polyposis colorectal cancer (HNPCC, Lynch syndrome) proposed by the International Collaborative group on HNPCC. Gastroenterology 116(6):1453–1456
9. Peterson G (1999) Genetic testings for cancer: the surgeon's critical role. Clinical cancer genetics: 1998 (what's available to you in your practice). J Am Coll Surg 188(1):89–93
10. Batra S, Valdimarsdottir H, McGovern M et al (2002) Awareness of genetic testing for colorectal cancer predisposition among specialists in gastroenterology. Am J Gastroenterol 97(3):729–733
11. Schroy PC, Barrison AF, Ling BS et al (2002) Family history and colorectal cancer screening: a survey of physician knowledge and practice patterns. Am J Gastroenterol 97:1031–1036
12. Schroy Lynch HT, Lynch JF (2000) Hereditary nonpolyposis colorectal cancer. Semin Surg Oncol 18(4):305–313
13. Jarvinen HJ (1995) Screening reduces colorectal cancer rates in families with hereditary non-polyposis colorectal cancer. Gastroenterology 108:1405–1411
14. de Vos tot Nederveen Cappel WH, Nagengast FM, Griffioen G et al (2002) Surveillance for hereditary nonpolyposis colorectal cancer: a long-term study on 114 families. Dis Colon Rectum 45:1588–1594
15. Scacheri PC, Davis S, Odom DT et al (2006) Genome-wide analysis of menin binding provides insights into MEN1 tumorigenesis. PLoS Genet 2(4): e51. DOI:10.1371/journal.pgen.0020051
16. Geerdink EAM, Van der Luijt1 RB, Lips CJM (2003) Do patients with multiple endocrine neoplasia syndrome type 1 benefit from periodical screening? Eur J Endocrinol 149:577–582
17. Schussheim DH, Skarulis MC, Agarwal SK et al (2001) Multiple endocrine neoplasia type 1: new clinical and basic findings. Trends Endocrinol Metab 12:173–178
18. Kopp I, Bartsch D, Wild A et al (2001) Predictive genetic screening and clinical findings in multiple endocrine neoplasia type 1 families. World J Surg 25:610–616
19. Marini F, Falchetti A, Del Monte F et al (2006) Multiple endocrine neoplasia type 2 Orphanet J Rare Dis 1:45
20. Lairmore TC, Wells SA Jr, Moley Jeffrey F (2003) Sindromi da neoplasie multiendocrine. In: Sabiston (ed) Trattato di chirurgia. Le basi biologiche della moderna pratica chirurgica, prima edizione italiana sulla sedicesima americana. Antonio Delfino Editore, Rome, pp 697–707
21. Robson ME (2002) Clinical considerations in the management of individuals at risk for hereditary breast and ovarian cancer cancer control. Cancer Control 9:457–465

22. Botkin JR, Smith KR, Croyle RT et al (2003) Genetic testing for a BRCA1 mutation: prophylactic surgery and screening behavior in women 2 years post testing. Am J Med Genet 118A:201–209
23. Schmeler KM, Sun CC, Bodurka DC et al (2006) Prophylactic bilateral salpingo- oophorectomy compared with surveillance in women with BRCA mutations. Obstet Gynecol 108:515–520
24. Jacobs IJ, Skates SJ, MacDonald N et al (1999) Screening for ovarian cancer: a pilot randomised controlled trial. Lancet 353:1207–1210
25. van Nagell JR Jr, DePriest PD, Reedy MB et al (2000) The efficacy of transvaginal sonographic screening in asymptomatic women at risk for ovarian cancer. Gynecol Oncol 77:350–356
26. Vasen HF, van der Luijt RB, Slors JF et al (1996) Molecular genetic tests as a guide to surgical management of familial adenomatous polyposis. Lancet 348(9025):433–435
27. Nugent KP, Philips RKS (1992) Rectal cancer risk in older patients with familial adenomatous polyposis and an ileorectal anastomosis: a cause for concern. Br J Surg 79:1204–1206
28. Renda A, Izzo P, D'Armeinto F et al (2004) Chirurgia oncologica "Dna-guidata". Archivio e Atti SIC, vol. 1. Pozzi, Rome, pp 141–172
29. Church JM (1995) The ileal pouch-anal anastomosis in challenging patients: stretching the limits. Aust N Z J Surg 65(2):104–106
30. Huls G, Koornstra JJ, Kleibeuker JH (2003) Non-steroidal anti-inflammatory drugs and molecular carcinogenesis of colorectal carcinomas. Lancet 362(9379):230–232
31. Sandler RS, Halabi S, Baron JA et al (2003) A randomized trial of aspirin to prevent colorectal adenomas in patients with previous colorectal cancer. N Engl J Med 348(10):883–890
32. Waddell WR, Loughry RW (1983) Sulindac for polyposis of the colon. J Surg Oncol 24(1):83–87
33. Giardiello FM, Hamilton SR, Krush AJ et al (1993) Treatment of colonic and rectal adenomas with sulindac in familial adenomatous polyposis. N Engl J Med 328:1313–1316
34. Giardiello FM, Yang VW, Hylind LM et al (2002) Primary chemoprevention of familial adenomatous polyposis with sulindac. N Engl J Med 346:1054–1059
35. Annie Yu HJ, Lin KM, Ota DM et al (2003) Hereditary nonpolyposis colorectal cancer: preventive management. Cancer Treat Rev 29(6):461–470
36. Karnes WE Jr, Shattuck-Brandt R, Burgart LJ et al (1998) Reduced COX-2 protein in colorectal cancer with defective mismatch repair. Cancer Res 58:5473–5477
37. Sinicrope FA, Lemoine M, Xi L et al (1999) Reduced expression of cyclooxygenase 2 proteins in hereditary nonpolyposis colorectal cancers relative to sporadic cancers. Gastroenterology 117:350–358
38. Toledo SPA, Cortina MA, Toledo RA, Lourenço DM (2006) Impact of RET proto-oncogene analysis on the clinical management of multiple endocrine neoplasia type 2. Clinics 61(1):59–70
39. Cohen MS, Moley JF (2003) Surgical treatment of medullary thyroid carcinoma. J Intern Med 253:616–626
40. Modigliani E, Coben R, Campos JM et al (1998) Prognostic factors for survival and for biochemical cure in medullary thyroid carcinoma: results in 899 patients. The GETC Study Group. Groupe d'étude des tumeurs à calcitonine. Clin Endocrinol (Oxf) 48:265–273
41. Gill JR, Reyes-Mugica M, Iyengar S et al (1996) Early presentation of metastatic medullary cancer on multiple endocrine neoplasia, type IIA: implications for therapy. J Pediatr 129:459–464
42. Stjernholm MR, Freudenbourg JC, Mooney HS et al (1980) Medullary carcinoma of the thyroid before age 2 years. J Clin Endocrinol Metab 51:252–253
43. Kaufman FR, Roe TF, Isaacs Jr H, Weitzman JJ (1982) Metastatic medullary thyroid carcinoma in young children with mucosal neuroma syndrome. Pediatrics 70:263–267
44. Samaan NA, Draznin MB, Halpin RE et al (1991) Multiple endocrine syndrome type IIb in early childhood. Cancer 68:1832–1834

45. Skinner MA, DeBenedetti MK, Moley JF et al (1996) Medullary thyroid carcinoma in children with multiple endocrine neoplasia types 2A and 2B. J Pediatr Surg 31:177–181
46. Smith VV, Eng C, Milla PJ (1999) Intestinal ganglioneuromatosis and multiple endocrine neoplasia type 2B: implications for treatment. Gut 45:143–146
47. Brandi ML, Gagel RF, Angeli A et al (2001) Guidelines for diagnosis and therapy of MEN type 1 and type 2. J Clin Endocrinol Metab 86:5658–5671
48. Lerman C, Hughes C, Croyle RT et al (2000) Prophylactic surgery decisions and surveillance practices one year following BRCA1/2 testing. Prev Med 31:75–80
49. Rebbeck TR, Friebel T, Lynch HT et al (2004) Bilateral prophylactic mastectomy reduces breast cancer risk in BRCA1 and BRCA2 mutation carriers: the PROSE Study Group. J Clin Oncol 22(6):1055–1062
50. Kauf ND, Satagopan JM, Robson ME et al (2002) Risk-reducing salpingo-oophorectomy in women with a BRCA1 or BRCA2 mutation. N Engl J Med 346:1609–1615
51. Olivier RI (2004) Clinical outcome of prophylactic oophorectomy in BRCA1/BRCA2 mutation carriers and events during follow-up. Br J Cancer 90(8):1492–1497
52. Iglehart JD, Kaelin CM (2003) Malattie della mammella. In: Sabiston (ed) Trattato di chirurgia. Le basi biologiche della moderna pratica chirurgica, prima edizione italiana sulla sedicesima americana. Antonio Delfino Editore, Rome, pp 555–590
53. Burke W, Daly M, Garber J et al (1997) Recommendations for follow-up care of individuals with an inherited predisposition to cancer: II. BRCA1 and BRCA2. Cancer Genetics Studies Consortium. JAMA 277:997–1003
54. Hartmann LC, Schaid DJ, Woods JE et al (1999) Efficacy of bilateral prophylactic mastectomy in women with a family history of breast cancer. N Engl J Med 340:77–84
55. Hartmann LC, Sellers TA, Schaid DJ et al (2001) Efficacy of bilateral prophylactic mastectomy in BRCA1 and BRCA2 mutation carriers. J Natl Cancer Inst 93:1633–1637
56. Meijers-Heijboer H, van Geel B, van Putten WL et al (2001) Breast cancer after prophylactic bilateral mastectomy in women with a BRCA1 or BRCA2 mutation. N Engl J Med 345:159–164
57. Hartmann LC, Degnim A, Schaid DJ (2004) Prophylactic mastectomy for BRCA1/2 carriers: progress and more questions. J Clin Oncol 22(6):981–983
58. Julian-Reynier CM, Bouchard LJ, Evans DG et al (2001) Women's attitudes toward preventive strategies for hereditary breast or ovarian carcinoma differ from one country to another: differences among English, French, and Canadian women. Cancer 15:959–968
59. Renda A, Romano G, Carlomagno N et al (1992) Il follow-up degli operati per poliposi familiare del colon. Atti della SIC, vol. 3. Pozza, Rome, pp 229–252
60. Lynch HT, Lynch JF (2000) Hereditary nonpolyposis colorectal cancer. Semin Surg Oncol 18(4):305–313
61. Rodriguez-Bigas MA, Vasen HF, Pekka-Mecklin J et al (1997) Rectal cancer risk in hereditary nonpolyposis colorectal cancer after abdominal colectomy. Ann Surg 225:202–207
62. Hahn M, Saeger HD, Schackert HK (1999) Hereditary colorectal cancer: clinical consequences of predictive molecular testing. Int J Colorectal Dis 14:184–193
63. Weber T (1996) Clinical surveillance recommendations adopted for HNPCC. Lancet 348:465
64. National Comprehensive Cancer Network (2003) Clinical practice guidelines in oncology. Available at: www.nccn.org
65. Del Vecchio Blanco C, Renda A (1999) Il trattamento dei tumori del colon-retto. Conferenza Regionale Campana. Giuseppe de Nicola Editore, Naples
66. Schmeler KM, Lynch HT, Chen LM et al (2006) Prophylactic surgery to reduce the risk of gynecologic cancers in the Lynch syndrome. N Engl J Med 354(3):261–269
67. Jimenez C, Gagel RF (2004) Genetic testing in endocrinology: lessons learned from experience with multiple endocrine neoplasia type 2 (MEN2) Growth Horm IGF Re, 14(Suppl A):S150-S157
68. Eccles DM (2004) Hereditary cancer: guidelines in clinical practice. Breast and ovarian cancer genetics. Ann Oncol 15(Suppl 4): iv133-iv138

69. Elit L (2001) Familial ovarian cancer. Can Fam Physician 47:778–784
70. Eisinger F (1998) Recommendations for medical management of hereditary breast and ovarian cancer: The French National Ad Hoc Committee. Ann Oncol 9:939–950

Chapter 18
Chemoprevention

Pietro Lombari, Gaetano Aurilio, Fernando De Vita, Giuseppe Catalano

Prevention represents an absolutely relevant area of oncology, its aim being to prevent the onset of cancer and to reduce mortality. The goal is to re-balance the factors that promote and inhibit carcinogenesis, including the countless exogenous (environmental) and endogenous (genetic) mechanisms. In the field of prevention, it is possible to distinguish four broad areas of research: primary prevention, secondary prevention, tertiary prevention, and chemoprevention.

The first one addresses the healthy population and consists of eliminating or reducing the exposure to risk factors. The second one deals with the early detection of preneoplastic lesions or of tumors in the preclinical stage. The third one includes measures to reduce the morbidity associated with a developing neoplasm, as well as complications and relapses after initial treatment, but also the development of multiple primary malignancies (MPM). The fourth area concerns anticancer chemoprevention, i.e., pharmacological intervention by the administration of chemically synthetic compounds or natural substances in order to stop or reverse carcinogenesis and thereby prevent the development of invasive tumors.

Cancer control must take into account two fundamental concepts: "multiphasic cancerogenesis" and "district cancerization." The former refers to a chronic process characterized by the accumulation of specific genetic and phenotypic alterations that can exert their effects for more than 10–20 years following the first initiating event. The latter concerns patients at high risk of epithelial cancer who have a wide spectrum of cancerous tissue changes, diagnosed at either the macroscopic (precancerous oral lesions, polyps), microscopic (metaplasia, dysplasia), or molecular (genes loss or amplification mechanisms) level [1]. These patients will develop multiple epithelial neoplastic lesions, the clinical importance of which is confirmed by the pattern of multicentrality, a phenomenon frequently observed in malignant tumors of the upper digestive tract, but also in the colon, breast and skin.

Individuals at risk of developing tumors, especially those with a previous history of tumor development, are candidates for chemoprevention. In fact, it is well-established that patients who have had a malignant neoplasm are at a two-fold risk of developing a second neoplasm (compared to age-matched controls). This review evaluates the role and potential of chemoprevention in the management of MPM, the drugs of interest, and the further risk factors for the development of second tumors. Interesting correlations regarding subsequent tumor formation comes out from several collections of case histories (Table 18.1).

In a recent trial involving 14,181 male cancer patients, 204 cases of MPM were observed. Multivariate analysis showed that the development of MPM (lung, esophagus, larynx, oral cavity, kidney, bladder, pancreas, liver cancer) was significantly associated with antecedent tobacco use at first evidence of the tumor (independent risk factor); obese patients (BMI ≥25 kg/m^2) had a significantly high relative risk (RR) for colorectal and urogenital MPM (bladder, kidney, and prostate); patients with serum glucose ≥126 mg/dl had a higher RR for tobacco-related and hepatopancreatobiliary MPM [2]. Moreover, it has been demonstrated that high serum levels of insulin-like growth factor (IGF)-1 and its binding protein IGFBP-3 are associated with an increased risk of developing MPM. Thus a simple measurement suggests the need for closer monitoring [3].

Several studies have concluded that smoking and alcohol intake, continuing after diagnosis of the first tumor, represent independent predictive factors for developing MPM [4]. The relationship between the patient's age at first diagnosis of cancer and the onset of MPM is another interesting aspect. In a study by Gao et al., consisting of 20,074 patients with survival from laryngeal tumor of at least 3 months, advanced age was associated with increased overall risk of MPM ($p = 0.0001$) and very poor survival ($p = 0.0001$) [5]. In the presence of the above-cited risk factors, some evidence suggests that genetic susceptibility contributes to the development of MPM. An association between expression of the gene encoding glutathione S-transferase polymorphism M1 and the development of MPM has been shown in patients previously treated for early-stage head and neck squamous cell carcinoma (HNSCC) [6]. The correlation between MPM and previous testicular cancer must be noted as well. In this regard, Travis et al. examined 40,576 testicular cancer patients from 1943 to 2001, identifying 2,285 cases of MPM. In particular, among 10-year survivors diagnosed for testicular cancer at age 35 years, the risk of developing MPM increased (RR = 1.9, 95% confidence interval = 1.8–2.1) and remained significantly high for 35 years (RR = 1.7, 95% CI = 1.5–2.0; p <0.001). High-risk sites were the pleura (mesothe-

Table 18.1 Risk factors for the development of multiple primary malignancies (MPM)

- Tobacco habit
- Alcohol consumption
- Obesity ≥25 kg/m^2
- Glycemia ≥12 6mg/dl
- IGF-1 and IGFBP-3 concentrations
- Age at the time of first tumor diagnosis
- Genetic susceptibility

lioma, RR = 3.4, 95% CI = 1.7–5.9), bladder (RR 2.7, 95% CI = 2.2-3.1), pancreas (RR 3.6, 95% CI = 2.8–4.6), and stomach (RR = 4.0, 95% CI = 3.2–4.8). It also should be underlined that an increased risk of MPM was observed in patients treated with radiotherapy (RR = 2.0, 95% CI = 1.9–2.2), chemotherapy (RR = 1.9, 95% CI = 1.3–2.5), or both (RR = 2.9, 95% CI = 1.9–4.2) [7].

Numerous chemopreventative agents are potentially effective in the treatment of premalignant and malignant lesions (Table 18.2). Epidemiological studies showing a correlation between vitamin A (the first essential nutrient identified, in 1913) consumption and the impact of cancer date from 1970, this finding is particularly relevant for lung cancer. Retinoids are natural derivatives and synthetic analogues of vitamin A. One member of the carotenoid class, β-carotene, was and still is one of the most intensively studied agents in chemoprevention, either alone or in combination with other such drugs.

Phase I–II trials provide useful information about the toxicity, feasibility, and potential activity of chemopreventative biomolecules. Nevertheless, for a strict evaluation of effectiveness, randomized phase III studies are clearly necessary. This is especially true for the analysis of intermediate targets, as the results are very difficult to interpret and may not be reliable in uncontrolled studies. Such targets include genetic markers (micronuclei, ploidy and DNA content, chromosomes, oncogenes and suppressor genes), markers of differentiation (epidermoids and blood-group antigens), and markers of proliferation (nuclear proliferation antigens, thymidine index, nuclear receptors for retinoid acid, and the epidermal growth factor and transforming growth factor-β receptors). The systematic use of these markers must take into account their specificity for cancerogenesis, qualitative and quantitative correlation with degree of disease progression, measurable on very small samples, and modulated by the substance used for prevention. Assays that are based on these markers provide fast answers, in contrast to the long-term outcomes of classical clinical studies.

Table 18.2 Potential agents in chemoprevention

Vitamin A and retinoids	Antioxidants	Antihormones	NSAIDs	Micronutrients
Retinol	β-Carotene	Tamoxifen	Sulindac	Calcium
Retinyl palmitate	Vitamin C	Raloxifene	Piroxicam	Selenium
Retinal	Vitamin E	Finasteride	Acetylsalicylic acid	Zinc
Fenretinide	N-acetyl-cysteine	Aromatase inhibitors	Selective inhibitors of COX-2	–
13-cis-retinoic acid				

During the last 10 years, our knowledge of the mechanism of action of retinoids has significantly increased, but this is not the case for carotenoids, which require further study.

Retinoids have been evaluated for their role in chemoprevention, especially in preclinical models in which the regulation of cell growth, differentiation, and apoptosis by these agents was examined. They act primarily at the level of post-initiation of tumor promotion and progression, which are the most relevant stages for chemoprevention. The mechanism of action of retinoids is similar to that of steroids and thyroid hormones. In fact, retinoid nuclear receptors are members of the steroid receptor superfamily, although they exhibit distinctive features. There are two receptor classes, retinoic acid receptors (RARs) and retinoid X receptor (RXRs). Each receptor contains α, β, and γ subtypes and many of the members of these subclasses have multiple isoforms. Retinoid receptors are DNA-binding transcription factors; they can activate or suppress the expression of many genes, the products of which mediate the effects of retinoids on cell growth, differentiation, and apoptosis. Different retinoids bind several classes and subclasses of receptors with variable affinities. This receptor complexity and diversity in ligand-binding, activation, and receptor function have important implications in prevention and therapy. Retinoid receptors are active only as dimers, and two types have been identified: RAR/RXR heterodimers and RXR/RXR homodimers. One part of the retinoid receptor binds to the ligand and the other to specific DNA sequences (RARE or RXRE), resulting in gene suppression or transcription (Tables 18.3, 18.4).

Carotenoids play a role in the prevention of photosensitization and some of them have well-characterized provitamin A activity. However, the mechanisms behind many of the biological actions of carotenoids, such as antioxidant activity, immunoenhancement, inhibition of mutagenesis, transformation, and regression of premalignant lesions are still far from clear. Some of these effects,

Table 18.3 Retinoid receptors

RAR receptors for all-*trans* retinoic acid	RXR receptors for 9-*cis* retinoic acid
RARα	RXRα
RARβ	RXRβ
RARγ	RXRγ

Table 18.4 Receptor domains

- DNA-binding domain
- Hormone-binding domain
- Heterodimerization-binding domain
- One or more transcription-activating domains

including regression of premalignant lesions, are shared with those of retinoid. Since the cleavage products from carotenoids have retinoid-like activity, there may well be a functionally interacting network based on structural-molecular sharing. The antioxidant activity of carotenoids as their mechanism of prevention has been discussed for many years. While there is now clear evidence of chemopreventative efficacy of β-carotene in some animal models of carcinogenesis, it is not yet clear whether antioxidant activity is responsible for the chemoprotective effects observed in vivo.

The chemopreventative effects of retinoids, carotenoids, and micronutrients with respect to tumors of the head and neck, lung, digestive system, skin, breast, bladder, prostate, uterus and cervix are under intensive investigation. Although many of these substances prevent or to reverse carcinogenesis and to modulate epithelial cell differentiation, especially in precancerous oral lesions, studies evaluating the impact of chemoprevention in MPM have not yielded analogously favorable results. This apparent dichotomy suggests that several factors, including patient selection, habits such as smoking or alcohol intake, tumor site, histopathological characteristics of the tumor, and the choice, dose, duration, and beginning of administration of chemopreventative drugs, play a decisive role in determining the effectiveness of these agents.

Of the several trials addressing MPM chemoprevention with results reported in the literature, the most considerable scientific evidence has been gathered for head and neck, lung, breast, skin and bladder cancers (Table 18.5). About 40–50% of HNSCC are diagnosed at stage I or II. Even if these patients have a good prognosis, the benefit of treatment, usually surgery, is often compromised by the occurrence of MPM, which develop in 15–20% of patients during the first 5 years after diagnosis, usually following cancers of the aero/upper digestive tract and usually associated with chronic exposure to alcohol and tobacco. Even if long-term survival is moderately improved, the main cause of morbidity and mortality in patients already treated for early-stage HNSCC is the development of second tumors. Accordingly, during the last 20 years, remarkable efforts have been aimed at determining whether chemopreventative agents, such as retinoids and antioxidants, can reduce the risk of new tumors.

In 1990, results of the first randomized phase III trial were published. In that study, 103 patients disease-free after primary treatment for squamous cell cancers of the larynx, pharynx, or oral cavity were randomized to receive isotretinoin (50–100 mg/day) or placebo for 12 months. The MPM rate was significantly lower in the arm with high-dose retinoids than in the placebo arm ($p = 0.005$). Although severely limited by the small sample size, and thus a very low statistical power, this is one of the few studies to report positive findings [8]. In fact, from 1994 to 2006, randomized trials with wider samples have not confirmed that study's conclusions.

In 1994, a multicentric double-blind randomized trial involving 316 patients demonstrated that, compared to placebo, etretinate, a second-generation retinoid, did not prevent the development of MPM in patients treated for squamous cell carcinoma of the oral cavity and oropharynx [9]. Following that result,

Table 18.5 Examined studies

Study (year) [reference]	N. of patients	Disease	Treatment	Statistical significance	Adverse effects
Hong et al. (1990) [8]	103	HNSCC	Isotretinoin vs. placebo	Yes	–
Bolla et al. (1994) [9]	316	HNSCC	Etretinate vs. placebo	No	–
Zandwijk et al. (2000) [10]	2,592	HNSCC and lung cancer	Vitamin A and/or N-acetyl-cysteine vs. placebo	No	–
Mayne et al. (2001) [11]	264	HNSCC	β Carotene vs. placebo	No	↑ Risk of lung MPM
Bairati et al. (2005) [12]	540	HNSCC	α-Tocopherol and β-carotene vs. placebo	No	↑ Impact of MPM
Khury et al. (2006) [13]	1,190	HNSCC	Isotretinoin vs. placebo	No	↑ Impact of MPM in smokers
ATBC trial (1994) [14]	29,133	Lung cancer	β-Carotene or α-tocopherol or both vs. placebo	No	↑ Lung and prostate cancer impact with β-carotene
CARET trial (1996) [15]	18,314	Lung cancer	β-Carotene plus retinol vs. placebo	No	↑ Impact of lung MPM
Lippman et al. (2001) [16]	1,166	Lung cancer	Isotretinoin vs. placebo	No	↑ Risk of lung MPM
Veronesi et al. (2006) [18]	1,739	Breast cancer	Fenretinide vs. placebo	Yes	–
Bertelsen et al. (2008) [19]	1,792	Breast cancer	CT vs. placebo TAM vs. placebo	Yes	–
Tangrea et al. (1992) [20]	981	Skin cancer	Isotretinoin vs. placebo	No	Significant systemic adverse events

continue ↑

continue **Table 18.5**

Levine et al. (1997) [21]	525	Skin cancer	Retinol or 13cRA or placebo	No	–
Moon et al. (1997) [22]	2,297	Skin cancer	Retinol or placebo	Yes for SCC, no for BCC	–
Clark et al. (1996) [23]	1,312	Skin cancer	Selenium vs. placebo	No for MPM	–
Duffield-Lillico et al. (2003) [24]	1,312	Skin cancer	Selenium vs. placebo	No	↑ risk of MPM
Pedersen et al. (1984) [25]	73	Bladder cancer	Retinoid etretinate vs. placebo	Not conclusive	–
Alfthan et al. (1983) [26]	30	Bladder cancer	Retinoid etretinate	Not evaluable	–
Studer et al. (1984) [27]	–	Bladder cancer	Retinoid etretinate	Yes	–

CT, Chemotherapy; *TAM*, tamoxifen; *SCC*, squamous cell carcinoma; *BCC*, basal cell carcinoma; *HNSCC*, head and neck squamous cell carcinoma the EUROSCAN trial evaluated the prophylactic role of vitamin A and *N*-acetylcysteine in 2,592 patients treated with curative aim for head and neck cancer or lung cancer. After 2 years of administration of retinol or antioxidant, no significant benefit in overall survival, event-free survival, or MPM prevention was noted. Moreover, paradoxically, there was a lower impact of MPM in the arm without treatment [10]. Likewise, in the series of Mayne et al., consisting of 264 patients administered β-carotene vs. placebo, a not significant benefit on head and neck MPM, but a possible increase in the risk of lung tumors was observed [11]. Another discouraging finding is the increased incidence of MPM in patients treated with α-tocopherol, which could imply that supplementation with antioxidants accelerates neoplastic progression [12].

Recently, a study of 1,190 patients treated for stage I–II HNSCC and randomized to receive low doses of isotretinoin (30 mg/day) vs. placebo for 3 years did not show a reduction in MPM (HR = 1.06) or increased survival in the isotretinoin arm. The MPM onset sites were, in order of occurrence, lung, oral cavity, larynx, pharynx, and esophagus, according to the usual presentation. The statistically significant increase in MPM and death in smokers compared to people who never smoked implicates tobacco habit as an important risk factor [13].

The results have also been disappointing for lung cancer. In patients with stage I disease whose tumors were resected, relapses of the primary tumor occurred in 20–30%, MPM was diagnosed in 10–20%, no benefits for chemoprevention in inhibiting MPM could be established whatsoever.

The authors of the ATBC Finnish trial followed 29,133 male smokers between the ages of 50 and 69 years. A 2 × 2 factorial design was used and participants were randomized to receive β-carotene (20 mg/day), α-tocopherol (50 mg/day), a combination of both, or placebo, for 5–8 years. Unexpectedly, participants receiving β-carotene (alone or with α-tocopherol) showed a statistically significant increase in the incidence of lung cancer, equal to 18% (RR 1.18; 95% CI 1.03–1.36) and an increase of 8% in total mortality (RR 1.08; 95% CI 1.01–1.16). Interesting observations emerged from this trial regarding vitamin E and prostate cancer. Participants who received α-tocopherol showed a reduction in the incidence of prostate cancer equal to a 32 and 41% decrease in cancer-related mortality. By contrast, among the subjects who received β-carotene, the incidences of mortality and prostate cancer were, respectively, 15 and 23% higher than in subjects who did not receive this treatment [14].

The CARET trial evaluated 18,314 smokers and workers exposed to asbestos. These subjects were randomized to receive β-carotene (30 mg/day) plus retinol (25000 IU/day) or placebo. However, the study was precociously closed, because preliminary analysis indicated that those in the β-carotene and retinol arm had an increased incidence of second lung tumors [15].

The "Lung Intergroup Trial" examined 1,166 patients with stage I non-small-cell lung cancer (NSCLC) who were treated with definitive surgery. Patients were randomized to receive isotretinoin (30 mg/day) or placebo. After a median follow-up of 3.5 years, there were no statistically significant differences between the two arms regarding MPM, the primary endpoint. No relationship between

MPM and tobacco use or relapses or mortality was found [16].

The era of chemoprevention in the treatment of breast cancer historically began in 1998, when tamoxifen, a first-generation selective estrogen receptor modulator, became the first drug approved by the FDA for breast cancer prevention. Approval was granted on the basis of the BCPT trial results, which showed that the drug reduced the incidence of breast cancer by 49% in women at increased risk. Raloxifen, a second-generation selective estrogen receptor modulator (SERM), was compared to tamoxifen in a large randomized trial (STAR TRIAL) and showed equal efficacy in breast cancer risk reduction, but without a clear effect on endometrial cancer [17]. Likewise, the aromatase inhibitors have been shown to reduce the incidence of contralateral breast cancer in the adjuvant setting; their efficacy is under investigation.

Veronesi et al. evaluated 1,739 patients with early breast cancer who were randomized to receive oral fenretinide (a synthetic derivative of *trans*-retinic acid) at a dose of 200 mg/day for 5 years (872 patients) or no treatment (867 patients). With a median follow-up of 14.6 years, the results showed a statistically significant lasting reduction in the incidence of breast MPM. Stratifying the analysis for menopause, a statistically significant reduction of breast MPM of 38% in premenopausal women was demonstrated, and the protective effect persisted for over 15 years, until 10 years after the interruption of retinoid administration. Such effects in premenopausal women could be related to a reduction in the number of breast cells at risk of transformation and/or to a hormone-mediated mechanism. Compared to tamoxifen, which inhibits only ER-positive tumors, fenretinide induces apoptosis in breast cancer cell lines, either ER-positive or ER-negative, although it is more effective in the former. Since in that study fenretinide reduced the incidence of MPM in premenopausal women, independent of the expression of hormonal receptors, the benefits of its use in combination with a SERM seem intuitive [18].

A study published this year on 1,792 patients with unilateral (1,158) and contralateral (634) breast MPM evidenced a statistically significant association between chemotherapy and a reduction in the risk of contralateral breast cancer. The effect was observed for more than 10 years after diagnosis of the first breast cancer, and the association was stronger in women who entered menopause within one year after diagnosis of the first breast tumor (RR = 0.28, 95% CI = 0.11–0.76). Moreover, the use of tamoxifen compared to non-use was associated with a reduction of contralateral breast cancer risk (RR = 0.66, 95% CI = 0.5–0.88). The association was statistically significant for 5 years after first diagnosis of the tumor [19].

Fenretinide inhibits breast carcinogenesis in animal models. It selectively accumulates in human breast tissue and can induce apoptosis in vitro, with a favorable toxicity profile in clinical studies.

In the treatment of skin cancer, several large randomized phase III trials assessing the preventative effects of retinoids have been carried out. Trials of low-dose 13cRA (10 mg/day) and retinol (25,000 IU/day) or 13cRA (5–10 mg/day) vs. placebo in patients with previous skin cancer did not show chemopreventative effect [20, 21]. A third trial, in which retinol was administered to patients with previous actinic keratoses, highlighted a significant reduction in squamous but not in basal cell carcinoma [22]. These contrasting results suggest the need for further analysis on the dose, optimal timing of administration, and appropriate histopathological target of retinoid.

Selenium is another molecule under investigation in the prevention of skin MPM. Clark et al. examined 1,312 patients with a history of non-melanoma skin cancer. Subjects were randomized to receive 200 µg/day of selenium or placebo. Selenium supplementation did not influence the incidence of skin MPM (RR = 1.10 for basal cell carcinoma; 1.14 for squamous cell carcinoma) but there was a significant reduction in total mortality (RR 0.50; 95 % CI, 0.31–0.80), connected mainly to reductions in the incidence of lung, colorectal, and prostate cancers [23]. The same study, examined with a longer follow-up by Duffield-Lillico et al., showed that supplementation with selenium was ineffective in preventing basalioma and significantly increased the risk of squamous cell carcinoma risk (HR 1.25) and the global risk of non-melanoma skin cancer (HR 1.17) [24].

Epidemiologic studies and data obtained in vitro and in vivo have suggested the efficacy of retinoids in the prevention of bladder cancer. Three randomized trials evaluated the use of the retinoid etretinate in patients who underwent resection of a superficial (noninvasive) bladder tumor. Relapses were observed in 40–90% of the patients and all patients experienced mucocutaneous toxicity [25–27]. In two of these three trials, prolonged low-dose etretinate (25 mg/day) was effective. These promising results must be interpreted with caution because of the small number of patients and the short follow-up.

Great emphasis is currently being placed on the role of non-steroid anti-inflammatory drugs (NSAIDS) in the treatment of colorectal tumors, especially regarding secondary prevention. In experiments performed on mice genetically modified mice so that they exhibited familiar adenomatous polyposis (FAP)-like disease, NSAIDS were shown to reduce the incidence and relapses of colorectal adenomas. In particular, prolonged use of sulindac seemed to be effective in polyps regression and in preventing relapses of high-grade adenomas in patients with ileorectal anastomosis after total colectomy for FAP [28]. In FAP management, with extension to gastric and duodenal polyposis, chemoprevention with NSAIDS can be considered after initial prophylactic surgery, supporting endoscopic surveillance by reducing the number and/or dimensions of polyps. Therefore, the use of either sulindac or acetyl-salicylic acid may be associated with a reduction in the number of polyps but there are no indications for their role in the therapy of malignant neoplastic lesions [29].

Many of the chemopreventative agents examined thus far act by modulating cell proliferation or differentiation through a cytostatic effect, stopping or retarding the progression of transformed cells. For this reason, they should be administered over a long period of time; however, both toxicity and resistance, which are often non-predictable, may well be associated with long-term use. These are the principal obstacles that may limit the use and the success of chemopreventative agents. An alternative may be substances that induce apoptosis rather than intervene in proliferation and/or differentiation. This would avoid chronic exposure and limit both the risk of long-term toxicity and the development of chemoresistance [30]. Based on this assumption, several chemopreventative molecules are currently in the preclinical phase of testing (Table 18.6).

In conclusion, with the exception of the role of tamoxifen in breast cancer and sporadic reports on effective chemoprevention of other tumors (vitamin E and prostate cancer, and retinol and squamous cell skin cancer), chemoprevention is not yet an effective therapy for MPM in routine clinical practice. In our opinion, candidates for chemoprevention studies must be patients who are at high risk of developing second tumors.

Progress in scientific research, through molecular studies, will eventually lead to the identification of specific targets for chemoprevention agents. This will no doubt be accompanied by a shift from cytotoxic agents (chemotherapy) to biological drugs (target therapy); that is, the transition from empirical experimentation with a single agent to treat various tumors to the identification of selective tissue targets (chemoprevention target). Some examples are provided by the potential use of gefitinib, a selective inhibitor of the tyrosine kinase activity of the epidermal growth factor receptor, and tipifarnib, which inhibits farnesyltransferase. Both drugs prevent the progression of premalignant lung lesions in patients with a history of tobacco-related cancer. Similar developments and investments in clinical and basic research will constitute the hub of the future of chemoprevention.

Table 18.6 Chemopreventative agents inducing apoptosis in malignant and premalignant cells in vitro

Class/agent	Cells in vitro
Retinoids	
Trans-retinoic acid	Breast cancer
N-(4-hydroxyphenyl) retinamide	Squamous cell skin, cervical and prostate cancer
Nonsteroidal antinflammatory drugs (NSAIDs)	
Acetylsalicylic acid	Gastric cancer
Sulindac	Hepatocarcinoma, prostate and colorectal cancer
Celecoxib	Prostate cancer
Polyphenols	
Resveratrol	Colorectal cancer
Epigallocatechin gallate	Prostate and skin cancer
Anti-estrogens	
Tamoxifen	Breast cancer
Rotenoids	
Deguelin	Colorectal and squamous cell skin cancer

References

1. De Vita VT, Hellman S Jr, Rosenberg SA (eds) (2005) Cancer, principles e practise of oncology. 7th edition. Lippincott Raven, Philadelphia
2. Park SM, Lim MK, Jung KW et al (2007) Prediagnosis smoking, obesity, insulin resistance, and second primary cancer risk in male cancer survivors: National Health Insurance Corporation Study. J Clin Oncol 25:4835–4843
3. Wu X, Zhao H, Do KA et al (2004) Serum levels of insulin growth factor (IGF-I) and IGF-binding protein predict risk of second primary tumors in patients with head and neck cancer. Clin Cancer Res 10:3988–3995
4. Do KA, Johnson MM, Doherty DA et al (2003) Second primary tumors in patients with upper aerodigestive tract cancers: joint effects of smoking and alcohol (United States). Cancer Causes Control 14(2):131–138
5. Gao X, Fisher SG, Mohideen N, Emami B (2003) Second primary cancers in patients with laryngeal cancer: a population-based study. Int J Radiat Oncol Biol Phis. 56(2):427–435
6. Minard CG, Spitz MR, Wu X et al (2006) Evaluation of glutathione S-transferase polymorphisms and mutagen sensitivity as risk factors for the development of second primary tumors in patients previously diagnosed with early-stage head and neck cancer. Cancer 106:2636–2644
7. Travis LB, Fosså SD, Schonfeld SJ et al (2005) Second cancers among 40,576 testicular cancer patients: focus on long-term survivors. J Natl Cancer Inst 97(18):1354–1365
8. Hong WK, Lippman SM, Itri LM et al (1990) Prevention of second primary tumors with isotretinoin in squamous-cell carcinoma of the head and neck. N Engl J Med 323(12):795–801
9. Bolla M, Lefur R, Ton Van J et al (1994) Prevention of second primary tumours with etretinate in squamous cell carcinoma of the oral cavity and oropharynx. Results of a multicentric double-blind randomised study. Eur J Cancer 30A(6):767–772
10. van Zandwijk N, Dalesio O, Pastorino U et al (2000) EUROSCAN, a randomized trial of vitamin A and N-acetylcysteine in patients with head and neck cancer or lung cancer. J Natl Cancer Inst 92(12):977–986
11. Mayne ST, Cartmel B, Baum M et al (2001) Randomized trial of supplemental β-carotene to prevent second head and neck cancer. Cancer Research 61:1457–1463
12. Bairati I, Meyer F, Gélinas M et al (2005) A randomized trial of antioxidant vitamins to prevent second primary cancers in head and neck cancer patients. J Natl Cancer Inst 97(7):481–488
13. Khuri FR, Lee JJ, Lippman SM et al (2006) Randomized phase III trial of low-dose isotretinoin for prevention of second primary tumors in stage I and II head and neck cancer patients. J Natl Cancer Inst 98(7):441–450
14. Anonymous (1994) The effect of vitamin E and beta carotene on the incidence of lung cancer and other cancers in male smokers. The Alpha-Tocopherol, Beta Carotene Cancer Prevention Study Group. N Engl J Med 330(15):1029–1035
15. Omenn GS, Goodman GE, Thornquist MD et al (1996) Effects of a combination of beta-carotene and vitamin A on lung cancer and cardiovascular disease. N Engl J Med 334(18):1150–1155
16. Lippman SM, Lee JJ, Karp DD et al (2001) Randomized phase III intergroup trial of isotretinoin to prevent second primary tumors in stage I non-small-cell lung cancer. J Natl Cancer Inst 93(8):605–618
17. Bevers TB (2007) The STAR trial: evidence for raloxifene as a breast cancer risk reduction agent for postmenopausal women. J Natl Compr Canc Netw 5(8):719–724
18. Veronesi U, Mariani L, Decensi A et al (2006) Fifteen-year results of a randomized phase III trial of fenretinide to prevent second breast cancer. Ann Oncol 17:1065–1071
19. Bertelsen L, Bernstein L, Olsen JH et al (2008) Effect of systemic adjuvant treatment on risk for contralateral breast cancer in the women's environment, cancer and radiation epidemiology study. J Natl Cancer Inst 100:32–40

20. Tangrea JA, Edwards BK, Taylor PR et al (1992) Long-term therapy with low-dose isotretinoin for prevention of basal cell carcinoma: a multicenter clinical trial. J Natl Cancer Inst 84:328–332
21. Levine N, Moon TE, Cartmel B et al (1997) Trial of retinol and isotretinoin in skin cancer prevention: a randomized, double-blind, controlled trial. Southwest Skin Cancer Prevention Study Group. Cancer Epidemiol Biomarkers Prev 6:957–961
22. Moon TE, Levine N, Cartmel B et al (1997) Effect of retinol in preventing squamous cell skin cancer in moderate-risk subjects: a randomized, double-blind, controlled trial. Cancer Epidemiol Biomarkers Prev 6:949–956
23. Clark LC, Combs GF Jr, Turnbull BW et al (1996) Effects of selenium supplementation for cancer prevention in patients with carcinoma of the skin. A randomized controlled trial. Nutritional Prevention of Cancer Study Group. JAMA 276:1957–1963
24. Duffield-Lillico, Slate EH, Reid ME AJ et al (2003) Selenium supplementation and secondary prevention of non melanoma skin cancer in a randomized trial. J Natl Cancer Inst 95:1477–1481
25. Pedersen H, Wolf H, Jensen SK et al (1984) Administration of a retinoid as prophylaxis of recurrent non-invasive bladder tumors. Scand J Urol Nephrol 18:121–123
26. Alfthan O, Tarkkanen J, Groehn P et al (1983) Tigason (etretinate) in prevention of recurrence of superficial bladder tumors. Eur Urol 9:6–9
27. Studer UE, Biedermann C, Chollet D et al (1984) Prevention of recurrent superficial bladder tumors by oral etretinate: preliminary results of a randomized, double blind multicenter trial in Switzerland. J Urol 131:47–49
28. Cruz-Correa M, Hylind LM, Romans KE M et al (2002) Long-term treatment with sulindac in familial adenomatous polyposis: a prospective cohort study. Gastroenterology 122 (3): 641–645
29. Asano TK, McLeod RS (2004) Non steroidal anti-inflammatory drugs (NSAID) and aspirin for preventing colorectal adenomas and carcinomas. Cochrane Database of Systematic Reviews 2004, Issue 1, CD004079. DOI:10.1002/14651858.CD004079.pub2
30. Sun SY, Hail N Jr, Lotan R (2004) Apoptosis as a novel target for cancer chemoprevention. JNCI 96:662–672

Conclusions

Andrea Renda

This monograph has analyzed many aspects of multiple primary malignancies (MPM) and several interesting conclusions concerning the epidemiology, guidelines, diagnosis, therapy, and legal issues have been drawn, even if definitive data are not yet available on every aspect of this problem.

Scientific interest in MPM is steadily increasing. On the one hand, the survival of cancer patients has improved as a result of therapeutic advances, but on the other, drug toxicity and prolonged exposure to risk factors has resulted in the possibility to develop a second primary cancer.

MPM are certainly underestimated because of the difficulty in obtaining exact information on each patient and the absence of up-to-date tumor registries in many countries and/or regions. However, nowadays, the overall incidence of MPM can be assessed at 10–15% of all malignant tumors. While a certain fraction of cancers would be expected to arise at the same rate as in the general population, the patterns of excess risk that have emerged are sufficiently distinctive to suggest certain factors that are shared by the primary and subsequent tumors, as well as effects of therapies that are potentially carcinogenic. In survivors who have changed their high-risk behaviors, the incidence of second cancers decreases, testifying to the importance of behavioral research, educational programs, and lifestyle changes. If 30-year follow-up series were available for several tumors, the data would no doubt show that one in three patients is at risk of developing a second cancer.

A distinction must be drawn between inherited codified syndromes and "sporadic" ones. In some organs (colon-rectum, breast) hereditary tumors are relatively frequent (~15%) and specific syndromes have been described. The genes involved in such diseases have been identified and cloned and their mechanisms of cancer induction have been clarified. In some cases, genetic data have greatly influenced clinical decision-making, in terms of screening, DNA-guided therapy, and surveillance programs. Mutational analyses can identify subjects at risk and prophylactic surgery is routinely adopted in familial adenomatous polyposis (FAP) and multiple endocrine neoplasia (MEN) 2A. For these syndromes, there are specific guidelines for each step of the clinical approach (screening, therapy, surveillance), allowing MPM in these patients to be foreseen. Based on geno-

A. Renda (ed.), *Multiple Primary Malignancies.*
©Springer-Verlag Italia 2009

type-phenotype correlations, patients at higher risk of developing dangerous alterations can be intensively followed and chemoprevention or other preventive therapies provided.

Some patients cured of a primary tumor have a high predisposition to develop a neoplasm in another body region. Many factors concur to yield multiple carcinogenesis, including prolonged exposure to radiation, lifestyle, endocrine correlations, virus and immunologic disorders. Yet, while these are recognized causes of cancer, their mechanisms of action remain to be fully analyzed.

Currently, some primary tumors are more likely to be "index tumors," i.e., they have a strict correlation with the onset of MPM. Some associations are so frequent that causality is obvious, as there is more than a simple statistical correlation; for instance, colorectal primary tumors with endocrine or urogenital neoplasm, and esophageal tumors and primary airways cancer. Such patients must be carefully followed. The literature has begun to report changes to traditional approaches, such as upper gastrointestinal UGI endoscopy, which is routinely suggested in the diagnosis of upper-airway tumors. Patients who have been treated with chemo- and/or radiotherapy have a significant predisposition to leukemia, lymphoma, or solid tumors and need to be followed with personalized surveillance programs.

There are no laboratory tests or imaging techniques able and specific enough to diagnose or predict MPM. A single, simple, inexpensive, robust, and reliable test to detect one or more neoplasms is desirable but remains elusive. As we have seen, the future of cancer prognosis will probably rely on a small panel of six to ten markers that allow accurate molecular staging to determine the likelihood of metastases, the involvement of the new neoplasia, and the best treatment response. We are rapidly approaching a time when the use of proper biomarkers will help to detect cancer and to monitor and manage progression of the disease.

Data collected for the gastrointestinal tract demonstrates the enormous potential of advanced endoscopy methods (chromoendoscopy, magnifying endoscopy, computed virtual chromoendoscopy, confocal laser endoscopy) as staging tools in the management of patients with suspected digestive-tract dysplasia or early cancer. These techniques increase the detection rate of diminutive or flat lesions and enhance the diagnosis and characterization of some mucosal lesions. Their role in the routine surveillance of patients with previously diagnosed primary malignancies (especially of the digestive tract) is very important and remains essential for reliability and accuracy.

As there is not yet a single ideal radiological examination that specifically detects synchronous cancers, a personalized diagnostic approach for each patient is needed. In this regard, the new imaging techniques (CT-PET, MRI-PET), especially, in combination with metabolic studies, can significantly increase specificity, sensitivity, and accuracy.

Once the etiopathogenesis is clear, the clinical approach may need to be drastically changed, as was shown for the inherited syndromes. To remove an organ before malignant transformation or development of a "cancer in situ" is a rational approach to treatment and prevention. Prophylactic surgery in hereditary forms of MPM is an example – and a consideration for some "sporadic" tumors as well. For now, its use is restricted to those diseases with biomolecular alterations. Preventive colectomy and thyroidectomy for FAP and MEN2 represent the prototype of "DNA-guided" surgery, while for other cancers (HBOC and HNPCC) there is no unanimous consensus but it remains a valid option in selected cases. In HNPCC, preventive hysteroannexectomy can be suggested in women aged >50 or in youngsters who do not wish further pregnancies.

The association of tumors in several organs requires rigorous surveillance. Knowledge of specific genetic mutations can be applied to design personalized schemes, thereby sparing patients useless investigations. Ultimately, knowledge of the biomolecular mechanisms behind tumor formation will lead to the adoption of chemoprevention to inhibit and/or limit neoplastic proliferation.

Medical care based on specific guidelines and genetics will also greatly modify clinical approaches, with subsequent ethical, legal, and psychological implications. Surgeons must actively participate in and be informed of emerging technologies since the management of specific problems will be greatly changed by this new knowledge and will challenge the existing dogma.

Likewise, physicians should quickly adopt and be thoroughly familiar with revised guidelines so as to avoid omissions or mistakes in caring for patients at risk of MPM. The introduction of molecular diagnostic tests into clinical practice to identify patients with inherited tumors who are at risk will bring many advantages, but is fraught with ethical and medicolegal problems, of relevant interest to physician and patient. Obviously the emergence of technologies that allow genetic evaluation makes it indispensable that the patient provides informed consent, but only after extensive and accurate discussions and equipped with written documentation of the risks, benefits, and limitations of the test. Such documentation must be one of the first acts of the consultation between the parties and, above all, serve as an informative instrument for the patient. Briefly, the informed consent must include: a description of the objectives of the test, the significance of a positive or negative test, a valuation of the risks of the illness, and the possibility that the test may not be informative. Moreover, the confidentiality of the test is indispensable to avoid discrimination at work and abuse by insurers. The patient must be informed about all possible medical options and the importance of surveillance and prevention in case of a positive test. Finally, it is necessary to inform individuals in whom the test is negative that they carry the same risk as the general population of contracting a sporadic tumor. An incorrect diagnosis can cause grave damage. A false-positive result wrongly exposes the patient to the sequelae of an unnecessary prophylactic operation, including its side effects. A false negative result may dissuade a person from undertaking a preventive program and/or complimentary treatments. In fact, in the USA, law suits have been brought in cases of diagnostic errors regarding hereditary diseases and for improper mastectomies.

Research may lead to the recognition of new syndromes and tumor types, and thus modify the Diagnostic Related Groups (DRG), which currently addresses MPM only superficially. Revisions of traditional staging systems and other diagnostic classifications are likely as well. A more careful codification could improve the dissemination of information about MPM, facilitate epidemiological evaluation, and perhaps alter the nature and quality of health services.

While many of the concepts discussed herein are based on assumptions, nonetheless, one of our tasks is to stimulate researchers to improve their knowledge about MPM. A greater effort is required to improve the collection of data by involving not only tumor registries and clinical specialists but also general practitioners. The identification of different patient groups will allow comparisons of experiences and of patients with diverse prognostic implications. Large series or Regional and National Tumor Registries could participate in highlighting the associations of particular parameters that for better or worse influence survival.

Subject Index

α-Tocopherol 272, 274

β-Carotene 269, 271, 272, 274

AIDS 84, 93
Alkylating agents 63–67
Antioxidants 56, 269, 271, 274
APC 55, 107, 114–116, 118, 120, 121, 123, 159–165, 172, 179, 256, 249
Apoptosis 54, 56, 65, 114, 270, 275, 277
Ataxia-telangiectasia 84–86, 115, 131, 144

Basal cell carcinoma 273, 276
Basalioma 276
Biomarkers 211, 212, 215–219, 282
Bladder carcinoma 68, 97
BRCA1 113, 114, 117, 120, 143–146, 149, 150, 152, 153, 206, 214, 217, 249, 254, 255, 257
BRCA2 113–115, 117, 120, 143–145, 149, 150, 152, 153, 206, 217, 249, 254, 255, 257, 258
Bruton's disease 84, 85, 86

Cancer of the larynx 24, 91, 97, 180, 196, 199, 268, 271, 274
Cancer registries 7–25
Cancer spectrum 143–153
Carboplatin 63
Carcinogens 53, 55, 59, 157, 169, 175, 199
Caretaker 54
Carotenoids 270, 271
Cervical cancer 97, 103, 207
Chemotherapy 78, 157, 158, 167, 168, 195, 206, 269, 273, 275, 277
Chromatin assembly factor 98, 102, 103

Chromoendoscopy 221, 223, 227–230, 282
Cisplatin 63
Colon cancer 3, 11, 32, 33, 34, 37, 41, 47, 146, 158, 167, 168, 185, 203, 208, 211, 216, 233
Computed tomography colonography 232
Computed tomography positron emission tomography 232, 234, 237–242
Computed virtual chromoendoscopy 227, 228, 282
Confocal laser endoscopy 229, 282
Congenital hypertrophy of retinal pigmented epithelium 122, 160, 161, 246
Contralateral breast cancer 69, 144, 275
c-RET 116, 252, 253

Disease-free survival (DFS) 69

Early gastric cancer 201, 202, 204, 215, 237
Endocrine correlation 192
Endometrial cancer 110, 216, 247, 257, 275
Epstein-Barr virus 84, 86, 93, 102
Esophageal cancer oppure Esophagus cancer 30, 36, 37, 67, 151, 195–199, 202, 205, 209, 236
Estrogen 69, 145, 172,
Etretinate 271–273, 276

Familial adenomatous polyposis 3, 107, 108, 124, 158, 161, 245, 247, 281
Fenretinide 269, 272, 275
FICE 227, 228
Fluorodeoxyglucose positron emission tomography 236, 241

Gastric cancer 3, 115, 131, 172, 200–205

Gastric tubulization 199, 200
Gastrointestinal cancer 86, 207
Gatekeeper 54
Gene polymorphism 64
Genotype-phenotype correlations 124, 160, 161
Glucagonomas 111
GTBP (hMSH6) 116

Head and neck squamous cell carcinoma 268, 271–274
Hepatoblastoma 160, 161, 256, 260
Hereditary breast and ovarian cancer 107, 113
Hereditary cancer syndrome 114
Hereditary nonpolyposis colorectal cancer 256–258, 260–262, 283
Herpesvirus 86, 93
hMSH3 54, 116
HNPCC 256–262, 283
Hodgkin's disease 63, 67, 77–79, 86, 94
Hormonal factors 55
hPMS2 54, 115, 116
Human papilloma virus 93, 97–103, 207, 208
Hyperparathyroidism 111, 112, 119, 212, 253, 256

Immunodeficiencies 63, 64, 83–87, 89, 93
Insulinomas 111
Intraductal mucinous carcinoma 204, 205
Isotretinoin 192, 218, 257, 275
Isotretinoin 271, 272, 274

Kaposi sarcoma 31, 33, 36, 37, 39
Kidney cancer 79, 151, 218

Leukemia 3, 8, 10–16, 64–69, 71, 85, 115, 131, 151–153, 158, 165, 166, 171, 188–190, 206, 282
Li-Fraumeni syndrome 144, 158
Linear energy transfer 70, 73
Lung cancer 3, 14, 35, 42, 67–69, 151, 153, 166, 202, 269, 272, 274

Magnifying endoscopy 224, 227, 282
Mantle therapy 68, 78, 79
Medullary thyroid cancer (MTC) 107, 111–113, 116, 117, 119, 140, 212, 213, 249, 252, 253, 261

Melanoma 8–16, 23, 32, 39, 90, 91, 100, 115, 145, 146, 166, 185, 189, 190, 202, 207, 240, 276
MEN1 111–113, 115, 116, 119, 252, 262
MEN2 107, 112, 113, 115, 116, 119, 249, 252, 262, 283
Menin 116
Meningioma 116
Metachronous tumors 90, 180, 191, 221
Metastasis 1, 57, 58, 112, 130–132, 137–139, 168, 195, 231, 234, 237, 240, 249, 253, 282
Mismatch repair gene 159, 207, 216
MOPP scheme 67, 68
MSH2 119, 120, 122, 207, 248
Multiple carcinogenesis 282
MYH 116, 120, 123, 164, 246, 252

N-acetyl-cysteine 269, 272
Neoangiogenesis 57
Neurofibromatosis 115
Nitrosification 204
Non-Hodgkin's lymphoma 63, 67, 68, 79, 86, 93, 171
Normal tissue complication probability 69

Oncogene 54, 55, 116, 119, 130, 217, 249
Onco-suppressor gene 54, 55, 116
Oncovirus 92
Oophorectomy 249, 254
Osteogenic sarcoma 109
Osteomas 109, 118, 121, 14, 246, 259
Ovarian cancer 47, 63, 113, 114, 143–146, 150, 153, 206, 207, 210, 213, 214, 216, 217, 219, 249, 250, 253, 254, 257, 263
Overall survival 63, 69, 114, 274
p53 55, 80, 102, 114, 120, 133, 134, 140, 141, 144, 199

Pancreatic cancer 49, 145, 146, 168, 204, 205, 215, 216, 258
PCR 99, 120, 139, 185, 190
Periampullary carcinoma 260
PET-CT colonography 234
Peutz-Jeghers syndrome 109, 118, 144,
Pheocromocytoma 115
Pituitary adenoma 111, 212
Platinum compounds 63
Polymorphism 158, 215
Proctocolectomy 160, 251, 258

Subject Index

Prolactinomas 111
Prophylactic surgery 3, 60, 250–254, 256, 257, 262, 276, 281, 282
Prostate cancer 22, 23, 35, 37, 40–42, 44, 46, 74, 75, 145, 153, 211, 216–218, 237, 258, 274, 277
Proto-oncogenes 54, 133, 140

Radiotherapy 3, 7, 29, 57, 64, 67–79, 84, 85, 157, 158, 168, 195, 206–208, 239, 253, 269, 282
Rectal cancer 12, 34–36, 74, 76, 234
Rectal stump cancer 251, 255, 256, 258
Relative biological effectiveness 70
Relative risk 22, 23, 28–30, 49, 77, 79, 143, 145, 14, 160, 192, 207, 268
Restorative proctocolectomy 258
RET 119, 137, 140, 163, 249, 252, 253
Retinoblastoma 54, 115, 151, 152, 158, 165, 166,
Retinoids 269–271, 275–277
Risk factor 94, 132, 135, 143, 256, 268, 274

Sarcoma 31, 33, 36, 37, 39, 109, 118, 166, 206
Screening 30, 76, 79, 98, 101, 103, 146, 148, 150, 164, 165, 179, 198, 207–209, 211, 212, 215, 216, 231, 237, 239, 240, 245–253, 257, 258, 261, 262, 281
Second multiple tumor 11–16, 66, 97, 205, 206
Second tumor prediction 35, 37, 38, 41, 42, 44, 46, 49
SEER database 17, 22, 29–32
SEER program 22, 27
Selenium 56, 269, 273, 276
Seminoma 66, 94, 186, 197
Simultaneous tumors 1, 5, 59, 68, 129, 140, 190, 199, 204, 205, 234, 239, 260, 261

Somatostatinoma 111
Sporadic tumor 161, 163, 283
Squamous cells cancer 91, 97, 100–102, 172, 181, 196–198, 268, 271, 273, 276, 277,
Standardized incidence ratio 29, 30, 32, 35–49
Stochastic effects 71, 73
Stochastic forecasting 71–73
Stomach cancer 136, 145, 153, 199, 200, 203, 208
Synchronous tumors 1, 5, 59, 68, 129, 140, 190, 199, 204, 205, 234, 239, 260, 261

Tamoxifen 57, 64, 69, 192, 193, 206, 269, 273, 275, 277
Target organs 198, 204
Thyroid cancer 7, 107, 137–139, 206, 249, 253, 256
Thyroidectomy 119, 139, 249, 252, 253, 257, 260, 262, 263
Time to second tumor 30
Total body computed tomography 241
Total body imaging 232, 234–237, 241, 242
Total body magnetic resonance 239–242
Transplant 68, 87, 88–92, 94
TSH secreting adenoma 111
Tumor control probability 69

Urinary cancer 44–48, 64, 92, 97, 100, 110, 180, 196, 216, 231, 247, 256,
Uterine cancer 3, 47, 48, 151

VIPomas 111
Vitamin A 269, 272, 274
Von Hippel Lindau disease 115, 213

Wiskott-Aldrich syndrome 84–86, 131

Printed in Italy in September 2008